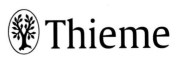

The Practice of Mammography

Pathology – Technique – Interpretation – Adjunct Modalities

Daniël J. Dronkers, MD, Radiologist

Jan H. C. L. Hendriks, MD, Radiologist

Roland Holland, MD, Professor of Pathology

Gerd Rosenbusch, MD, Professor Emeritus
of Radiology

University Medical Center St. Radboud, Nijmegen,
The Netherlands

with contributions by

H. Aichinger
L. V. A. M. Beex
Carla Boetes
Petra A. M. Bun
D. J. Dronkers
J. H. C. L. Hendriks
Sylvia H. Heywang-
   Köbrunner
R. Holland
J. Hoogenhout
W. J. Hoogenraad
N. Karssemeijer
Natalie McGauran

J. W. Th. Muller
Henny Rijken
B.-P. Robra
G. Rosenbusch
M. Säbel
A. Stargardt
M. A. O. Thijssen
A. L. M. Verbeek
T. von Volkmann
Th. Wobbes
Harmine M. Zonder-
   land

488 illustrations
18 tables

Technical editor
Peter F. Winter, MD, Peoria, IL., USA

Thieme
Stuttgart · New York

Library of Congress Cataloging-in-Publication Data

Radiologische Mammadiagnostik. English
   The practice of mammography : pathology,
   technique, interpretation, adjunct modalities /
Daniel J. Dronkers ... [et al.].
      p. cm.
   Includes bibliographical references and index.
   ISBN 3-13-124371-6 – ISBN 1-58890-004-5 (U.S.)
   1. Breast—Radiography. 2. Breast – Cancer – Diagnosis.
   I. Dronkers, Daniël J. II. Title.
   [DNLM: 1. Mammography – methods.
   2. Breast Neoplasms – radiography.
   WP 815 R1294 2001a]
RG493.5.R33R3413 2001
616.99'44907572 – dc21

2001041467

This book is an authorized translation of the German edition published and copyrighted 1999 by Georg Thieme Verlag, Stuttgart, Germany. Title of the German edition: Radiologische Mammadiagnostik.

© 2002 Georg Thieme Verlag
Rüdigerstraße 14, D-70469 Stuttgart, Germany
Thieme New York, 333 Seventh Avenue,
New York, N.Y. 10001, U.S.A.

Typesetting by Druckhaus Götz GmbH,
D-71636 Ludwigsburg

Printed in Germany by Staudigl-Druck, Donauwörth

ISBN 3-13-124371-6 (GTV)
ISBN 1-58890-004-5 (TNY)   1 2 3 4 5

Preface

When Thomas Scherb, MD, from Thieme Publishers approached us for a German textbook on mammography, we readily accepted this opportunity.

We deemed it prudent not to rely exclusively on the knowledge and experience from Nijmegen, The Netherlands, but to use a broader basis by including experts from other mammographic centers in the Netherlands and Germany. We wanted to create a short new textbook on clinical mammography.

Based on the anatomy and pathology of the breast, the radiological findings are presented plainly and clearly, with emphasis on instruction as found in a teaching book rather than on completeness as expected from a reference text. We have tried to accommmodate the underlying physics and the importance of positioning in mammography.

Mammography is one of the best-perfected conventional radiographic methods. Even after the advent of newer techniques, such as sonography (ultrasound) and MRI (magnetic resonance imaging), mammography remains the most important radiological examination of the breast. Radiological imaging of the breast is primarily directed at discovering breast carcinoma, which forms the core of this book. Nonimaging aspects of breast carcinoma, such as clinical diagnosis, treatment, epidemiology, and risk factors, are also discussed. Certain details are covered in more than one chapter, which should make it easier to study each chapter separately.

Mammographic screening is discussed in addition to diagnostic mammography. After the screening trials in Nijmegen and Utrecht in 1975, national screening began in the Netherlands in 1988. The LRCB (National Expert and Training Center for Breast Cancer Screening) was established in Nijmegen for this purpose. Besides their commitment to scientific research, LRCB experts conduct technical quality control of all 60 screening centers in the Netherlands, as well as postgraduate training of all radiologists, pathologists, and radiologic technologists involved in national breast cancer screening. The experience of the LRCB is incorporated into this book.

We would like to thank all contributors for their cooperation, especially Horst Aichinger, PhD, who coordinated Chapter 5. We are grateful for the support of the Stichting Vroege Opsporing Kanker Oost-Nederland (SVOKON). K. Siekman and W. Veldkamp, both from LRCB in Nijmegen, provided the digitization of the mammographic images. Cooperation with the publisher and its co-workers on this edition was as good as it was for the German edition; special thanks go to Clifford Bergman, MD, Ms. Annie Hollins, and Gert A. Krüger for their support. F. Hartmann provided the instructive illustrations and graphics. When the publisher decided on an English edition of this book, we updated the text. Ms. Annelies Schef and Johan Schouten supported us in the translation of some of the chapters. Peter Winter, MD, was responsible for the final English version.

The German edition was dedicated to Professor W. H. A. M. Penn, former head of the Department of Radiology of the University Hospital St. Radboud, Nijmegen, the Netherlands, and a great advocate of screening for breast carcinoma in the Netherlands, and to the late professor W. Höffken, Cologne, Germany, one of the pioneers of mammography. We dedicate this English edition to our wives.

Nijmegen, Fall 2001   The Editors

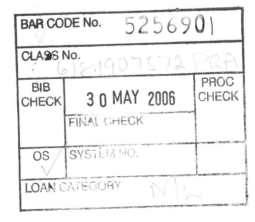

Contributors

Aichinger, H., PhD
Formerly: Siemens AG
Medical technology, basic research
Erlangen, Germany

Beex, L. V. A. M., MD
UMC St. Radboud
Dept. Oncology
Nijmegen, Netherlands

Boetes, Carla, MD
UMC St. Radboud
Dept. Radiology
Nijmegen, Netherlands

Bun, Petra A. M., MD
UMC Leiden
Dept. Radiology
Leiden, Netherlands

Dronkers, D. J., MD
Radiologist
Velp, Netherlands

Hendriks, J. H. C. L., MD
UMC St. Radboud
Dept. Radiology and LRCB
Nijmegen, Netherlands

Heywang-Köbrunner, Sylvia H., MD
Professor of Radiology
Martin-Luther-Universität
Klinik für Radiologische Diagnostik
Halle, Germany

Holland, R., MD
Professor of Pathology
UMC St. Radboud
LRCB
Nijmegen, Netherlands

Hoogenhout, J., MD
UMC St. Radboud
Dept. Radiotherapy
Nijmegen, Netherlands

Hoogenraad, W. J., MD
UMC St. Radboud
Dept. Radiotherapy
Nijmegen, Netherlands

Karssemeijer, N., PhD
UMC St. Radboud
Dept. Radiology
Nijmegen, Netherlands

McGauran, Natalie, MD
Otto-von-Guericke-Universität
Institut für Sozialmedizin
Magdeburg, Germany

Muller, J. W. Th., MD
Diakonessen Ziekenhuis
Dept. Radiology
Utrecht, Netherlands

Rijken, Henny,
Chief technologist
UMC St. Radboud
LRCB
Nijmegen, Netherlands

Robra, B.-P., MD
Professor of Epidemiology
Otto-von-Guericke-Universität
Institut für Sozialmedizin
Magdeburg, Germany

Rosenbusch, G., MD
Professor Emeritus of Radiology
Nijmegen, Netherlands

Säbel, M., PhD
Professor of Medical Physics
Universitäts-Frauenklinik
Medizinische Physik
Erlangen, Germany

Stargardt, A., PhD
Klinikum der RWTH
Klinik für Radiologische Diagnostik
Aachen, Germany

Thijssen, M. A. O., PhD
UMC St. Radboud
Dept. Radiology and LRCB
Nijmegen, Netherlands

Verbeek, A. L. M., MD
Professor of Epidemiology
UMC St. Radboud
Dept. Epidemiology
Nijmegen, Netherlands

von Volkmann, T., PhD
Kodak AG
GB Medizin
Stuttgart, Germany

Wobbes, Th., MD
Professor of Surgery
UMC St. Radboud
Dept. Surgery
Nijmegen, Netherlands

Zonderland, Harmine M., MD
UMC Leiden
Dept. Radiology
Leiden, Netherlands

Contents

Abbreviations

CC	Craniocaudal
CIS	Carcinoma in situ
DCIS	Ductal carcinoma in situ
FNA	Fine-needle aspiration for cytology
IDC	Invasive ductal carcinoma
ILC	Invasive lobular carcinoma
LCIS	Lobular carcinoma in situ
MLO	Mediolateral oblique
TDLU	Terminal ductal lobular unit

1 Clinical Characteristics of Breast Cancer

Th. Wobbes

To a woman, any change in the breast is cause for concern. The fear of breast cancer makes most breast complaints a great emotional burden on the patient. The omnipresent possibility of breast cancer means that any breast complaint, even if it is only pain or swelling, should be taken seriously. The adage that any lump in the breast is malignant until proven otherwise still holds true today. Modern diagnostic modalities almost always enable the distinction between a benign or a malignant lump, though only histological biopsy can provide the final diagnosis.

To avoid missing a malignancy, it is necessary to know the limitations of the various diagnostic methods.

The typical complaints encountered in daily practice and their underlying clinical findings are summarized in Table 1.**1**.

Table 1.**1**   Typical complaints and specific pathological condition

- Physiologic lumps and tenderness
  - Mastalgia (mastodynia)
- Nodularity
- Dominant lumps
  - Breast cancer
  - Fibroadenoma
  - Cysts
- Nipple discharge
- Inflammation and infections
  - Lactation
  - (Peri-)Subareolar
  - Mondor disease
- Skin and nipple changes
  - Eczema
  - Retraction
  - Edema

Physiological Lumps and Tenderness

■ Mastalgia

During a woman's menstrual years, the breasts are continuously under the influence of cyclic hormonal stimulation. Almost half of all women experience some pain during the luteal phase of their cycle, often associated with some swelling.

The normal nodularity is often rather pronounced, particularly in the upper outer quadrants. This is a physiological condition with no increased incidence of breast cancer. Up to half of women older than 30 years complain of some breast pain (mastalgia) in the period preceding menstruation. This pain is not necessarily accompanied by the nodularity mentioned earlier, and may be diffuse throughout the breasts as well as local in the outer halves. Sometimes the pain is unilateral. Mastalgia is probably caused by parenchymal swelling during the luteal phase of the cycle because of increased water retention (Milligan et al., 1975). This cyclic painful swelling is commonly regarded as physiological, but is reported as something abnormal or pathological in 5 % of women. Besides cyclic mastalgia, noncyclic breast pain can be experienced, particularly by women after age 40, and is described as a continuously burning or shooting sensation.

Nodularity

Swelling that may fluctuate with the menstrual cycle is physiological, but some women have a definite nodularity that is always present. The irregular lumps are mostly in the upper outer quadrants and are frequently painful. It is difficult to distinguish a normal finding from a pathological condition. Some consider such a nodularity pathological if it lasts for more than a week (Love et al., 1987). The clinician has to be concerned not to overlook an early carcinoma, although nodularity as such has no direct relationship with the development of a carcinoma. It is difficult to detect a malignancy in these breasts with either palpation or mammography. A discrete palpable lump that does not change during the menstrual cycle should be biopsied and examined histologically.

Dominant Lumps

Dominant lumps always need close attention. It is important to realize that breast cancer may present at any age. Fibroadenomas are found particularly in young women (age 20–30 years), and cysts are mostly found in older women (age 35–50 years). In pubertal girls, a giant fibroadenoma is sometimes diagnosed as a palpable firm lump in a unilaterally enlarged breast.

■ Breast Cancer

Breast cancer presents mostly as a painless lump and is difficult to separate from surrounding tissue. Almost 70% of carcinomas are located centrally or in the upper outer quadrants. Most women have no visible signs of the tumor. Cutaneous changes may occur if the tumor is located just beneath the skin, and nipple retraction is seen if the tumor is located in the nipple area. In addition, skin changes, nipple retraction, and edema (peau d'orange) with or without erythema or red to blue discoloration may be present as signs of cutaneous infiltration. Sometimes even ulceration can be seen. In some patients, breast cancer presents as diffuse induration of the gland, together with some shrinking of the breast. A special manifestation of breast cancer is the inflammatory carcinoma, a locally advanced stage with erythema of the skin, edema, and induration, but without a palpable dominant lump. The erythema is caused by tumorous infiltration of the skin.

If breast cancer is suspected, the regional lymph nodes should be palpated (axilla, supraclavicular and infraclavicular region).

Paget disease of the nipple is an eczematoid change of the nipple, sometimes preceded by itching and/or a pain sensation. This is at least the manifestation of a ductal in situ carcinoma (microcalcifications), and sometimes that of an invasive carcinoma.

■ Fibroadenoma

The fibroadenoma is a painless, circumscribed, mobile lump, usually measuring not more than 1–3 cm, although a giant fibroadenoma that exceeds 5 cm can occur in young girls. Histologically, the lump consists of both epithelial and stromal tissue. In case of a lump larger than most fibroadenomas found in women who are about 30 years of age, a phyllodes tumor should be considered. This tumor usually is benign but may display malignant behavior.

■ Cysts

Cysts are found primarily in perimenopausal women. It is frequently difficult to differentiate a cyst from a carcinoma despite its smooth surface. Fluctuation may be felt with superficial cysts. Often, additional cysts can be found in the same breast as a manifestation of cystic disease. Cysts are generally asymptomatic, but rapidly expanding cysts may be painful. A definitive diagnosis can be made by aspirating the contents.

Nipple Discharge

Several types of nipple discharge are encountered in clinical practice. A mostly bilateral milky discharge (galactorrhea) is physiological. A clear, but usually discolored (green, black, brown), discharge indicates ectasia of the major subareolar ducts; it also has no pathological significance. A bloody or serosanguinolent discharge may indicate intraductal pathological changes:

• Duct ectasia
• Benign intraductal epithelial proliferations
• Breast cancer.

It is important to search for a palpable lump as indication for an underlying malignant tumor. Mammography may disclose clinically occult pathology by displaying microcalcifications. A carcinoma is found in not more than 5% of patients with bloody nipple discharge.

Inflammation and Infections

Breast infections are common, especially during lactation. Almost 10% of nursing women encounter a more or less severe infection of the breast, mostly occurring within six weeks after delivery. The infections present with pain, fever, and malaise. While the early phase of the infection might not have visible signs, full-blown mastitis presents with redness and swelling. Fluctuation may be elicited in superficially located abscesses. Antibiotic treatment of mastitis over a longer period of time may mask the abscess, which is then detectable only by sonography.

Out of the lactation period, periareolar or subareolar infections occur and are mostly seen in women between ages 30 and 35 years. The infection is located behind or just around the areola and causes erythema. It is attributed to an obstructed lactiferous duct, and in the early phase there is usually no sign of microorganisms. The infection frequently recurs even with adequate treatment. Smoking seems to be a predisposition. Mastitis is occasionally seen in women with cystic disease and presents clinically as an abscess.

Mondor disease is an inflammation of a superficial vein (thrombophlebitis) and is mostly located in the upper outer quadrant. It occurs primarily in older women. Redness and a cordlike painful infiltration develop along the involved vein. Thrombophlebitis may also be present in other parts of the body.

A special type of inflammation is the inflammatory carcinoma of the breast. This is an aggressive breast cancer that infiltrates the overlying skin. The breast may show redness and feel warmer than the contralateral breast. The skin shows edematous thickening, characteristically presenting as peau d‹orange. In contrast to a true mastitis, this neoplastic manifestation is not associated with fever.

Skin and Nipple Changes

Changes of the skin and/or the nipple may reflect an infection but can indicate an underlying carcinoma.

- **Eczema.** Eczema of the nipple is called Paget disease. It is usually a manifestation of an underlying malignancy, but a real eczema can occur, mostly arising in the areola. The underlying carcinoma is generally a ductal carcinoma in situ, but invasive breast cancers also may induce this finding.
- **Retraction**. Retraction of the nipple and/or the skin or asymmetry of the breasts are suspicious for underlying breast cancer. If the tumor infiltrates the underlying muscle, the retraction characteristically appears more pronounced, with muscle contraction or elevation of the ipsilateral arm.
- **Edema.** Edema of the skin (peau d'orange) is almost always a sign of breast cancer. It frequently is associated with redness.

References

Hughes, L. E., R. E. Mansel, D. J. T. Webster: Benign Disorders and Diseases of the Breast. Baillière Tindall, London 1989

Love, S. M., S. J. Schnitt, J. J. Connolly, R. L. Shirley: Benign breast disorders. In Harris, J. R., et al.: Breast Diseases, Lippincott, Philadelphia 1987 (pp. 15–53)

Milligan, D., J. O. Drife, R. V. Short: Changes in breast volume during normal menstrual cycle and after oral contraceptives. Brit. med. J. 4 (1975) 494–496

2 Anatomy

J. H. C. L. Hendriks, D. J. Dronkers and G. Rosenbusch

The glandular tissue of the breast changes not only during pregnancy and in the lactation period but also, to a lesser degree, during the menstrual cycle. Furthermore, breast tissue undergoes changes over the woman's life. Normal breast anatomy, therefore, exhibits great variation, which is also reflected on mammograms.

The mammary structures are completely developed only after the first full-term pregnancy. In most women, fatty infiltration appears after the first lactation period. The breast arises on the curved thoracic wall and is movable against the major pectoral muscle. The highest mobility is inferior and lateral. This is an essential consideration when positioning the breast for mammography (see p. 101).

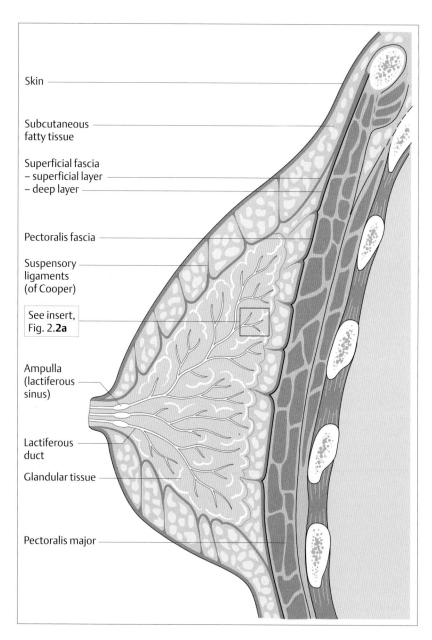

Skin

Subcutaneous
fatty tissue

Superficial fascia
– superficial layer
– deep layer

Pectoralis fascia

Suspensory
ligaments
(of Cooper)

See insert,
Fig. 2.**2a**

Ampulla
(lactiferous
sinus)

Lactiferous
duct

Glandular tissue

Pectoralis major

Fig. 2.1 a, b Glandular and connective tissue with fasciae of the breast
a Schematic drawing
b Galactography with filling of two segments of the lactiferous ductal system

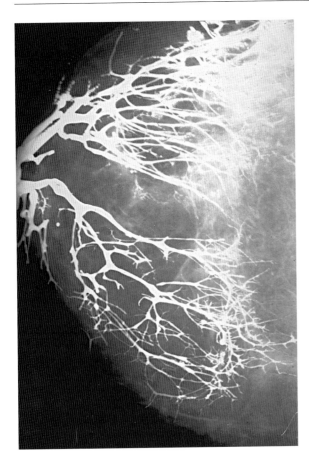

Fig. 2.**1 b**

Mammary Gland (Fig. 2.**1**)

The breast consists of 15 – 20 lobes or segments, each with one lactiferous duct. Two or three lactiferous ducts unite to form a total of five to eight lactiferous sinuses, which exit at the nipple. On mammograms the lactiferous ducts appear as linear or slightly nodular densities, radiating from the nipple into the breast. The ducts have a diameter of 1 – 2 mm. Ampullae or lactiferous sinus are local dilatations up to 4 mm of these ducts, just behind the mamilla. The lactiferous ducts are formed by uniting lactiferous ductules. The active secretory glandular tissue is located in the periphery of the breast.

The TDLU (terminal ductal lobular unit) (Fig. 2.**2**) is the basic histological unit. It consists of the extra- and intralobular terminal ducts and the blind ending acinar ductules. A lobule consists of 25 – 35 acini. *Fibrofatty tissue* surrounds the ductular and lobular structures, forming the major component of breast tissue. *Cuboid epithelial cells* line the ducts. *Myoepitheliocytes* form a discontinuous layer between lining cuboid cells and basement membrane. The myoepitheliocytes transport the milk through the ducts. The basement membrane separates the epithelial cells from the connective tissue. Evaluation of the basement membrane is important because its interruption by malignant cells means that the carcinoma is invasive. Toward the nipple, the cuboid cells of the ducts change to squamous cells. The lobules measure 0.5 to 1(or 2)mm and are visible on mammograms as small nodules as long as they are separated from each other in the encompassing adipose tissue. Superimposition makes them appear confluent, resulting in densities of various sizes and forms. Several hundred lobules form a lobe at the time of sexual maturity.

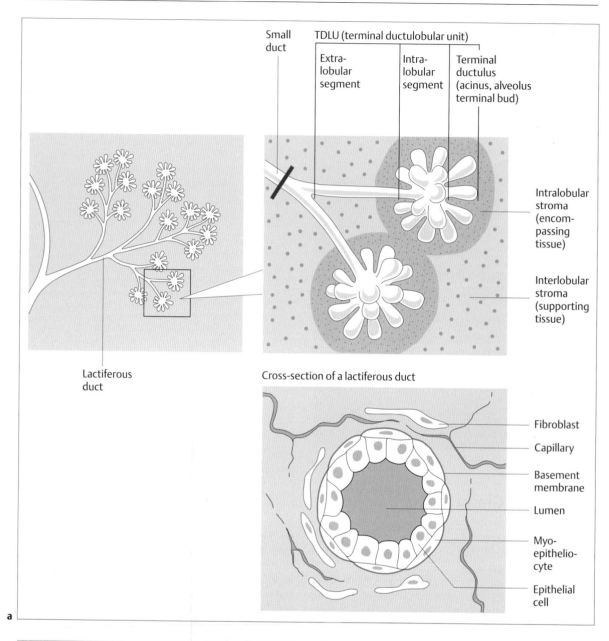

Small duct

TDLU (terminal ductulobular unit)

Extra-lobular segment

Intra-lobular segment

Terminal ductulus (acinus, alveolus terminal bud)

Intralobular stroma (encompassing tissue)

Interlobular stroma (supporting tissue)

Lactiferous duct

Cross-section of a lactiferous duct

Fibroblast

Capillary

Basement membrane

Lumen

Myo-ep.helio-cyte

Epithelial cell

a

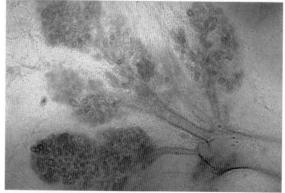

b

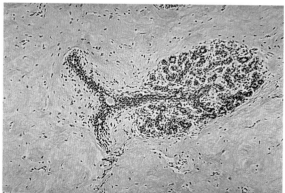

c

Fig. 2.2 a – c   **Anatomy of the lobe**
a Schematic drawing
b Several TDLUs. Three-dimensional specimen
c A single TDLU (HE)

Fasciae and Connective Tissue

The glandular body is enveloped by the deep and superficial layers of the superficial fascia. A thin layer of loose adipose and connective tissue behind the deep layer provide a connection with the fascia of the pectoral muscle. The connective tissue of the breast consists of interlobular and intralobular components. Cooper ligaments are delicate septa of the superficial layer of the superficial fascia and run through the breast to act as suspensory ligaments for the breast tissue. Along the superficial layer, the Cooper ligaments follow a scalloped course and are anchored in the subcutaneous fatty fibrous tissue and the skin.

Under normal conditions the Cooper ligaments are not thickened and exhibit a regular pattern. The connective tissue determines form and consistency of the breast.

The intralobular connective tissue surrounds the TDLU. It is the active component of the connective tissue. Under hormonal influence of the menstrual cycle it shows edematous changes. It is the zone of ductal growth by cellular proliferation, the site of inflammatory reaction, and the origin of mesenchymal tumors such as fibroadenoma and sarcoma.

The lobules also enlarge in adenosis, sclerosing adenosis, and fibrocystic changes. The single lobules are mammographically visible only along the border of involuted glandular tissue. In the center they look bigger or even may form a homogeneous density due to superimposition.

The TDLU is the region where most of the benign and malignant tumors originate, apparently related to the functional and morphological changes the cells are subjected to during the menstrual cycle and pregnancy.

Normally the glandular tissue is relatively symmetrical in both breasts, but asymmetry does occur, sometimes requiring further examination. With increasing age the glandular parenchyma is replaced by adipose tissue.

Parenchymal Pattern and Skin Pattern

On the basis of the relative amount of epithelial and connective tissue, J. N. Wolfe (1976) divided the parenchyma on mammograms into four groups (Tab. 2.1), with the groups P2 and DY presumably having a 3–4 times greater cancer risk. The breast density is expressed in percentages on the CC-projection. The parenchymal pattern is almost always symmetrical.

A parenchymal pattern with a higher risk for carcinoma is found more often in nulliparous than in multiparous women. With increasing number of full-term pregnancies the pattern changes to one with a lower cancer risk.

The skin (epidermis and corium syn. dermis) is 0.5–2 mm thick, and increases inferiorly and at the transition to the axillary fold to 2–4 mm. In the less dense parts of the breast the skin can produce a reticular structure on the mammogram. This is not caused by skin pores but probably by dermal papillae and epidermal ridges (Fig. 2.3). The dermal papillae consist of relatively radiolucent, vascularized connective tissue and the epidermal ridges of less radiolucent, squamous cells around the papillae. The papillae correspond to the central radiolucencies on the mammogram, and the epidermal ridges to the more reticular radiodensities. As the result of the projection geometry, the reticular structure usually originates from the skin nearest to the film.

Table 2.1 Parenchymal breast pattern classification according to Wolfe (from Byrne and colleagues).

Pattern	Mammographic features
N1	Normal aspect of the breasts, predominantly composed of fat with little, if any, dense areas. Low breast cancer risk. Dense area: 1–25% of the total breast area.
P1	Mainly composed of fatty tissue with dense areas of ductal prominence represented by nodular or linear densities, predominantly in the anterior part of the breast. Dense area: 25–49% of the total breast area.
P2	Dense areas of ductal prominence. P1 and P2 reflect hyperplasia of connective tissue around the ducts. Dense area: 50–74% of the total breast area.
DY	More or less general increase of parenchymal density, with homogeneous sheet–like areas of density, without recognizable ducts. Epithelial changes varying from hyperplasia to atypia. Dense area: >75% of the total area.

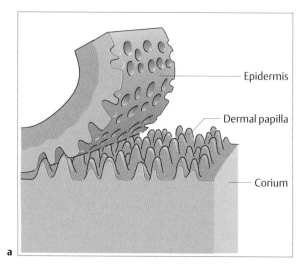

a

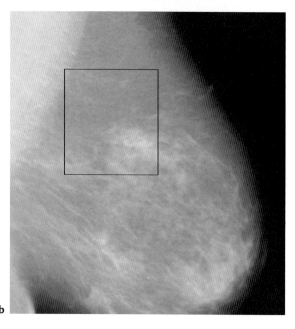

b

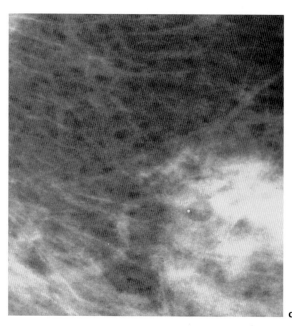

c

Fig. 2.**3** a – c   **Reticular structure on mammogram**
a Papillae of the corium, which are anchored in grooves of the epidermis, causing the reticular structure on mammograms. Schematic drawing
b Oblique view of the left breast
c Detail of (**b**) with the reticular structure

Arteries, Veins, Lymphatics

The arterial supply of the breast is derived from branches of the subclavian artery (internal mammary artery), axillary artery (lateral thoracic artery and intercostal arteries. Smaller branches often run along the major lactiferous ducts and form a capillary network around the lobules. Larger arteries can be seen on mammograms as linear densities that do not converge toward the nipple. Calcified vascular walls occur exclusively in arteries. Veins cross the breast as bands of 2 – 4 mm thickness.

Veins have a larger diameter in the upper outer quadrant than in the other quadrants. The superficial veins run in the subcutaneous fat and the deep veins are more deeply situated. The veins carry the blood mainly to the axillary vein (Fig. 2.**4**).

The more cellular and vascularized stroma contains lymph vessels (Fig. 2.**5**), which are not visible on mammograms. Their drainage occurs deeply in the glandular tissue into regional lymph nodes, at least in 75 % into the axillary lymph nodes and in the rest into parasternal lymph nodes (intrathoracic). An additional superficial lymphatic system with subareolar plexus is part of the subcutaneous plexus of the thoracic wall. The deep and superficial systems are connected. Intramammary lymph nodes can be found in 25 % of anatomic breast specimens, but only 5 % are seen on mammograms, more often in the upper outer quadrant than in the other quadrants. Multiple occurrence is possible. By definition, intramammary lymph nodes have to be surrounded by fibroglandular tissue to differentiate them

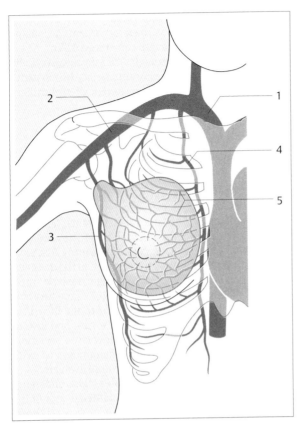

Fig. 2.**4**   **Veins of the breast**
1 Anonymous vein
2 Axillary vein
3 Thoracoepigastric vein
4 Internal mammary vein
5 Intercostal veins with perforating veins

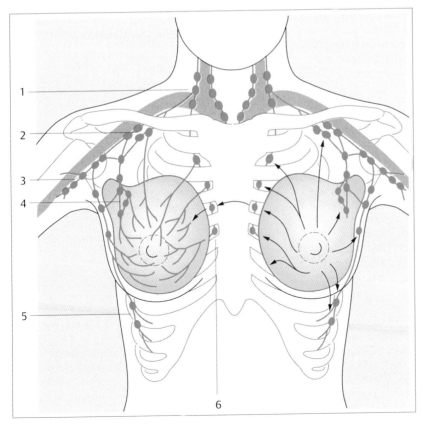

Fig. 2.**5**   **Regional lymph nodes and lymphatic drainage of the breast (according to Bässler)**
1 Deep cervical nodes
2 Infraclavicular nodes
3 Nodes along the axillary vein
4 Axillary nodes
5 Nodes to the abdominal wall
6 Parasternal nodes (intrathoracic location)

from axillary lymph nodes. On mammograms, intramammary lymph nodes display the typical appearance of lymph nodes: they are less than 0.5 to 1 (or 1.5) cm in diameter and, depending on the projection, they are oval or round. A small recess corresponds to the hilum. In the absence of the recess, fibroma, cyst, hemangioma, and carcinoma have to be considered. A central

radiolucency within a lymph node ("fatty degeneration") is a sign of benignity. The fatty content can enlarge the lymph node and its length can exceed 1.5 cm.

Intramammary lymph nodes can be metastatically involved. Metastases to the intramammary lymph nodes do not necessarily imply involvement of the axillary lymph nodes.

Physiological Changes of the Breast

- One to two years before *menarche*, enlargement of the breasts begins by an increase in connective tissue. With menarche, the gland buds branch and a greater number of TDLUs are formed. The TDLUs enlarge by proliferation of the epithelial cells that line the ducts of TDLUs.
- In *young women* before the first pregnancy, the lobules are not fully developed and fatty infiltration is low. The breasts consist mainly of connective tissue, and mammography shows homogenously dense breasts.
- At *menopause,* the glandular tissue involutes. The intralobular and interlobular connective tissue also becomes atrophic. At first the lower inner quadrant involutes, then the upper inner quadrant and finally the lower outer and upper outer quadrants. This occurs relatively symmetrically. In the sixth decade, the atrophy progresses and fat tissue becomes dominant. As the lactiferous ducts do not involute, they become more visible in the more adipose breasts. During hormone replacement therapy, the involution of the glandular tissue reverses to some extent in about 20% of women, indicating a reactivation of the mammary tissue.

- During the first half of *pregnancy,* the synergic effect of several hormones (estrogen, progesterone, prolactin) leads to growth and further branching of the TDLUs, with proliferation of the acini. The acini cells are cuboid and become columnar during *lactation.* They produce milk, which is secreted in the ductules. After lactation the epithelial cells resume their cuboid shape. In the growth period, i.e., the first half of the pregnancy, the enlargement of the breast reflects hypertrophy of the glandular cells and distension of the ductules caused by increased secretion. The breasts are very dense on mammograms, with the structures blurred and difficult to evaluate.
- During the *menstrual cycle* the breast also undergoes changes: early in the cycle the epithelial cells of the acini are reduced and form a more or less solid cord. Later in the cycle the cells of the acini become cuboid, a lumen appears and the connective tissue is more strongly vascularized. In the premenstrual phase, the breast may be tender. Proper compression might fail and the mammographic examination is best deferred until mid-cycle.

Embryology and Anomalies

In the second fetal month, an ectodermal ridge, the milk line, develops ventrolaterally at both sides of the fetus, running from the axilla to the groin. Buds branch out from the milk line. One bud on each side, usually the fourth bud, develops to form the breast and the milk line disappears, but supernumerary buds can remain and later appear as supernumerary nipples (hyperthelia) or breasts (hypermastia, polymastia). Typically, the supernumerary nipples are arranged along the original milk line (Fig. 2.**6**).

Accessory breast tissue. In about 2–3% of women, accessory mammary tissue occurs inferiorly or superiorly in the axilla as the axillary tail (or axillary process, tail of Spence). This accessory tissue has a duct, which drains into the ductal system of the major gland. Affected women notice an atypical intumescence during pregnancy as evidence of an axillary process. Accessory breast tissue rarely occurs below the breast. *Caution*: Ac-

cessory breast tissue should not be mistaken for a tumor, but may well harbor a cancer.

Accessory breast tissue seems to involute later than the breast itself and might then simulate a tumorlike process on the mammogram.

Besides the mentioned excess formations, defective breast development may occur.

Defective developmental anomalies

- Amastia (absence of the breast)
- Athelia (absence of the nipple, in the presence of mammary tissue)
- Micromastia (hypoplasia; bilateral symmetrical hypoplasia is found in gonadal dysgenesis with Turner syndrome)
- Anisomastia (unequally sized breasts by unilateral hypoplasia or macromastia)

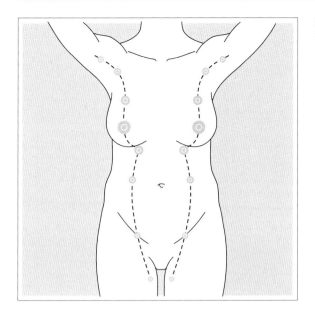

Fig. 2.**6** **Schematic drawing of the embryonal milk line, where accessory mammary tissue can occur**

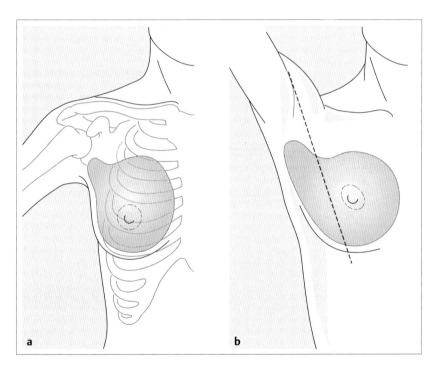

a   b

Fig. 2.**7 a, b** **Schematic drawing of the axillary process (tail of Spence)**

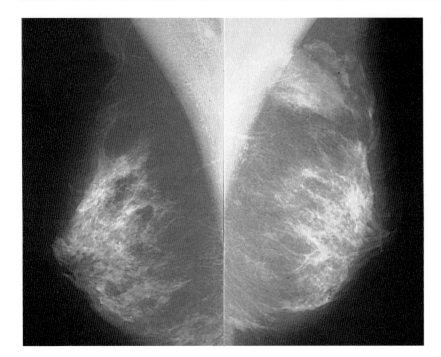

Fig. 2.8   **Ectopic glandular tissue cranially in the left breast**

References

Bässler, R.: Mamma. In Remmele, W.: Pathologie Band 3. Springer, Berlin 1984

Barth, V.: Die Feinstruktur der Brustdrüse im Röntgenbild. Thieme, Stuttgart 1979

Byrne, C., Schairer, C., Wolfe, J., Parekh, N., Salane, M., Brinton, L.A., Hoover, R.N., Haile, R.: Mammographic features and breast cancer risk: effects with time, age and menopause status. Journal of the National Cancer Institute 87 (1995) 1622–1629.

Cyrlak, D., C. H. Wong: Mammographic changes in postmenopausal women undergoing hormonal replacement therapy. Amer. J. Roentgenol. 161 (1993) 1177–1183

Egan, R. L.: Breast embryology, anatomy and physiology. In Eagan, R. L.: Breast Imaging: Diagnosis and Morphology of Breast Diseases. Saunders, Philadelphia 1988

Gils, van C. H., J. D. M. Otten, A. L. M. Verbeek, J. H. C. L. Hendriks: Short communication: breast parenchymal patterns and their changes with age. Brit. J. Radiol. 68 (1995) 1133–1135

Meyer, J. E., F. A. Ferraro, T. H. Frenna, P. J. DiPoro, C. M. Denison: Mammographic appearance of normal intramammary lymph nodes in an atypical location. Amer. J. Radiol. 161 (1993) 779–780

Osborne, M.: Breast development and anatomy. In Harris, J. R., et al.: Diseases of the Breast. Lippincott, Philadelphia, 1996 (pp. 1–14)

Page, D. L., T. J. Anderson: Diagnostic Histopathology of the Breast. Churchill Livingstone, Edinburgh 1987

Wellings, S. R., H. M. Jensen, R. G. Marcum: A hypothesis of the origin of human breast cancer from the terminal ductal lobular unit. Pathol. Res. Pract. 166 (1975) 515–535

Wolfe, J. N.: A study of breast parenchyma by mammography in the normal woman and those with benign and malignant disease of the breast. Radiology 89 (1967) 201–205

Wolfe, J. N.: Breast patterns as an index of risk for developing breast cancer. Amer. J. Radiol. 126 (1976) 1130–1139

Wolfe, J. N., A. F. Saftlas, M. Salane: Mammographic parenchymal patterns and quantitative evaluation of mammographic densities: a case-control study. Amer. J. Radiol. 148 (1987) 1087–1092

3 Benign and Malignant Disorders of the Breast

R. Holland, G. Rosenbusch , J. H. C. L. Hendriks, and
D. J. Dronkers

Benign Disorders

The breast can develop a variety of benign disorders. Some are easily recognizable as benign by mammography, whereas others may resemble breast cancer. The most important benign disorders will be described.

■ Fibrocystic Disease

Fibrocystic disease (synonyms: mastopathy, fibroadenosis, mastopathia cystica fibrosa, dysplasia) includes various changes of the breast that differ only slightly from the normal aging process and are often characterized by hyperplasia of the parenchymal tissue.

Fibrocystic Changes of the Breast

- Cysts
- Epitheliosis
- Adenosis
- Radial scar.

■ Cysts

Cysts are classified by their size as microcysts or macrocysts. Microcysts have a diameter of 3–5 mm. Secretion accumulates due to inadequate resorption by the epithelium or obliteration of the terminal duct by fibrosis or epithelial hyperplasia, leading to increased pressure in the TDLU (Fig. 3.**1**). With increasing size, adjacent acini become involved, and larger cysts may develop. The cysts are lined with flattened epithelium, often showing apocrine metaplasia.

Macrocysts

These cysts may reach 6–10 cm in diameter and are unilocular or multilocular. They are filled with cloudy or milky fluid that may contain calcium particles, which appear mammographically round (Fig. 3.**2**) or amorphous granular. With time, the color of the fluid of the cyst may change from bright yellow or bright green to black due to denaturation of the protein in the fluid. The cyst's contents then become hygroscopic, causing the cyst to be under tension. If the cyst ruptures, the denatured protein in the escaped fluid may induce a sterile inflammatory reaction of the stroma.

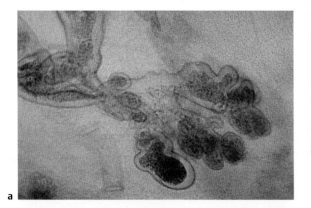

a

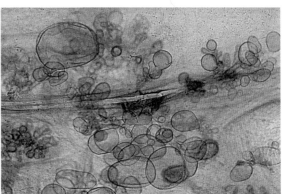

b

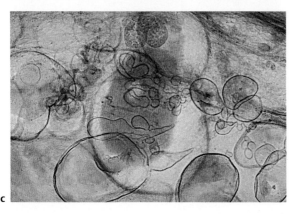

c

Fig. 3.**1 a – c   Development of cysts**
a TDLU. Initial dilation of lobule due to hypersecretion. 3-D preparation
b Multiple microcysts and a duct with fibrocystic changes. 3-D preparation
c Multiple cysts and fibrocystic changes. 3-D preparation

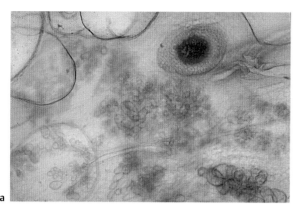

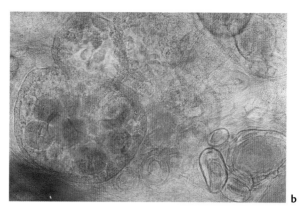

Fig. 3.2 a, b   Calcifications in cysts
a Microcysts with one solitary laminated calcification.

b Cysts with multiple crystalline calcifications

Larger cysts under high tension (tension cysts) are palpable and may become painful due to further fluid accumulation during the premenstrual phase. This occurs in about 7% of women diagnosed with cysts. Cysts may spontaneously decrease in size or even disappear, mainly around the menopause. Mammographically, the solitary larger cysts are round or oval, depending on their tension, and are well demarcated. A thin radiolucent zone (the so-called halo) is often visible around the cysts, representing compressed fat tissue or the Mach effect. Calcifications may appear in the walls of larger cysts.

Sonography usually provides quick and reliable information as to whether a mammographically detected mass is a cyst or a solid lesion: a cyst should be well-defined, lack internal echoes, and demonstrate dorsal acoustic enhancement due to increased transmission.

Microcysts

Mammographically, multiple small cysts (microcysts) produce a nodular image. It is only possible to differentiate these cysts from adenosis when they contain so-called "milk of calcium," which consists of numerous small calcium particles. On the CC view, the milk of calcium appears as round calcific densities (Fig. 3.**3a**). On the MLO view, it presents as upward concave, crescentic calcific densities due to sedimentation along the bottom of the cyst (described by Lányi as "teacup phenomenon") (Figs. 3.**3b**, 8.**15**).

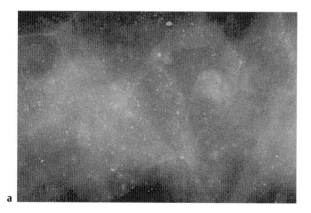

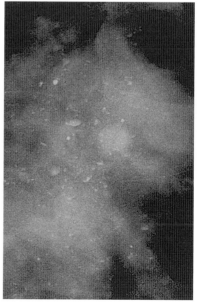

Fig. 3.3 a, b   Diffusely distributed calcifications in microcysts ("milk of calcium")
a CC view with punctate calcifications
b ML view with sedimentary microcalcifications, resulting in levels (so-called "teacup phenomenon")

Longitudinal sections	Transverse sections

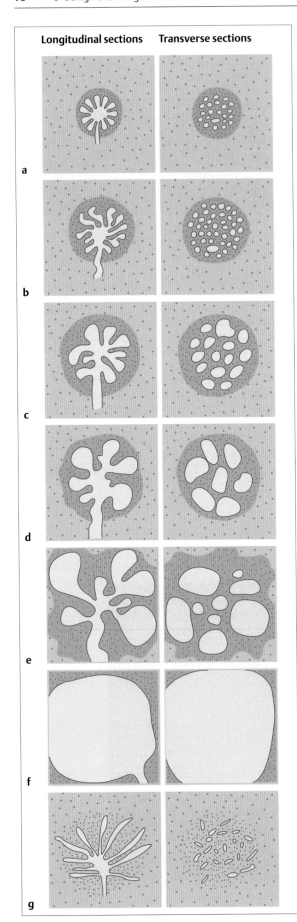

◀ Fig. 3.4 a – g   **Schematic representation of the types of adenosis (according to Lányi)**
  a Normal lobule
  b Simple adenosis
  c Blunt duct adenosis
  d Small or microcystic adenosis
  e Advanced small or microcystic adenosis
  f Tension cyst
  g Sclerosing adenosis

■ Epitheliosis

Epitheliosis (synonyms: ductal epithelial hyperplasia, papillomatosis) is an abnormal proliferation of epithelial and also myoepithelial cells within the ducts of the TDLU. The proliferating epithelial cells fill the lumen partly or entirely. The morphological features of some of these intraductal epithelial proliferations might be close to but not fully identical with those of a DCIS (so-called atypical ductal hyperplasia [ADH]). These lesions must be differentiated from DCIS. Epitheliosis, ADH, simple adenosis and blunt duct adenosis do not induce any mammographic signs.

■ Adenosis

Adenosis (Fig. 3.4) refers to an increase in the number of the acini within the lobules, which is sometimes associated with hyperplasia of the epithelial and myoepithelial cells. The hyperplasia develops in a relatively orderly way, or may be dominated by one of the components.

> **Types of adenosis**
>
> • Simple adenosis
> • Blunt duct adenosis
> • Microglandular (microcystic or small cystic adenosis)
> • Sclerosing adenosis

Simple Adenosis

In simple adenosis, the size and number of lobules are increased and the normal structure becomes accentuated. The lobules are about 1 mm in diameter.

Blunt Duct Adenosis

In blunt duct adenosis, proliferations in small ducts lead to dilation with hyperplasia of myoepithelial cells. Epitheliosis may exist at the same time and calcium may precipitate. The lobules measure about 1–2 mm.

Microglandular (microcystic or small cystic) Adenosis

In microglandular adenosis, the glandular parenchyma proliferates within the fibrous and adipose tissue, leading to cystic dilation of the terminal ductules (acini). Mammographically, 3–5 mm nodular densities are visible. A differentiation from microcysts can be made by sonography or identified mammographically by calcium content.

Sclerosing Adenosis

Sclerosing adenosis represents sclerosis around the ductules of the hyperplastic lobule and resultant luminal narrowing. This distorts the architecture on the microscopic level. Lumps are rarely palpable. Mammographically, this disorder shows an irregular density, a stellate lesion or a well-defined density, sometimes with typical small round calcifications.

■ Radial Scar

The radial scar (synonyms: radial sclerosing lesion, complex sclerosing lesion, non-encapsulated sclerosing lesion, benign sclerosing ductal proliferation) consists of a fibrotic core with radiating extensions. Different benign proliferations may be encountered within a radial scar.

Benign proliferations

- Sclerosing adenosis
- Cyst
- Obliterated ducts due to epitheliosis
- Ductal ectasia

Histologically, it may be difficult to differentiate the center of a radial scar from an invasive tubular carcinoma. For this reason, frozen sections should not be obtained from a mammographically suspected radial scar. The mammogram (Fig. 3.**5**) shows a stellate density without a distinct center, often containing radiolucent areas caused by adipose deposition or small cysts. Microcalcifications are rare. The differential diagnosis from invasive tubular carcinomas is almost impossible. The lesion is not palpable (see p. 212).

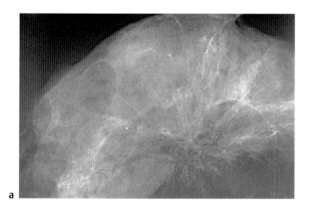

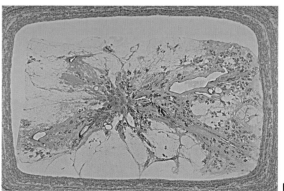

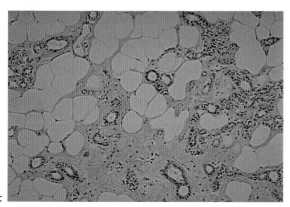

Fig. 3.**5 a – c   Radial scar**
a Stellate lesion without a central dense core. Relatively thin and long spicules. Magnification view
b True size of histological specimen
c The central part of the radial scar with benign adenosis resembling a tubular carcinoma, especially in frozen sections, leading to erroneous diagnosis and possible overtreatment

■ Benign Tumors

■ Fibroadenoma

Fibroadenoma is the most common circumscribed breast lesion before menopause. It occurs in more than 25% of all women, most frequently in the third decade. Pregnancy and lactation stimulate growth, and the lesion tends to regress during menopause. The lesion is a fibroepithelial proliferation and may lead to a palpable, elastically compressible, sometimes lobulated, freely movable tumor. The fibroadenoma varies in size (mostly 1–5 cm) (Fig. 3.**6**), can be painful, mostly occurs unilaterally (bilaterally in only 3–5% of cases), and is generally solitary, rarely multiple (10–17%). Fibroadenomas tend to become hyalinized and calcified, especially during menopause. Malignant change of a fibroadenoma is rather rare (1/1000 cases) and, if it occurs, it usually becomes a LCIS and very seldom a DCIS.

Mammographically, the fibroadenoma is round or oval, but can be lobulated, and is well defined. Calcifications are mostly coarse ("popcornlike"). Local blurring of the margin and spicules due to hyalinization can make the differentiation from a carcinoma difficult. The differential diagnosis includes the also well-defined mucinous and medullary carcinoma and a cyst. Sonography with core biopsy or fine-needle aspiration is needed for further evaluation.

■ Phyllodes Tumor

The phyllodes tumor (synonym: cystosarcoma phyllodes) differs from the fibroadenoma by a hypercellular stroma with characteristic epithelium-lined clefts. It occurs mainly in the fourth to fifth decade. These tumors are usually big, solitary and unilateral, and show rapid growth. Most phyllodes tumors are benign, but they tend to recur after incomplete resection. Metastases are found in about 3–12% of cases. Mammographically, phyllodes tumors are homogeneously dense, well defined and without calcifications. They may grow to 2–6 cm in size. Mitoses > 10/10 HPF (high power field) suggest malignancy, while mitoses < 3/10 HPF suggest a benign process.

■ Intraductal Papilloma

The intraductal papilloma (synonym: papillary adenoma) is a benign, often branching proliferation of the epithelium within a major mammary duct. Histologically, it has a fibrovascular center covered with a layer of epithelial cells. The papilloma may fill the duct completely and lead to retained secretion and ductal ectasia, resulting in a palpable lump. The *solitary intraductal papilloma* occurs most frequently toward the end of the fifth decade, is located in the subareolar region, manifests itself by serous or bloody nipple discharge, and may lead to sclerosis, calcification, and infarction. The *multiple intraductal papilloma* (papillomatosis) causes nipple discharge in only 20% of all cases, is located mostly peripherally and more often bilaterally, and occurs in women around the age of 40 years.

The solitary papilloma is a lesion with a low cancer risk, while papillomatosis has a higher cancer risk and may progress to a DCIS. Since an intraductal papilloma is only a few millimeters in diameter, it may at most induce a minor dilation of a retromamillary duct. When the

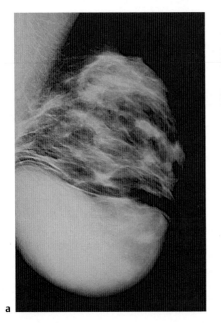

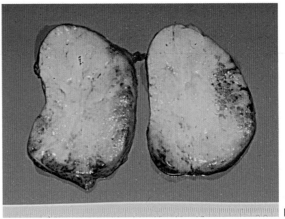

Fig. 3.**6 a, b   Giant fibroadenoma**
a Well-defined homogeneous round density on the MLO view
b Excised tumor after sectioning

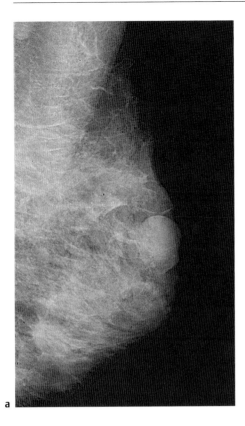

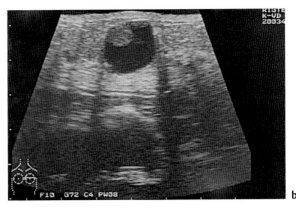

Fig. 3.**7 a, b   Intracystic solid lesion**
a Well-defined round density on the MLO view
b Intracystic proliferation on ultrasound. Histology: benign papilloma

papilloma reaches a certain size, it may appear as a longitudinal nodular density on the mammogram. Papillomas may also develop in cysts (Fig. 3.**7**).

Juvenile Multiple Intraductal Papilloma

The juvenile multiple intraductal papilloma (synonym: juvenile papillomatosis) occurs predominantly in young women (around the age of 20 years). It produces a palpable tumor and is unilaterally located. It is assumed to have precancerous potential.

Lipoma

Lipoma is soft at palpation and therefore difficult to define. Mammographically, it is a radiolucent round or lobulated mass. The tumor is enveloped by a pseudo-capsule and is easily recognized.

Fibroadenolipoma

Fibroadenolipoma (FAL) (synonym: hamartoma) is a mixed tumor showing features both of lipoma and fibroadenoma. Mammographically, the encapsulated radiolucent adipose tissue is traversed by densities caused by fibroglandular elements.

Rare Benign Tumors

> **Rare benign tumors of the breast**
>
> - (Adeno-)Myoepithelioma
> - Juvenile fibroadenoma
> - Lactating adenoma

These lesions appear mammographically as round opacifications and lack any characterizing features.

Inflammation and Abscesses

Inflammations. Acute mastitis mainly occurs during lactation (mastitis puerperalis) and easily is diagnosed clinically. The causative organism usually is *Staphylococcus aureus haemolyticus*. Acute mastitis unrelated to lactation is caused by inadequate draining resulting in retained secretion. It can even be seen in menopause (retention mastitis). Because of the increased parenchymal density, skin thickening, and enlarged axillary lymph nodes, the mammographic findings of mastitis may simulate breast cancer (mastitis carcinomatosa).
Abscesses. Abscesses appear mammographically as nodular densities with spicules or ill-defined margins. Treatment with antibiotics and puncture/drainage is effective, resulting in quick resolution.

■ Duct Ectasia

Chronic inflammation of the walls of the major mammary ducts and their adjacent tissue (*periductal mastitis*) (synonyms: plasma cell mastitis, mastitis obliterans) leads to dilation of the ducts through weakening of the walls, including loss of elasticity. Only one segment may be involved. Furthermore, papillomas or DCIS can cause duct ectasia. The secretion thickens, the walls become fibrotic, and the duct eventually obliterates (mastitis obliterans). Duct ectasia mainly occurs during menopause and may cause nipple retraction. Galactorrhea is observed in 20% of cases and patients may complain of retromamillary pain, but most patients are clinically asymptomatic. Any association with a breast carcinoma is incidental. Mammographically, the dilated, thickened mammary ducts appear in the retromammillar region as serpentine tubular structures, which converge toward the nipple.

Through periductal inflammatory reaction and fibrosis, duct ectasia evolves to plasma cell mastitis with histological predominance of plasma cells. Calcifications appear in the retained secretion within the dilated ducts and in their walls. The mammogram shows linear, well-defined, needlelike macrocalcifications, which may branch (Fig. 8.**17**). These calcifications can in the majority of cases be differentiated from the linear branching calcifications seen in DCIS. These comedo calcifications are irregular, smaller and of different densities.

■ Mondor Disease

Mondor disease is a local thrombophlebitis of the thoracoepigastric vein and its branches. The disease occurs between the ages of 20 and 55 years and usually affects the upper outer portion of the breast. A painful pencil-like thrombophlebitic cord is palpable immediately under the skin. A longitudinal retraction of the skin along the obliterated vein is pathognomonic. Most cases resolve spontaneously. The typical mammographic finding consists of a superficially located, often beadlike linear density. A carcinoma can be excluded by sonography (Fig. 8.**43 b**).

■ Hematoma

A hematoma may develop after needle biopsy, surgical procedure, or trauma (e.g., caused by safety belts in motor vehicle accidents). It also occurs spontaneously in thrombocytopenia and during anticoagulant therapy.

The mammographic finding of a hematoma is an ill-defined diffuse density. In advanced stages a hemorrhagic cyst can evolve, which has a higher density than a simple cyst due to the hemoglobin content. Spicules or microcalcifications as seen in a carcinoma are not present. The lesion regresses spontaneously, leaving behind scarring, distortion, or calcifications.

■ Fat necrosis

Fat necrosis may develop after needle biopsy, surgical biopsy, or trauma (see Hematoma) and may be solitary or multiple. Local destruction of adipose cells forms viscous lipidic fluid, in which giant cells and foamy histiocytes develop. The mammographic findings depend on the morphological stage. Fibrotic reaction in a later stage produces an ill-defined opacity that may simulate a carcinoma. When a central cavity is formed and filled with oily material, an oil cyst is present. The oil cyst has a thin capsule around a radiolucent center. Curvilinear calcifications in the wall or dystrophic calcifications are not infrequently seen. A fat necrosis located relatively close to the skin may cause retraction of the overlying skin.

Carcinoma in Situ and Invasive Carcinoma

It is essential to differentiate noninvasive cancer (CIS) from invasive cancer (Fig. 3.**8**) because of the difference in management. If invasive cancer is present, assessing the state of the axillary nodes is usually the next diagnostic step. It is generally assumed that all invasive cancers develop from noninvasive precursors (CIS), but not every CIS may progress to an invasive carcinoma in the patient's lifetime.

■ Carcinoma in Situ

Carcinoma in situ (CIS) of the breast is a preinvasive carcinoma characterized by proliferation of malignant-appearing cells found in either ducts (DCIS) or lobules (LCIS), without invasion of the surrounding connective tissue at histological examination, that is, the basement membrane of the duct or lobule is not interrupted. Excluding small areas of invasion requires careful review of the slides and, even then, the risk of sampling error remains due to unrecognized sites of microinvasion. This explains the nodal metastases found in about 1% of patients with the diagnosis of a DCIS.

■ Ductal Carcinoma in Situ (DCIS)

In the past, DCIS (synonym: intraductal carcinoma) was an incidental diagnosis (3–5% of breast malignancies), mainly diagnosed in patients with nipple discharge or a

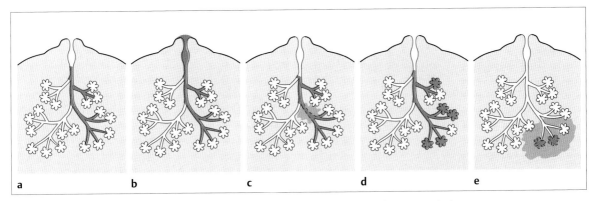

Fig. 3.**8 a – e**   **Schematic representation of ductal and lobular carcinoma (according to Bässler)**
a Noninvasive ductal carcinoma
b Noninvasive ductal carcinoma with Paget disease (Paget carcinoma)
c Invasive ductal carcinoma
d Ductal carcinoma with involvement of the lobule
e Invasive lobular carcinoma

palpable lump. Presently, screening mammography has made it a much more frequent diagnosis due to the detection of microcalcifications in clinically occult cases (15–20% of all malignancies detected by screening). Morphologically, DCIS is not a homogeneous disease but comprises a heterogeneous group of changes with differences in morphology and biological behavior (Table 3.**1**). The division into *comedo-* and *non-comedo* DCIS was an improvement, but is still inadequate because it reflects only the predominant growth pattern of the lesion and not its biological behavior. The term comedo is used for intraductal carcinoma with solid growth pattern and central necrosis. Pressure on the sectioned specimen can extrude necrotic tumor material like comedos on the skin. However, necrosis may also occur in other types of DCIS with various architectures.

Subdivision of non-comedo CIS

- Cribriform
- Micropapillary
- Solid
- Other types

The following classification was proposed on the basis of the cytonuclear and architectural differentiation and the biological behavior (Holland et al., 1994).

Poorly differentiated DCIS (Fig. 3.**9**). This consists of poorly differentiated cells containing pleomorphic nuclei, which show marked variation in size and shape. The nuclei have irregular contours, coarse clumped chromatin, and prominent, sometimes multiple, nucleoli. Mitoses are often evident. The architectural differentiation (cellular polarization) is usually absent. The cellular growth pattern is generally solid, but can be pseudo-cribriform and pseudo-micropapillary. A central necrosis often appears in the intraductal tumor cords, frequently with amorphous calcifications in the necrotic material.

Table 3.**1**   Features of DCIS

- DCIS is to be differentiated from infiltrating ductal carcinoma by the absence of histopathologic stromal invasion through the basement membrane.
- Incidence increases with the large-scale use of screening mammography.
- Not all lesions that are incompletely excised progress to invasive lesions.
- Lesions are almost always unicentric, arising in one area and not in two separated areas, however, the lesions can be very extensive.
- Treatment of regional lymph nodes is not necessary.
- DCIS refers to lesions with heterogeneous features:
  – histological
  – radiological
  – biological

(From EORTC Consensus Meeting 1992)

On the mammogram, the calcifications are linear (Fig. 3.**10**), branching, or coarse granular. The affected ducts often dilate and show extensive periductal fibrosis and lymphocytic reaction. Poorly differentiated DCIS has no recognizable pre-existing condition. Poorly differentiated DCIS has a high malignant potential, and most cases progress to a poorly or intermediately differentiated invasive ductal carcinoma (IDC).

Well-differentiated DCIS (Fig. 3.**11**). Well-differentiated DCIS is composed of cells with monomorphic, evenly arranged small nuclei, which contain fine chromatin, no suspicious-appearing nucleoli, and only few mitoses. The cells have a well-defined apex and show a definite polarization, with the apex oriented toward the ductal lumen, producing a cribriform, micropapillary or rosettelike pattern. Calcifications are not associated with necrosis. If calcifications are present, they are formed by crystallization in extracellular secretory material. Mammography shows clustered microcalcifications, which are usually fine and granular and appear benign. These

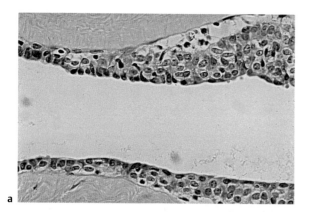

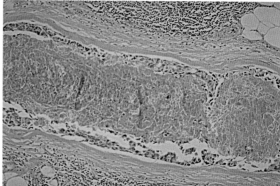

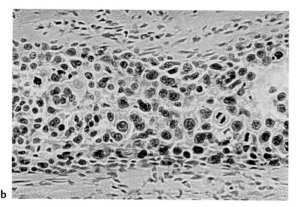

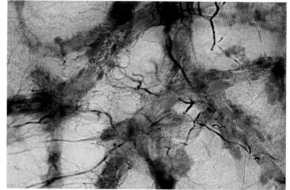

Fig. 3.9a–d Poorly differentiated DCIS
a Initial tumor development in duct epithelium
b Advanced tumor proliferation with obstruction of the ductal lumen

c The central part of the DCIS shows necrosis
d Poorly differentiated DCIS with continuous spread in the duct system. 3-D preparation

clusters are often multiple. The well-differentiated DCIS possibly develops from atypical hyperplasia. It is more often found together with invasive tubular, invasive lobular, and well-differentiated IDC. Not every well-differentiated DCIS will lead to an invasive cancer. Such a progression may take many years.

Intermediately differentiated DCIS. This category is composed of intermediately differentiated cells, with features intermediate between the other two groups. The nuclei of the cells are not as pleomorphic as they are in the poorly differentiated group. Shape, size, and irregular outline show moderate variation. Mitoses are rare. The architecture may be solid or nonsolid. An additional feature differentiating this group from the poorly differentiated category is the presence of polarization of cells, with orientation toward the intercellular spaces. Necrosis may or may not be present. Calcifications, when present, may be crystalline within secretions or amorphous particles within necrotic material. Mammographically, these calcifications are coarse granular or fine granular, but can be linear.

DCIS is almost always unicentric and segmental in distribution. Large lesions often involve the subareolar re-

gion. Mammographically, DCIS is usually detected by the microcalcifications but in few cases also by increased density. As microcalcifications are not in all parts of the DCIS, the mammographic extent is usually smaller than the true histopathological extent. In the study of Holland et al., (1994), about 15–20% of cases were found to have a difference of more than 2 cm between mammographic and histological extent.

■ Lobular Carcinoma in Situ (LCIS)

Lobular carcinoma in situ is a proliferation of small cells in the acini within a lobule. The cells have small round or oval nuclei. The cells fill and distend the ductules, occluding the lumen. The delineation from a well-differentiated solid DCIS is sometimes difficult. LCIS is often an incidental histological finding diagnosed in surgical specimens since it is not recognizable clinically or mammographically. It is multicentric in about 70% of cases, and bilateral in 30%. LCIS often occurs in the premenopausal phase.

The cumulative risk of progression into an invasive carcinoma is 1% per year. Both breasts are at almost equal risk. The cancer may not only be the invasive lobu-

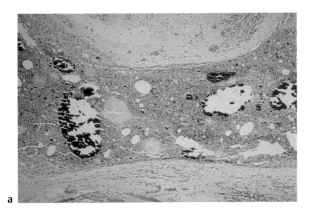
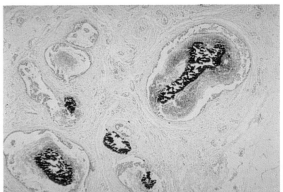
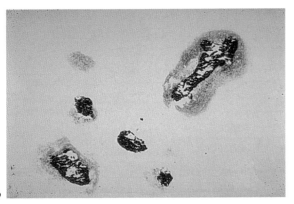

Fig. 3.**10 a – d**   **Calcifications in poorly differentiated DCIS**
a Coarse calcifications in the necrotic part of the DCIS, filling the entire duct (HE and von Kossa staining)
b Linear and coarse granular calcifications. Only calcifications are visible (von Kossa staining). This also shows deposits of very fine "calcium dust" in the necrotic material adjacent to the calcifications

c The same specimen as (**b**), with additional HE staining. The calcifications emerge from the necrotic areas of the DCIS. Their shape is irregular. The powdery calcium deposits around the calcifications are responsible for the slightly ill-defined outline of the calcifications on the mammogram
d Specimen radiograph. Multiple linear branching and coarse granular calcifications, typical of poorly differentiated DCIS

lar type (ILC), but can also be the invasive ductal type (IDC).

LCIS does not have any typical mammographic features. If microcalcifications have prompted the biopsy, calcifications are usually also found outside the LCIS.

■ Invasive Breast Cancer

Most invasive breast cancers are adenocarcinomas of the ductal or lobular type (Fig. 3.**12**).

Other invasive carcinomas

- Tubular carcinoma
- Medullary carcinoma
- Mucinous (colloid) carcinoma
- Papillary carcinoma

Table 3.**2** shows the histopathologically distinguishable types of invasive cancer.

■ Invasive Ductal Carcinoma (IDC)

Three-quarters of all invasive breast cancers are an IDC. In IDC, tumor cells proliferate not only in the ducts, as in DCIS, but also in the tissue surrounding the ducts. Macroscopically, IDC is often lobulated with spicules radiating from its center, producing a stellate configuration on the mammogram. The spicules consist not only of tumor cells but also of connective tissue (Fig. 3.**13**). Histologically, the carcinoma may be fibrotic, and often—but not invariably—shows a paucity of tumor cells, giving it a firm consistency. Retractile forces of the stroma might cause retraction of the skin or nipple. On the mammogram, the IDC appears as a density that is frequently ill-defined or has radiating spicules. Microcalcifications within or outside the IDC usually indicate an extensive intraductal component. Dense parenchyma makes it mammographically difficult to detect centrally located carcinomas.

Calcifications occur not only in the lumina of the ducts at the site of the original in situ elements but also in the invasive component of the tumor. These calcifica-

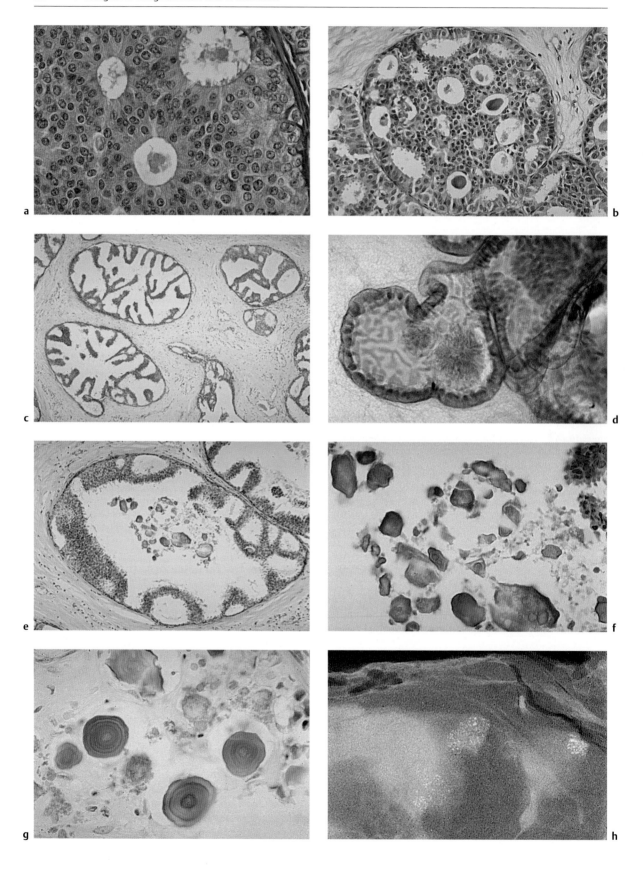

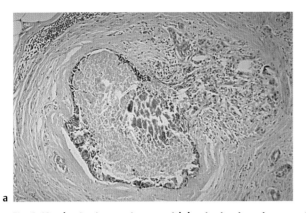
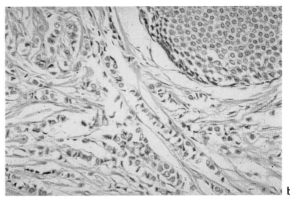

Fig. 3.**12a, b   In situ carcinoma with beginning invasive growth**
a DCIS with beginning penetration of tumor cells through the basement membrane
b ILC and its precursor LCIS in top right

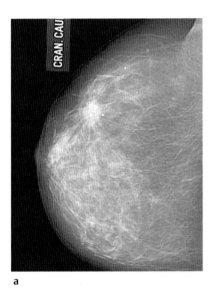
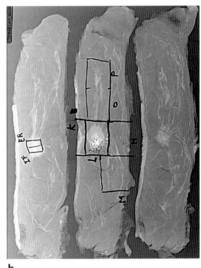

Fig. 3.**13a, b   Tumor with spicules in a 54-year-old woman**
a CC mammogram
b Radiograph of lamellated mastectomy specimen. Histology: IDC and intermediate type DCIS at the site of opacity. The spicules consist only of connective tissue. Typical DCIS calcifications are present. Four axillary lymph nodes positive

tions usually occur in necrotic areas due to an altered cellular milieu and are mostly amorphous.

◀ Fig. 3.**11a – h   Well-differentiated DCIS with calcifications**
a Well-differentiated (non-comedo) DCIS with rosettelike polarization and monomorphic small nuclei (HE)
b Well-differentiated (so-called cribriform) DCIS with multiple calcifications (HE)
c,d Well-differentiated (so-called micropapillary non-comedo) DCIS. c (HE); (d) (3-D preparation)
e Well-differentiated (so-called clinging non-comedo) DCIS with "Roman bridges"
f Central section (magnification of (e)) with crystalline calcifications
g Laminated round calcifications of a well-differentiated (non-comedo) DCIS. The calcifications have similar laminated structure as in microcysts (Fig. 3.2)
h Specimen radiograph with multiple clusters of fine granular microcalcifications with lobular distribution. Histology: well-differentiated (non-comedo) DCIS

■ **Invasive Lobular Carcinoma (ILC)**

About 10 – 15% of all invasive breast cancers are ILC, the second most frequent breast carcinoma. It infiltrates in thin cords along the ducts, ductules, and vessels within the stroma, thus preserving the original breast architecture. The monomorphic tumor cells have small nuclei. Some ILC are pleomorphic and have a poor prognosis, similar to that of IDC. The desmoplastic reaction is slight, making it difficult to detect early lesions by palpation or mammography. Since ILC induces only a moderate increase in the connective tissue, it is not easily delineated from adjacent parenchyma. Furthermore, the newly formed connective tissue resembles intralobular fibrotic tissue, accounting for the subtle mammographic density

Table 3.**2**   Types of invasive carcinoma

1 Not-otherwise-specified types (NOS) or no-special types (NST) (also "ductal type," "common types")
- They include the majority of invasive carcinomas.
- Often it is a diagnosis by exclusion; these are cancers that do not fit in special types.
- Mostly and especially in the radiological literature they are called invasive ductal carcinoma (IDC).
- Histologically a great variety of patterns exist without the uniformity that is noticed in special types.
- They have the worst prognosis of all invasive carcinomas: five-year survival rate < 60% (palpable, non-mammographically detected tumors).
- Often they are "true" interval cancers, i.e., carcinomas that are found clinically due to their fast growth during the interval of a biannual screening program.

2 Intermediate types
- These include the true medullary and lobular types, as well as the carcinoma with predominantly in situ components of the well-differentiated and intermediately differentiated types.
- They show a median degree of malignancy.

3 Special types
- They have a low malignancy potential and a relatively good prognosis: five-year survival rate of 90–95%.
- The special types include:
  - tubular carcinoma
  - mucinous (colloid) carcinoma
- They are often detected in screening programs.

(Holland et al., 1983). A well-circumscribed density is absent. ILC manifests itself as a palpable tumor in the majority of cases (Hilleren et al., 1991; Newstead et al., 1992), but even large tumors may not be palpable.

The essential diagnostic difference between ILC and IDC is that ILC is often better—or even only—seen on the CC view, which is attributed to the better compression achieved in this projection (9%). According to Hilleren et al. (1991), the relevant radiological signs are visible only half as often on the MLO view or lateral view as on the CC view. Furthermore, ILC is mammographically more often (6–16%) completely occult, ascribed mostly to its low density, poor demarcation and growth pattern along the trabecular structures About half of ILC cases show mammographic signs of malignancy, while a quarter exhibit changes that are only suspicious for malignancy. Malignancy cannot be excluded in 8% of cases, and 16% have a normal mammogram or only benign mammographic changes.

Most frequent mammographic signs of ILC, in decreasing frequency

- Ill-defined mass (density may be the same as the fibroglandular tissue)
- Mass with spicules
- Asymmetry
- Architectural distortion

Microcalcifications occur in only a quarter of the cases. They are not typical for ILC, as similar calcifications are also seen in benign lesions like sclerosing adenosis or in malignant tumors other than ILC, such as IDC. Microcalcifications should be considered as a nonspecific finding. Often ILC shows only indirect (secondary) signs of malignancy.

Indirect signs of malignancy in ILC

- Skin retraction (21%)
- Skin thickening (15%)
- Nipple retraction (12%)
- Axillary lymph nodes (1.5%)
- Diffuse edema (1.5%)

Many patients with ILC undergo a biopsy because of palpable findings suspicious for malignancy, but about one-third of the patients have tissue thickening as felt in fibrocystic changes or induration only.

Symptoms of locally advanced ILC

- Skin thickening
- Skin retraction
- Retraction of the nipple

ILC is often difficult to diagnose, and subtle and nonspecific signs have to be correlated with palpable findings.

For focal solid lesions, especially for palpable lesions that lack mammographic signs, sonography is helpful.

Assuming that 16% of all cases of ILC are mammographically occult and that 10% of all invasive breast cancers are an ILC implies that only 1.6% of all mammographically occult breast cancers are an ILC (Holland et al., 1983). Multicentricity is rare, while multifocality is characteristic for ILC:

- LCIS in > 75% of cases.
- Multiple invasive foci in 45% of cases.
- Bilaterality is a characteristic feature.

With increasing tumor size, positive axillary lymph nodes are found more often: with a tumor diameter of 21–30 mm they are found in 50% of cases, and with a diameter greater than 30 mm in 83% of cases (Hilleren et al., 1991).

■ Invasive Tubular Carcinoma (Fig. 3.**14**)

Invasive tubular carcinoma comprises 2–6% of all breast cancers. Because of its relatively slow growth, it is often detected by mammography, especially in screening programs. Microscopically, the highly differentiated tumor cells form tubules, consisting of one row of cells surrounded by connective tissue. In less than half of these

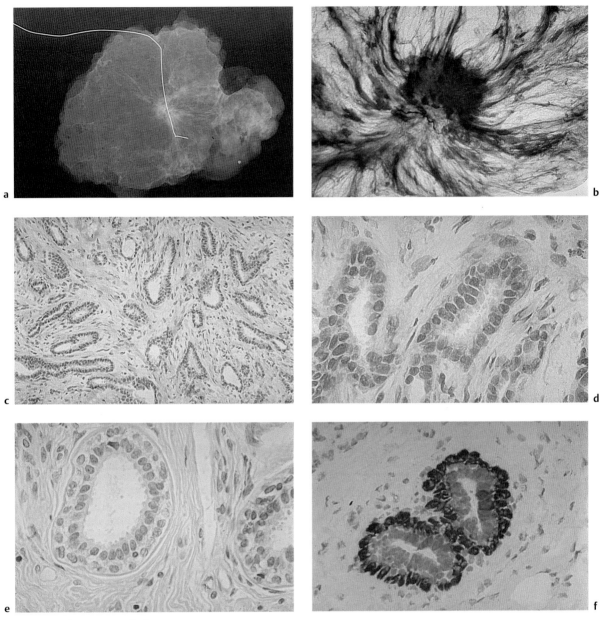

Fig. 3.**14 a–f   Invasive tubular carcinoma**
a Specimen radiograph. Tumor with spicules, preoperative marking wire
b 3-D preparation showing these longer spicules of the tumor
c Tubular carcinoma with ductules
d Tubular carcinoma resembles a normal ductulus; however, there is no outer layer of myoepithelial cells

e Normal ductulus with two layers of cells: inside epithelium and outside myoepithelial cells
f Demonstration of outer layer of cells by myoepithelial marker (α–SM 1) for excluding tubular carcinoma

patients a palpable mass is the indication for mammography. Mammography shows a small density with spicules. Microcalcifications are rare. Sonography is not very helpful for further clarification. Invasive tubular carcinoma has a better prognosis than IDC. The differential diagnosis must consider adenosis, radial scar and IDC.

◼ Invasive Medullary Carcinoma

Invasive medullary carcinoma accounts for 5–7% of all breast cancers. Histologically, it shows poorly differentiated tumor cells with highly polymorphic nuclei and numerous mitoses. Infiltration of lymphocytes and plasma cells are seen in typical cases. The tumor is usually well circumscribed without formation of spicules. Mammographically, this carcinoma manifests itself as a rather well-circumscribed oval to round, sometimes lobulated, density with smooth or indistinct margins. This makes its mammographic differentiation from a fibroadenoma or cyst difficult. A halo is partly present (Fig. 3.**15**). Sonography and core biopsy or FNA are necessary. Sonography shows internal echoes and occasionally en-

hanced sound transmission due to its high cellularity. Despite its fast growth, typical cases have a low tendency to metastasize.

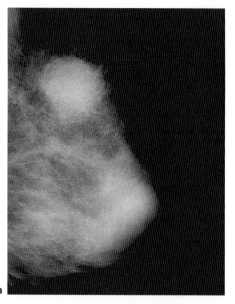

a

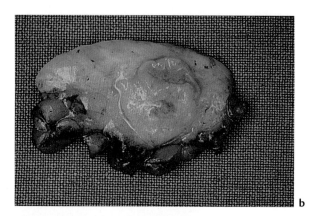

b

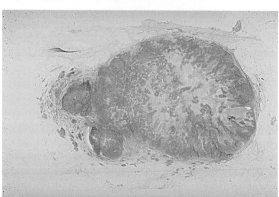

c

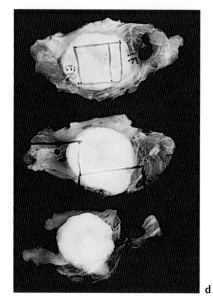

d

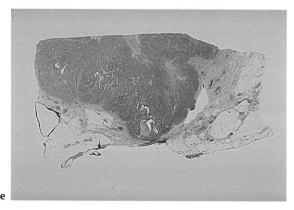

e

Fig. 3.**15 a – e** **Medullary carcinoma**
a Rather well-circumscribed round density on the CC-view
b Excision specimen with the tumor
c Histological specimen shows expansive invasive growth (HE)
d Radiograph of lamellated excision specimen
e Margin is histologically free of tumor (HE)

■ Invasive Mucinous (Colloid) Carcinoma
(Fig. 3.**16**)

Invasive mucinous carcinoma accounts for about 3% of all breast cancers. It is a large mucinous accumulation around clusters of tumor cells. It grows slowly and expansively, occurs frequently at a higher age. Mammography shows a circumscribed lobulated or microlobulated lesion of low density that is partly ill-defined and barely displays a halo. The size ranges between 1 and 3 cm. Calcifications are rare. Detection is common at screening. Only one-third of the tumors are palpable.

■ Rarely Occurring Carcinomas

■ Papillary Carcinoma, Intraductal

Papillary carcinoma constitutes up to 2% of all breast cancers. It grows relatively slowly in the mammary ducts and is located mostly central and subareolar. It has a soft consistency and often is hemorrhagic. Mammographically, it frequently appears as multinodular or solitary density. In about one-third of cases, microcalcifications are present. It cannot be differentiated from multiple papillomas.

■ Intracystic Carcinoma (Fig. 3.**17**)

The intracystic tumor is usually a papillary carcinoma. When the carcinoma does not permeate the cystic wall (= basement membrane), the process should be regarded as a CIS (intracystic CIS) and, in case of penetration, as an invasive carcinoma. The cyst can have a diameter of up to 10 cm. Less than 0.1 % of cysts are found to have an intracystic carcinoma. When sonography shows intracystic vegetation, the cyst should be excised and not aspirated. Negative FNA does not exclude a malignant process.

The intracystic carcinoma shows the expected well-defined mammographic contour of a cyst. If it is invasive, pericystic changes are present.

Intracystic hemorrhage increases the mammographic density of the cyst. Therefore, very dense cysts are suspicious for an intracystic process. Sonography

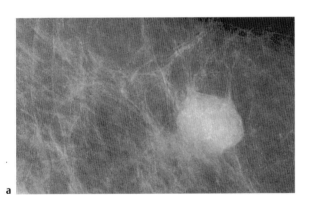
a

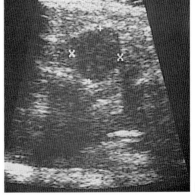
b

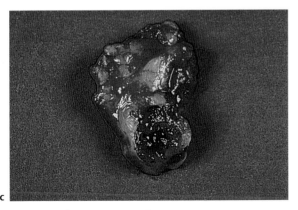
c

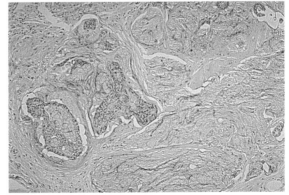
d

Fig. 3.**16 a – d   Mucinous carcinoma**
a MLO magnification view with partly ill-defined tumor mass
b Hypoechoic lesion with slightly increased sound transmission

c Excision specimen with the tumor
d Histological clusters of tumor cells surrounded by mucous material (Alcian blue)

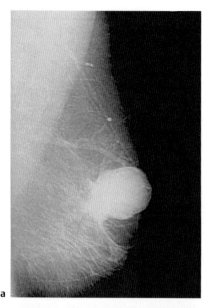

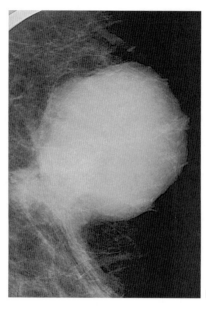

Fig. 3.17 a – d   Intracystic papillary carcinoma
a MLO view showing round lesion with local ill-defined protrusion
b Magnification view in MLO projection
c Sonography. Proof of intracystic proliferation with acoustic shadowing
d Sectioned excision specimen

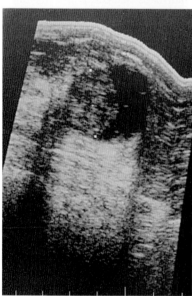

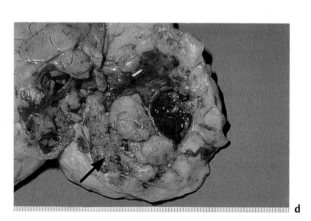

provides the decisive finding. Wall thickening of the cyst may also be caused by intracystic bleeding or secondary inflammation.

■ Paget Disease of the Nipple

Paget disease of the nipple is almost always a sign of underlying breast malignancy, with a poorly differentiated DCIS found in about 40% of cases and poorly differentiated IDC in 60%, but only 1–3% of all invasive breast cancers present as Paget disease. Carcinomatous cells migrate intraductally toward the nipple, infiltrate the epidermis, and produce an eczematous reaction. More than half of patients have nipple discharge as well as ery-

thema and ulceration of the nipple and areola. The average age of the patients is 60 years. Mammography is negative in about half of the cases, even if the DCIS is extensive, especially in the absence of microcalcifications. Retro-mamillary densities and, slightly more frequently, calcifications can be found mammographically. The microcalcifications may be linear, branching, granular, or punctuated. Different types of microcalcifications can exist simultaneously. Furthermore, mammographic thickening of the mamilla and areola necessitates further investigation by sonography and possibly biopsy to confirm or exclude Paget disease of the nipple.

■ Inflammatory Carcinoma of the Breast

Inflammatory carcinoma of the breast (synonyms: lymphangitis carcinomatosa, mastitis carcinomatosa) represents a superficial manifestation of an advanced invasive breast cancer, usually a poorly differentiated IDC with massive involvement of the dermal lymphatic vessels. Bilateral occurrence is not rare: 10 – 55 %! Its incidence is 1 – 4 % of all invasive breast cancers. Clinically, the skin of the affected breast is red, edematous, and warm. The "peau d'orange" is caused by edema of the skin, with the pores becoming more prominent due to apparent retraction. More than half of the patients have a palpable tumor, mostly diffuse and with retraction of the nipple. Histological sections of the skin show dilated dermal lymph vessels with tumor emboli and lymphocytic reaction around the blood vessels of the skin.

> **Mammographic signs**
>
> - Tumor mass
> - Microcalcifications
> - Blurred delineation of the skin from the subcutaneous tissue
> - Coarsening of trabecular structures
> - Thickening of Cooper ligaments
> - Increase of reticular pattern in subcutaneous fat tissue by dilated lymphatic vessels and/or increased density of the entire breast

The prognosis of inflammatory carcinoma is poor. Postradiation changes and breast abscesses/mastitis can be excluded by physical examination and histology.

■ Unilateral Multifocality and Multicentricity

Since the introduction of conservation therapy, it has become necessary to determine the extent of the tumor and to exclude additional carcinomatous foci outside the primary tumor. Incomplete resection with microscopic residual tumor (usually DCIS) may result in local recurrence, even after postsurgical radiation. *Multifocality* refers to additional foci that are directly related to the primary tumor, and *multicentricity* refers to additional foci that are unrelated to the primary tumor and separated from it by a distance of at least 3 – 4 cm. Using this definition, Holland and colleagues found multicentricity of breast cancers to be uncommon and multifocality common (Holland et al., 1985). They reviewed 399 cases of carcinoma, which would qualify for breast-preserving treatment by today's criteria, but which were treated with mastectomy during 1980 – 82. Cases already diagnosed clinically and/or mammographically as multicentric or fixed to the thoracic wall were excluded. Diffusely growing carcinomas were not analyzed further, since they were mainly an ILC consisting of multiple microscopic tumor foci and extending often beyond one quadrant. Holland et al. formed two groups: 282 invasive carcinomas (T1 – T2) and 32 intraductal carcinomas (CIS). The histopathological and mammographic analysis revealed that 37 % of the 282 invasive carcinomas did not have tumor foci around the primary tumor in the mastectomy specimen. Tumor foci within 2 cm of the primary tumor were present in 20 % of cases, and beyond 2 cm in 43 %. The tumor foci beyond 2 cm were noninvasive cancers in 27 % but 16 % contained also invasive foci. If the 264 invasive cancers smaller than 4 cm had been removed with a safety margin of 3 – 4 cm, invasive cancer would have been left behind in the breast in 7 – 9 % of the patients and foci of noninvasive cancer in 4 – 9 %.

It is noteworthy that the foci of intraductal carcinoma extended more than 2 cm beyond the invasive primary tumor in 10 %, and more than 3 cm in 5 % of cases..

Comparison of mammographic/clinical findings with the histological findings revealed that the maximal tumor size as determined by the extension of microcalcifications seen on the mammogram came close the histologically determined tumor size.

■ Bilateral Occurrence

Patients with a history of breast carcinoma are at high risk for developing a carcinoma in the other breast (5 – 15 %). *Synchronous* occurrence defines a second carcinoma detected within six months after the first tumor was diagnosed, and *metachronous* occurrence defines a second carcinoma detected in the contralateral breast later than six months. Bilateral carcinomas are synchronous in about 50 % of cases and metachronous in 50 % (Roubidoux et al., 1996). Two decades ago, a metachronous carcinoma was diagnosed more frequently. But improved mammography detects contralateral tumors earlier, with a corresponding increase in synchronous and a decrease in metachronous carcinomas.

There is no significant difference in the age of patients with unilateral and bilateral carcinoma, but the risk of a contralateral carcinoma increases when the first carcinoma was found at an early age.

Mammographic appearance and location of bilateral carcinomas do not differ significantly from those of unilateral carcinomas. More than 50 % of the contralateral carcinomas are located in the mirror-image quadrant of the first carcinoma. Synchronous carcinomas are similar in size, but the metachronous carcinoma is smaller than the first, probably due to its relatively early diagnosis during follow-up.

Bilateral occurrence of breast carcinoma does not change the prognosis. The prognosis is determined by the tumor with the least favorable stage.

A different histological type is a helpful criterion for the differentiation from metastases in the contralateral breast,. Also, the presence of CIS favors a second carcinoma over metastases.

■ Metastases in the Breast

Metastases in the Contralateral Breast

These account for most intramammary metastases. Metastases spread to the contralateral breast through the lymphatic system. They appear first medially in the breast in adipose tissue surrounding the breast parenchyma. Intraparenchymal metastases can be observed in hematogenous spread. They can be multiple or involve diffusely one segment of the breast. These criteria are helpful in differentiating metastases from a second primary carcinoma. In the presence of generalized distant metastatic disease, metastasis to the breast is more likely than a second primary tumor.

Intramammary Metastasis of Nonmammary Malignant Tumors

Every malignant tumor, especially those with widespread seeding, can metastasize to the breast, but most frequent are lung cancer, melanoma, and malignant lymphoma. Metastases frequently occur solitarily and localize in the upper outer quadrant.

Metastases are dense, round, slightly lobulated, often well-circumscribed or only slightly indistinct. Any possible spicules are short. Often they are confined to one breast, but one-third of melanoma metastases involve both breasts.

■ Locally and Regionally Recurrent Carcinomas

After Mastectomy

Local recurrence may occur in the scar, skin, and chest wall after incomplete resection of the carcinoma (retained lymphatic vessels with tumor cell thrombi). Regional recurrence refers to tumorous involvement of the axillary, supraclavicular, or parasternal lymph nodes. These recurrences can be traced to an advanced stage at the time of the mastectomy, with tumor or affected lymph nodes left behind.

Sonography is important for detecting recurrences in the chest wall and nodal metastases. Sonography, CT, MRI are indicated for suspicious findings in the mastectomy site.

After Breast-Conserving Surgery

As described in conjunction with multifocal carcinomas, breast-conserving surgery and inadequate radiation therapy run the risk of continuing proliferation of carcinomatous foci that were not excised. After breast-conserving surgery, the reported recurrence rate is up to 33% without and 2–21% with additional radiotherapy. About 30–50% of these recurrences are detected by mammography and the rest by palpation.

Recurrent carcinomas have the same mammographic appearance as primary carcinomas. A primary tumor characterized by microcalcifications or focal density usually has a recurrent tumor that displays the same finding. The first follow-up mammogram should be obtained six months after completion of the treatment, and the next mammogram at one year. Thereafter, mammography should be obtained annually. Any changes secondary to surgery and radiation can be recognized by comparison with previous films and should not be misdiagnosed as carcinoma. Radiation induces skin changes and increases the density of the fibroglandular structures. Postsurgical intramammary hematomas may lead to calcifications, focal lesions and distortions (see chapter 8).

Orel et al. (1993) studied 72 patients with recurrent carcinoma after lumpectomy, excision, segmental resection, and irradiation. The average interval until the development of a recurrence was 42.5 months (6–158). Most of the recurrences developed within the first five years. The relapse-free five-year survival rate was 73%. Recurrent tumors are detected in 47% of cases by mammography exclusively, in 33% by physical examination exclusively, and in 19% by both mammography and physical examination.

The recurrences detected by mammography had a more favorable stage, with 93% representing an CIS or found at stage T1. Patients with recurrent tumor exclusively found at physical examination more often had positive axillary lymph nodes. Both mammography and physical examination, therefore, are important in the follow-up of breast cancer patients. As to the contribution of dynamic MRI to the follow-up, especially in differentiating recurrent breast carcinoma from late radiation fibrosis, see p 176.

■ Pregnancy and Breast Cancer

Breast carcinoma is considered to be associated with pregnancy when it is diagnosed during or up to one year after pregnancy (lactation period). The incidence is 1 in 3000–10 000 pregnancies, and 1–2% of all breast carcinomas occur during pregnancy or in the lactation period. In women under the age of 35 years with breast carcinoma, an association with pregnancy and lactation, respectively, has to be considered. The prognosis of pregnancy-associated invasive breast carcinoma is poor. The five-year survival rate is 20% at most. The carcinoma in these patients is often discovered at an advanced stage.

Liberman et al. (1994) analyzed 23 breast carcinomas that occurred during pregnancy or lactation and recorded the following mammographic findings:

- Mass without calcifications: 17%.
- Mass with calcifications: 39%.
- Microcalcifications only: 17%.
- Diffusely increased density of parenchyma with skin thickening: 4%.

- No mammographic signs: 22%.
- Histopathological analysis of 23 cases revealed IDC in 22 cases and ILC in one case.

Sonography could be helpful for a palpable mass without corresponding mammographic findings. Whenever neither mammography nor sonography delineate a palpable mass, a biopsy should be performed.

■ Growth Rate of Breast Carcinoma

Only few studies address the clinical growth rate of breast cancer. The great variability in volume doubling time of tumors points to the heterogeneity of breast cancer. The very different behavioral pattern of the disease leads to the assumption that the genetic basis varies.

With a median volume doubling time of 150 days, the tumor needs 21 volume doubling times to grow from one tumor cell to a size of 5 mm and 25 doubling times to reach a size of 1 cm. However, the volume doubling time varies: it is less than 150 days (28%) for fast-growing carcinomas, 150–300 days (39%) for the average breast cancer, and longer than 300 days (33%) for slowly growing cancers. The median volume doubling time is 100–180 days. As shown in Table 3.**3**, recent studies have demonstrated that volume doubling time is age-dependent (Peer et al., 1993). A tumor can be palpable when it has a size of 1.5–2 cm, but can be detected by mammographic screening at a size of 0.5 cm. Under the most favorable circumstances, therefore, screening with mammography can detect a tumor two to three years earlier than physical examination.

■ Missed, Mammographically Occult and Interval Cancer

■ Missed Carcinoma

Reasons for carcinomas being missed on the mammogram are listed in the boxes below.

Table 3.**3** Tumor volume doubling time of primary breast cancer according to age

Age at diagnosis (years)	Geometric mean doubling time
< 50	80 days (2.6 months)
50–70	157 days (5.1 months)
> 70	188 days (6.1 months)

Positioning and technical shortcomings

The suspicious lesion is not discernible:
- Lesion not imaged: incorrect positioning.
- Faulty exposure: incorrect position of automatic exposure control (AEC) detector.
- Faulty development: incorrect adjustment of processor.

Observer errors

The carcinoma is visible on the mammogram but is not detected or recognized as carcinoma by the observer:
- Insufficient experience in mammography.
- External distraction during viewing.
- Loss of concentration.
- Superficial viewing, especially failure to compare images of both breasts.
- Difficult to recognize, i.e., no distinct signs; refers to subtle mammographic signs only recognized by experienced observers:
  - asymmetry of glandular tissue, slight distortion of the architecture,
  - density in its incipient stage.
- clusters of microcalcifications interpreted as benign but later found to be malignant.

The number of observer errors can be reduced by double reading (independent reading of two observers).

Indirect mammographic signs of carcinoma

These signs frequently are very subtle and, therefore, quite often remain unrecognized:
- Solitary dilated duct behind the areola or unusual complex of dilated ducts.
- Clusters of microcalcifications (intraductal, intralobular).
- Increasing density.
- Increasing asymmetry of glandular tissue.
- Caution: every asymmetry on both views is a suspicious sign.
- Density with benign aspect in one view may be a fibroadenoma since fibroadenomas arise in the same part of the parenchyma as carcinomas; a fibroadenoma may mask a carcinoma; a circumscribed carcinoma, especially medullary and mucinous carcinoma (colloid carcinoma), may be misinterpreted as fibroadenoma.

■ Mammographically Occult Carcinoma

Almost all carcinomas smaller than 0.5 cm are not detectable with present mammographic technique. Even larger carcinomas may be invisible in dense glandular tissue, which especially applies to the large diffusely growing ILC, which may not be visible even with optimal examination technique.

When a carcinoma is palpable and not visible mammographically, it is called mammographically occult. About 5% of all breast cancers are mammographically occult:

- The average age of patients with mammographically occult carcinoma is 50 years, while the average age of patients with mammographically detectable carcinomas is 61 years.
- Already 6% of the patients have positive axillary lymph nodes.
- It mostly represents an IDC, less frequently an ILC, and sometimes a mucinous carcinoma (Dronkers, 1985).

ILC is relatively often mammographically occult. Hilleren et al. (1991) analyzed 22 cases (16%) of ILC that were mammographically occult on all three standard views in a series of 137 cases.

■ Interval Cancers

Interval cancer is defined as a carcinoma that is discovered during the interval between two screening examinations after a negative screening examination, often by the woman after it has become clinically manifest.

In The Netherlands, the annual incidence of breast cancer in the age group of 50–69 years is 2.25/1000 women, corresponding to a two-year incidence of 4.5/1000 women. The national screening program detects about 70% of these carcinomas, which translates to 3–3.5/1000 women. The undetected 30% equal the number of interval cancers: approximately 1–1.5/1000 women per two years. In a more detailed analysis of interval cancers, 50% are true interval cancers, 30% have minimal signs on the preceding screening mammogram, and 5% are not visible on the screening examination because of technical shortcomings or occult mammographic presentation. Observer errors account for 15–20% of missed cancers.

Reviewing the mammographic findings of interval cancers by the readers of both mammograms is absolutely essential for quality assurance of a screening program.

References

Bässler, R.: Mamma. In Remmele, W.: Pathologie, Band 3. Springer, Berlin 1984

Burhenne, H. J., L. W. Burhenne, F. Goldberg et al.: Interval breast cancers in the screening mammography program of British Columbia: analysis and classification. Amer. J. Roentgenol. 162 (1994) 1067–1071

Burrell, H. C., D. M. Sibbering, A. R. M. Wilson et al.: Screening interval breast cancers: mammographic features and prognostic factors. Radiology 199 (1996) 811–817

Ciatto, S., D. Morrone, S. Catarzi et al.: Radial scars of the breast: review of 38 consecutive mammographic diagnoses. Radiology 187 (1993) 757–760

Dongen, van J. A., I. S. Fentiman, J. R. Harris et al.: In situ breast cancer. The EORTC consensus meeting. Lancet 334 (1989) 25–27

Dongen, van J. A., R. Holland, J. L. Peterse et al.: Ductal carcinoma in-situ of the breast; second EORTC consensus meeting. Europ. J. Cancer 28 (1992) 626–629

Dronkers, D. J.: Mammografisch occult mammacarcinoom. Ned. T. Geneesk. 129 (1985) 1632–1635

Faverly, D., R. Holland, L. Burgers: An original stereomicroscopic analysis of the mammary glandular tree. Virchows Arch. Abt. A 421 (1992) 115–119

Feig, S. A.: Breast masses: mammographic and sonographic evaluation. Radiol. Clin. N. Amer. 30 (1992) 67–92

Gils, van C. H., J. D. M. Otten, A. L. M. Verbeek, J. H. C. L. Hendriks: Short communication: breast parenchymal patterns and their changes with age. Brit. J. Radiol. 68 (1995) 1133–1135

Harris, J. R., M. E. Lippman, M. Morrow, S. Hellman: Diseases of the Breast. Lippincott, Philadelphia 1996

Helvie, M. A., C. Paramagul, H. A. Oberman, D. D. Adler: Invasive lobular carcinoma: imaging features and clinical detection. Invest. Radiol. 28 (1993) 202–207

Hilleren, D. J., T. T. Anderson, K. K. Lindholmn et al.: Invasive lobular carcinoma: mammographic findings in a 10 year experience. Radiology 178 (1991) 149–154

Holland, R., J. H. C. L. Hendriks: Microcalcifications associated with ductal carcinoma in situ: mammographic pathologic correlation. Semin. diagn. Pathol. 11 (1994) 181–192

Holland, R., M. Mravunac, J. H. C. L. Hendriks, B. V. Bekker: Socalled interval cancers of the breast. Pathologic and radiologic analysis of sixty-four cases. Cancer 49 (1982) 2527–2533

Holland, R., J. H. C. L. Hendriks, M. Mravunac: Mammographically occult breast cancer. A pathologic and radiologic study. Cancer 52 (1983) 1810–1819

Holland, R., J. Connolly, R. Gelman et al.: The presence of an extensive intraductal component (EIC) following a limited excision correlates with prominent residual disease in the remainder of the breast. J. clin. Oncol. 8 (1990) 113–118

Holland, R., J. L. Peterse, R. R. Millis u. Mitarb.: Ductal carcinoma in situ: a proposal for a new classification. Semin. diagn. Pathol. 11 (1994) 167–180

Homer, M. J.: Imaging features and management of characteristically benign and probably benign breast lesions. Radiol. Clin. N. Amer. 25 (1987) 939–951

Ikeda, D. M., I. Andersson, C. Wattsgard, L. Janzon, F. Linell: Interval carcinomas in the Malmö mammographics screening trial: radiographic appearance and prognostic considerations. Amer. J. Roentgenol. 159 (1992) 287–294

Ikeda, D. M., M. A. Helvie, T. S. Frank, K. L. Chapel, I. T. Andersson: Paget disease of the nipple: radiologic-pathologic correlation. Radiology 189 (1993) 89–94

Lanyi, M.: Diagnosis and Differential Diagnosis of Breast Calcifications. Springer, Berlin 1986

Liberman, L., C. S. Giess, D. D. Dershaw, B. M. Deutch, J. A. Petrek: Imaging of pregnancy-associated breast cancer. Radiology 191 (1994) 245–248

Mellink, W. A. M., R. Holland, J. H. C. L. Hendriks, P. H. M. Peeters, E. J. T. Rutgers, W. A. J. van Daal: The contribution of routine follow-up mammography to an early detection of asynchronous contralateral breast cancer. Cancer 67 (1991) 1844 – 1848

Mendelsohn, E. B., K. M. Harris, N. Doshi et al.: Infiltrating lobular carcinoma: mammographic pattern with pathologic correlation. Amer. J. Roentgenol. 153 (1989) 265 – 271

Mitnick, J. S., M. F. Vazquez, M. N. Harris, S. Schechter, D. F. Roses: Invasive papillary carcinoma of the breast: Mammographic appearance. Radiology 177 (1990) 803 – 806

Moskowitz, M.: Interval cancers and screening for breast cancer in British Columbia. Amer. J. Roentgenol. 162 (1994) 1072 – 1075

Murphy, T. J., E. F. Conant, C. A. Hanau, S. M. Ehrlich, S. A. Feig: Bilateral breast carcinoma: mammographic and histologic correlation. Radiology 195 (1995) 617 – 621

Newstead, G. M., P. B. Baute, H. K. Toth: Invasive lobular and ductal carcinoma: mammographic findings and stage at diagnosis. Radiology 184 (1992) 623 – 627

Orel, S. G., B. L. Fowble, L. J. Solin, D. J. Schultz, E. F. Conant, R. H. Troupin: Breast Cancer recurrence after lumpectomy and radiation therapy for early-stage disease: prognostic significance of detection method. Radiology 188 (1993) 189 – 194

Page, D. L., T. J. Anderson: Diagnostic Histopathology of the Breast. Churchill Livingstone, Edinburgh 1987

Peer, P. G. M., J. A. A. M. van Dijck, J. H. C. L. Hendriks, R. Holland, A. L. M. Verbeek: Age-dependent growth rate of primary breast cancer. Cancer 71 (1993) 3547 – 3551

Peer, P. G. M., A. L. M. Verbeek, H. Straatman, J. H. C. L. Hendriks, R. Holland: Agespecific sensitivities of mammographic screening for breast cancer. Breast Cancer Res. Treatm. 38 (1996) 153 – 160

Prechtel, K.: Pathologie der Mastopathie und des Mammakarzinoms. Radiologe 33 (1993) 236 – 242

Roubidoux, M. A., M. A. Helvie, N. E. Lai, C. Paramagul: Bilateral breast cancer: early detection with mammography. Radiology 196 (1995) 427 – 431

Roubidoux, M. A., N. E. Lai, C. Paramagul, L. K. Joynt, M. A. Helvie: Mammographic appearance of cancer in the opposite breast: comparison with the first cancer. Amer. J. Roentgenol. 166 (1996) 29 – 31

Sewell, C. W.: Pathology of benign and malignant breast disorders. Radiol. Clin. N. Amer. 33 (1995) 1067 – 1080

Sickles, E. A.: The subtle and atypical mammographic features of invasive lobular carcinoma. Radiology 178 (1991) 25

Sickles, E. A.: Nonpalpable, circumscribed, noncalcified solid breast masses: likelihood of malignancy based on lesion size and age of patient. Radiology 192 (1994) 439 – 442

Stomper, P. C., J. L. Connolly: Ductal carcinoma in situ of the breast: correlation between mammographic calcification and tumor subtype. Amer. J. Roentgenol. 159 (1992) 483 – 485

Tabár, L., N. Faberberg, E. Day et al.: Breast cancer treatment and natural history: new insights from the results of screening. Lancet 339 (1992) 412 – 414

Tinnemans, J. G. M., T. Wobbes, J. H. C. L. Hendriks, R. Holland, R. F. van der Sluis, H. H. M. de Boer: The role of mammography in the detection of bilateral primary breast cancer. Wld J. Surg. 12 (1988) 382 – 388

Trojani, M.: A Colour Atlas of Breast Histopathology. Chapman and Hall Medical, London 1991

Tulusan, A. H.: Breast cancer pathology. In Burghardt, E., M. J. Webb, J. M. Monaghan, G. Kindermann: Surgical Gynecologic Oncology. Thieme, Stuttgart 1993 (pp. 542 – 560)

4 Epidemiology and Treatment of Breast Cancer

Epidemiology and Risk Factors

B.–P. Robra, A. L. M. Verbeek and Natalie McGauran

■ Epidemiology

Breast cancer is the most frequent malignant tumor among women in most European countries, North America, and most of South America, Australia, and New Zealand. This malignancy is also the most common cause of death in women between the ages of 35 and 55 in these countries (Baum and Schipper, 1998), affecting approximately one in eight females. In the United States alone, an estimated 176 300 new cases were diagnosed and 43 700 women died of the disease in 1999 (American Cancer Society, 1999).

Incidence rates (the number of new cases per year per 100 000 women) have steadily increased over the past decades, especially in postmenopausal women. Figure 4.2 displays the age-specific incidence, the incidence per 100 000 women of a specified age group, which increases with age. There is a further rise before the menopause; the peak of this curve is referred to as Clemmesen's hook (Clemmesen 1948). The curves refer to different periods of registration and show a significant increase in the incidence of breast cancer in the 1986 –

90 period compared to the period from 1978 to 1981. Since incidence rates rose before the introduction of screening programs (which led to a rise in incidence due to earlier tumor detection) and improved registration for new breast cancer cases, other external factors such as lifestyle and environmental features seem to be responsible for this development.

There are extreme geographical variations in the frequency of breast cancer. The countries with the highest incidence rates are displayed in Figure 4.1. The lowest incidence rates are observed in Asia, where the rates are only about 25 % of those in the United States. However, incidence and mortality (the number of deaths per year per 100 000 women) have increased steeply in some industrialized Asian regions. In Japan and Singapore, the incidence rates doubled and mortality rates rose by 50 – 60% in women aged 35 – 44 years from 1960 to 1985 (Ursin et al., 1994). Incidence rates of Japanese immigrants in the United States approach local levels by the second generation, indicating a strong association between nonhereditary lifestyle factors and breast carcinogenesis (Spratt et al., 1995).

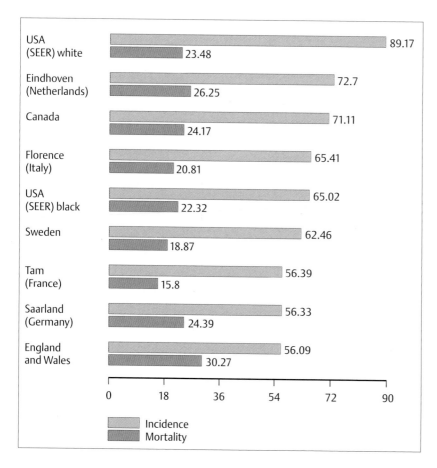

Fig 4.1 **Breast cancer incidence and mortality rates per 100 000 women in the United States and Europe between 1983 and 1987** (age-standardized for the world population, according to Parkin, 1992)

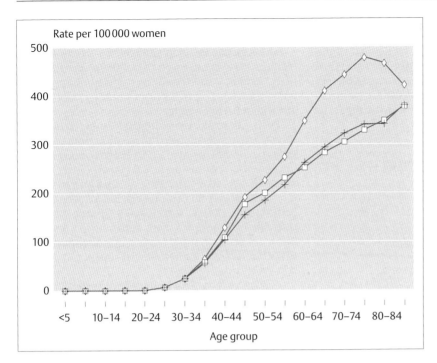

Rate per 100 000 women

Fig. 4.**2   Average age-specific
breast cancer incidence rates for
women in the United States.**
Rates per 100 000 women within
the respective age group (according to Feur, 1992)
☐ 1986 – 1990
+ 1978 – 1981
◇ 1973 – 1977

Ethnic differences within countries have been observed. In the United States, breast cancer incidence
rates are higher among white women (>40 years) compared to African-American women, possibly due to reproductive factors (fewer births, older age at first birth),
but lower among younger white women (Brinton et al.,
1997). Mortality rates for African-American women have
exceeded those for white women. Previously published
lower mortality rates may have been due to incomplete
reporting. Social factors such as limited access to medical facilities and diagnosis at an advanced stage of disease with poor survival prospects could also contribute
to this discrepancy.

Women from higher socioeconomic classes (who
show different reproductive patterns compared to
women from low-income groups) are more commonly
affected but have better survival rates. Women from low
social classes have a lower attendance at screening programs and are diagnosed at a later stage (Garvican,
1998).

Since 1990, mortality rates in developed countries
have remained stable or declined slightly despite increasing incidence rates (Fig. 4.**3**). This discrepancy can
be attributed to the introduction of widespread mammographic screening, earlier diagnosis with detection of
tumors at a curable stage, and the introduction of more
effective therapies with improved survival prospects
(Mettlin, 1999). An additional factor is the detection of
tumors that are not always fatal, such as the well-differentiated DCIS and tubular and mucinous carcinomas.
Currently, Great Britain has the highest breast cancer
mortality rate, followed by The Netherlands and Germany.

■ Risk Factors

Population-based studies have characterized factors associated with greater breast cancer risk, leading to a better understanding of mammary carcinogenesis. Breast
cancer has been the subject of intensive research.
Though a variety of well-established risk factors have
been identified, the role of other etiological factors is still
controversial as study results are inconsistent.

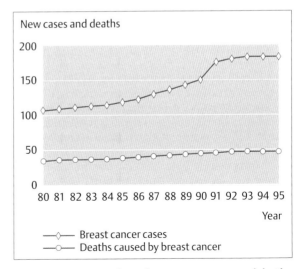

Fig. 4.**3   Estimation of new breast cancer cases and deaths
caused by breast cancer per 100 000 women in the United
States between 1980 and 1995** (American Cancer Society,
1995)

The detection of specific risk factors offers possibilities for risk reduction, such as changes in lifestyle. Furthermore, high-risk women can be advised to undergo regular screening. The relative risk (the strength of a risk factor) is defined as the incidence among persons possessing a characteristic in question divided by the incidence among otherwise similar persons without the characteristic (Harris et al., 1992).

Factors associated with increased breast cancer risk

- Aging
- Prior diagnosis of breast cancer
- Genetic predisposition
- Estrogen dominance
- Nutritional and other lifestyle factors
- History of benign breast disease
- Exposure to irradiation

Aging. Old age is the greatest risk factor for nonhereditary breast cancer. The incidence rate steadily increases from age 25 onwards. In past years (1986–1990) the postmenopausal leveling of the incidence curve has decreased (Fig. 4.**2**, 1986–90 period).

Prior diagnosis of breast cancer. Women with a prior breast cancer diagnosis have a threefold to fourfold increase in risk of a second primary breast tumor of the contralateral or affected breast after breast conservation surgery. These tumors sometimes occur only shortly after diagnosis of the first tumor.

Genetic predisposition. Specific breast cancer susceptibility genes induce alterations of the chromosomal DNA. Mutated tumor suppressor genes result in a defective control of DNA replication, enabling cell division to continue before repair of damaged DNA and consequent transcription of abnormal DNA. Little additional DNA damage is necessary in order to generate malignancy, meaning an increased breast cancer risk for gene carriers.

A hereditary component exists for about 10% of all breast cancer cases (up to 25% of cases diagnosed before the age of 40 years). A first-degree relative with premenopausal breast cancer is a significant risk factor. The existence of a genetic mutation is likely in families with multiple first-degree relatives with premenopausal onset (occasionally with bilateral manifestation). The relative risk for female family members with two affected first-degree relatives is fourfold to sixfold and exceeds 50% in women who have a sister with bilateral breast cancer before the age of 50 years (Gail et al., 1989).

The majority of these cases are attributed to distinct germline mutations of the tumor suppressor genes *BRCA 1* and *BRCA 2*. An estimated 1 : 500 of the general population are carriers of these mutated genes, which are inherited in an autosomal-dominant mode. The frequency of gene carriers in women of Ashkenazi-Jewish descent is approximately five times higher (Coughlin et al., 1999).

Although families with multiple first-degree affected relatives have an increased risk of these specific mutations, cancer clustering was detected in pedigrees without such genes, indicating the existence of at least one additional *BRCA* gene.

Exact risk prediction is difficult due to the mutation variety. Studies of families with identified mutated *BRCA* genes (i.e., Lancaster et al., 1997) have predicted a lifetime possibility exceeding 80% for breast cancer for mutated *BRCA 1* and *BRCA 2* gene carriers, and an ovarian cancer risk of over 50% for mutated *BRCA 1* gene carriers. Both breast cancer susceptibility genes show unfavorable prognostic factors, such as an increased frequency of bilateral and multicentric disease, more invasive tumors, and earlier onset of illness compared to non-gene carriers.

Carriers of the ataxia-telangiectasia gene who have a reduced DNA repair capacity and an increased sensitivity to irradiation have an elevated cancer risk, especially of breast cancer (Inskip et al., 1999).

Other genetic defects such as Li-Fraumeni syndrome, Cowden disease (Mann and Borgen, 1998) and Peutz–Jeghers syndrome (Boardman et al., 1998) play a minor role in the overall incidence of breast cancer, but gene carriers are at a significantly higher risk compared to non-gene carriers.

Estrogen dominance. A number of factors associated with hormonal stimulation of breast glandular tissue (estrogen dominance) are also significantly associated with the risk of developing breast cancer. An increased lifetime exposure to menstrual cycles (premature menarche, late menopause) leads to an excess risk. Ovariectomy before menopause is a protective factor.

Harris et al. (1992) reported increases in the risk associated with age at menarche, menopause, and first pregnancy. Menopause after the age of 55 means a doubling of risk compared to menopause before the age of 45, and menarche before the age of 12 a relative risk of 1.2 of developing breast cancer compared to menarche after the age of 14 (this could partially explain the international differences in breast cancer rates: the average age of menarche is 17 years in China, compared to 12.8 years in the United States). Nulliparity and late first full-term pregnancy are also significant predictive factors. Women who give birth after the age of 30 years for the first time have a twofold breast cancer risk compared to women who give birth before the age of 20 years (first pregnancy at a young age leads to early differentiation of glandular tissue).

Earlier reports postulated a connection between induced abortion and excess breast cancer risk, but recent literature does not confirm this hypothesis (Bartholomew and Grimes, 1998).

Lactation as a preventive factor seems to have been overrated in the past. Recent data suggest only a weak protective effect (Furberg et al., 1999).

The use of oral contraceptives and hormone replacement therapy (HRT) and the risk of breast cancer have been studied extensively because of the association between sex hormones and breast cancer risk. Both the estrogen and progestin components are potential risk modifiers. The combination of both components (progestin reduces the risk of endometrial cancer) apparently has no decreasing effect on the elevated breast cancer risk.

A meta-analysis of data from 54 studies involving over 150000 women concluded that women who had taken contraceptives within the previous ten years had a small increased risk of developing breast cancer (relative risk 1.24, 95% CI 1.15 – 1.33); the risk was higher for women who had begun to use contraceptives before age 20 (Collaborative Group on Hormonal Factors in Breast Cancer, 1996).

Concerning the role of HRT, a meta-analysis of 51 epidemiological studies involving over 150000 women described an increased risk for women who were on current or recent HRT. The risk increased with duration of use. The relative risk was 1.35 (95% CI 1.21 – 1.49) for women who were on HRT for more than five years (Collaborative Group on Hormonal Factors in Breast Cancer, 1997).

The excess risk decreases rapidly after cessation of both HRT and oral contraceptives and reaches normal levels after about 10 years.

Considering the fact that millions of women are currently participating in an exposition experiment with external sex hormones, further risk differentiation is an urgent necessity. This should include a woman's age, reproductive history, and hormonal status as well as composition of the hormone preparations, their dose and duration of use.

Nutritional and other lifestyle factors. A comparison of international mortality and incidence rates with the average consumption of fat and other nutritional components indicates a positive correlation between breast cancer and high-fat, high-calorie, and low-vitamin diets. Studying the epidemiology of the nutritional aspects involves considerable methodological demands as regards to estimating the contribution of the different nutrients to a diet and to the total calorie intake. So far, epidemiologic studies have produced inconsistent results.

The role of dietary fat remains unclear. An English case-control study involving over 1500 women (breast cancer patients and controls) could not detect differences in fat intake between affected and healthy women (Cade et al., 1998). A prospective study involving nearly 90000 American nurses failed to link a lower intake of total or specific types of fat to a decreased breast cancer risk (Holmes et al., 1999). In contrast, a meta-analysis of 12 case-control studies found a statistically significant positive correlation between breast cancer risk and saturated fat intake (Howe et al., 1990). A prospective Japanese study associated excess consumption of animal fat with an increased breast cancer risk (Hirayama, 1990).

Previous reports that linked frequent meat consumption to increased breast cancer risk have not been confirmed. Recent studies conclude that a high dietary intake of vegetables or a vegetarian diet does not at all or only minimally decreases mortality (Key et al., 1999).

A number of studies have recently been performed concerning the role of vitamins. Some demonstrate that the intake of vitamin C (Howe et al., 1990), vitamin D (John et al., 1999) and beta-carotene (Jumaan et al., 1999) is inversely correlated with breast cancer, but the findings have not been consistent.

Specific phytoestrogens (naturally occurring chemicals with a structure similar to estrogen) have also been identified as protective factors (Ingram et al., 1997).

Various researchers have displayed a modest positive association between alcohol consumption and breast cancer (Bowlin et al., 1997; Tseng et al., 1999). This may be explained by the inhibiting effect of alcohol on estrogen metabolism and a subsequent increase in blood estrogen levels, or by an inadequate folate intake of alcohol consumers. Zhang et al. (1999) found a negative association between a high folate intake and the risk of breast cancer.

Studies investigating the role of smoking and the risk of breast cancer do not provide conclusive evidence. One of the largest prospective studies in Sweden conducted on 26,000 women negated a significant connection (Nordlund et al., 1997). However, female smokers with low-activity *N*-acetyltransferase genotypes may have an increased risk (Ambrosone et al., 1996).

Relative overweight (as determined by the body mass index in kg/m^2) has been strongly linked to breast cancer in postmenopausal women, particularly among women who were not taking hormones (Huang et al., 1997). The excess risk associated with adult obesity is attributed to the production of sex hormones in fat tissue. A negative association has been implied in premenopausal women (Peacock et al., 1999). Teenage obesity appears to be a protective factor, possibly due to more frequent anovulation in overweight adolescents compared to their normal-weight peers (Stoll, 1998). Further research is needed concerning the association between obesity and breast cancer and other outcomes such as atypia, benign breast disease and specific (i.e., ER+ [estrogen receptor]) types of mammary carcinoma.

Height, which is variably dependent on genetic and adolescent nutritional factors, has also been described as risk factor in studies incorporating height measurements (Wang et al., 1997). The increased risk for tall women could be explained by the effect of a high-calorie diet on the adolescent breast gland. Animal experiments show a significant reduction in mammary tumors in animals given a restricted diet in adolescence (Welsch, 1992).

Physical activity has been inversely associated with breast cancer in postmenopausal women, but no association with premenopausal breast cancer has been confirmed (Sesso et al., 1998). These findings could be explained by the influence of exercise on body fat stores and by irregular ovulatory activity induced by physical exertion, especially at a strenuous level.

A positive association between a high bone mass density and breast cancer has been identified (Zhang et al., 1997). However, this correlation has no causal implications, as bone mass density is an indicator of cumulative exposure to estrogen.

History of benign breast disease. Chronic cystic mastopathy is a premalignant condition. Women with increasing epithelial dysplasia (diagnosed by biopsy) have an increased breast cancer risk. Compared to women with no proliferative disease, women with proliferative epithelial changes have a relative risk of 1.6 (95% CI 1.0–2.5) and women with atypical epithelial hyperplasia a relative risk of 3.7 (95% CI 2.1–6.8) of developing breast cancer (London et al., 1992).

Older studies did not associate cysts or fibroadenomas with an increased breast cancer risk, but this has been contradicted by recent studies. A prospective study that enlisted nearly 1400 women with solitary benign breast cysts in Scotland (Dixon et al., 1999) found an increased risk for this cohort, independent of the cyst type. Women with a prior diagnosis of mammary fibroadenoma have also been identified as a group with an elevated risk (Dupont et al., 1994).

Women with mammographically dense breast tissue have been reported as having an increased risk for breast cancer (Boyd et al., 1995). Furthermore, cancers diagnosed in this cohort are more advanced, as early tumor detection is difficult. In general, studies associating benign breast disease with an increased breast cancer risk should be interpreted cautiously, as surveillance bias (an increase in incidence due to an increase in screening of women in whom benign breast disease has been diagnosed) has to be taken into account.

Exposure to radiation. Exposure to ionizing radiation (whole-body or thorax radiation, single high-dose or frequent low-doses) is an established risk factor for breast cancer, with a linear dose-response. Women who underwent radiation therapy (e.g., for mastitis or Hodgkin lymphoma) or had multiple diagnostic radiographic examinations for pulmonary or cardiac disorders had an elevated risk, especially if examinations were performed without image intensifiers. Women with the highest risk were exposed to radiation during puberty, with women irradiated at the age of 15 years at maximum risk (Spratt et al., 1995).

■ Other Possibly Causal Factors

Environmental carcinogens. The role of organochlorines as an etiological agent of breast cancer remains controversial. A Danish study found a positive association between some organochlorine compounds and breast cancer (Hoyer et al., 1998), while other researchers have

not identified these chemicals as a predictive factor (Zheng et al., 1999).

Studies suggesting electromagnetic radiation (Hansen, 1999) and organic solvents (Kliuckiene et al., 1999) as potential mammary carcinogens need further evaluation.

Psychological factors. Bleiker et al. (1996) found a weak correlation between the development of breast cancer and a so-called antiemotional personality structure (lack of appropriate emotional behavior). No significant associations have been found regarding the influence of stressful life events on breast cancer risk (Roberts et al., 1996).

■ Prevention

A better understanding of the association between specific dietary factors and breast cancer could lead to the introduction of potentially protective eating habits (a prudent diet) as a preventive measure. A healthy diet and regular exercise should always be recommended. Besides probably reducing the incidence of breast cancer, such a lifestyle also decreases the incidence of other widespread diseases (cardiovascular and degenerative disorders).

A more effective way to reduce breast cancer mortality would be the introduction of standardized screening mammography together with an intensive education campaign that actively encourages women to participate. By offering comprehensive information, this would decrease anxiety and aversion. In 1987, a nationwide mammography-based screening program was introduced in Finland. The nearly 90 000 women who participated had a significantly reduced breast cancer mortality rate compared to the nearly 70 000 nonparticipants (Hakama, 1997). The fact that Finland has the highest breast cancer survival rate in Europe (Sant et al., 1998) underlines the potentially life-saving aspect of regular mammography.

Incorporating genetic testing for women with a family history of breast cancer should be discussed critically, as no standardized guidelines exist for women who test positive. This group may also be discriminated by insurance companies and exposed to severe psychological strain. Women from cancer-prone families should be under intensive surveillance. Annual mammography plus a semiannual breast and ovarian ultrasound and measurement of CA 125 are currently recommended by the 10 German centers involved in testing patients for mutated *BRCA 1* and *BRCA 2* genes (Schmutzler et al., 1999). The first studies of prophylactic mastectomy show at least a 90% decline in the breast cancer rate for high-risk women who underwent prophylactic surgery compared to their sisters who did not (Hartmann et al., 1999), but the hazards of such a radical intervention have to be considered.

Another future prevention scheme could include chemoprevention with selective estrogen receptor modulators. High-risk women using tamoxifen showed a 45% reduction in the risk of postmenopausal breast cancer. Women suffering from osteoporosis taking raloxifene had an even more significant risk reduction of about 50% (Jordan, 1999). Whether this risk reduction is permanent and whether women with a genetic susceptibility to premenopausal breast cancer also benefit from this prevention scheme needs to be evaluated in prospective trials. In addition, the possible beneficial effects (decreasing the risk of fractures and heart disease) and adverse effects (endometrial cancer/tamoxifen, thromboembolic disease/tamoxifen and raloxifene) need further investigation. The STAR Trial (Study of Tamoxifen and Raloxifene) is ongoing.

Summary

Besides reproductive and genetic factors, the most important breast cancer risk factors are external determinants such as lifestyle, environment and socioeconomics. A high-calorie diet and the suppression of infectious diseases have led to an optimal physical development and an earlier onset of sexual maturity, and a resultant longer exposition to sexual hormones. Several studies imply that dietary factors are a significant contributor to the rise in incidence of breast cancer, but more long-term intervention studies are needed to differentiate the incriminating nutritional components beyond the high calorie content. Modifiable dietary risk factors offer a preventive potential for reducing the risk of breast cancer.

Recent reports on the protective effect of chemoprevention promise progress in primary cancer prevention. High-quality comprehensive mammography screening could lead to an improvement in secondary prevention, resulting in further reduction of mortality.

Treatment

J. Hoogenhout, Th. Wobbes, W. J. Hoogenraad and L. V. A. M. Beex

Staging

Adequate staging and treatment of breast cancer requires interdisciplinary cooperation between radiologist, pathologist, surgeon, radiation oncologist, and medical oncologist.

Before surgery, the stage of disease is determined by the TNM classification. The letters T, N, and M indicate the extension of the primary tumor (T1–4), the spread to regional lymph nodes (N1–3), and the absence or presence of distant metastases (M0–1), respectively.

The notation pTNM refers to the surgical and postoperative histopathological results of investigation. Unless the prefix p is included, the classification refers to the preoperative staging (Table 4.**1**).

Treatment of the Primary Tumor

The treatment of an invasive breast cancer may be curative or palliative. If the disease is beyond cure, palliative treatment aims to reduce symptoms and to maintain quality of life. After adequate local and regional therapy and, if indicated, adjuvant systemic therapy, cure can be expected in less extensive tumor stages (pT1–2; N0–1; M0). The prospect is less favorable in more advanced stages (pT3; N2–3; M0). For locally advanced tumors (T4) or generalized disease (M1), treatment is no longer curative but palliative. The purpose of local and regional surgical treatment and radiation is tumor control, including prevention of local and regional recurrent disease. Axillary node dissection removes possible metastases and contributes to staging of the disease. Screening for metastases is indicated in patients with locally advanced disease (pT4; pN2–3) or with physical signs suggestive of metastases. No reliable method of demonstrating micrometastases has yet been found.

■ Curative Therapy

The standard treatment for small tumors (T1 and small T2) is a breast conservation procedure. Larger tumors (large T2 and T3) are treated with modified radical mastectomy, unless signs of metastases are found.

Breast conservation therapy. Breast conservation surgery encompasses a wide local excision of the tumor, an axillary node dissection, and radiation of the breast. The ultimate goal is local tumor control while retaining a cosmetically acceptable breast.

Randomized studies have shown that for small tumors, breast conservation treatment offers the same local control and life expectancy as a mastectomy. The cumulative risk of local or regional recurrence is 10% in the first 10 years after the primary treatment (Veronesi et al., 1993, Fisher et al., 1985, 1995).

Indications for Breast Conservation Surgery

- Histologically invasive breast carcinoma, inclusive of all subtypes.
- Stage pT1–2; pN0–1; M0.
- Local excision with a tumor-free margin of 1–2 cm around the tumor is acceptable from a cosmetic point of view.

Table 4.**1** TNM classification of breast tumors (Sobin LH, Wittekind Ch, 1997)

Tis	In situ		
T1	≤ 2 cm		
T1mic	≤ 0.1 cm		
T1a	> 0.1 to 0.5 cm		
T1b	> 0.5 to 1 cm		
T1c	> 1 to 2 cm		
T2	> 2 to 5 cm		
T3	> 5 cm		
T4	Chest wall/skin		
T4a	Chest wall		
T4b	Skin edema/ulceration, satellite skin nodules		
T4c	Both 4a and 4b		
T4d	Inflammatory carcinoma		
N1	Movable axillary lymph nodes		
		pN1	
		pN1a	Micrometastasis only, ≤ 0.2 cm
		pN1b	Gross metastasis
			(i) 1–3 nodes/ > 0.2 to < 2 cm
			(ii) ≥ 4 nodes/ > 0.2 to < 2 cm
			(iii) through capsule/< 2 cm
			(iv) ≥ 2 cm
N2	Fixed axillary lymph nodes	**pN2**	
N3	Internal mammary lymph nodes	**pN3**	
M1	Distant metastases		

Contraindications for Breast Conservation Surgery

Absolute contraindications:
- Tumor larger than 5 cm
- Extensive microcalcifications on the mammogram
- Multifocal tumor localizations in more than one quadrant
- Personal preference of the patient for breast amputation

Relative contraindications:
- Very small or very large breasts
- Very peripheral or subareolar tumor location
- Pregnancy or lactation
- Familial history of breast cancer
- *BCRA 1* and *BCRA 2* carriers
- Tumor larger than 3 cm

Surgical aspects of breast conservation:
In a breast conservation procedure, the surgical treatment consists of local excision of the tumor with a safety margin of 1 – 2 cm (lumpectomy, quadrantectomy). An axillary node dissection is still part of the standard treatment, although nowadays the tendency is strong to perform a sentinel node biopsy first to prevent the complications of resecting tumor-negative axillary nodes. For a tumor located in the upper quadrants, a semicircular incision is advised. For a tumor located in the lower quadrants, a radial incision produces better cosmetic results. The axillary node dissection is performed through a separate axillary incision. Lymph nodes are removed at all levels (I–III) and marked for pathological investigation. The receptor status of the primary tumor should be established.

Sentinel lymph node biopsy:
Axillary node dissection is a staging procedure but also removes tumor to achieve better regional control. Side effects such as loss of optimal shoulder and arm function or lymphedema may cause a considerable burden to the patient. Sentinel node biopsy is advocated to distinguish between patients who may benefit from a node dissection and those who may not.

The procedure consists of the injection of ^{99m}Tc-labeled colloid into the skin overlying the tumor or into the periphery of the lesion, possibly in combination with Patent Blue-V. During the operation the radioactively labeled (or blue-stained) lymph node is located with a gamma probe or identified visually and excised.

Pathological examination may reveal metastases by conventional or immunohistochemical staining. Submicroscopic disease may be demonstrated by polymerase chain reaction technology. The failure rate of this procedure is 5 – 10% in experienced hands (Borgstein et al., 1998; Cox et al., 1999).

Radiotherapy in breast conservation:
For optimal tumor control and cosmetically acceptable result, a homogeneous dose distribution is necessary. The three-dimensional form of the breast requires an individually adapted technique of radiation for each patient. The department of radiotherapy should have a modern simulator, a computerized planning system, and, if possible, both a low and high-energy linear accelerator. Radiation therapy after breast conservation surgery consists of two phases: radiation of the entire breast, and a boost to the site of the primary tumor excision.

- *Principles of radiotherapy:* By histological examination of amputated breasts, Holland et al. (1985) found foci of invasive and noninvasive cancers at sites more than 2 cm outside the original T1 and T2 tumor in 43% of cases. Only 37% of the patients with T1 and T2 tumors had no additional carcinomatous foci. Rosen et al. (1975) detected residual carcinoma in the breast after a simulated partial mastectomy in 26% of patients with tumors smaller than 2 cm and in 38% of patients with tumors larger than or equal to 2 cm. These clinical studies prove that microscopic tumor foci can be found in the entire breast, but especially directly around the primary tumor. Several nonrandomized clinical studies on breast conservation surgery without radiation showed that the frequency of local recurrence varied from 15% to 37% after 8–10 years (Montgomery et al.; 1978, Freeman et al., 1981; Lagois et al., 1983; Greening et al., 1988; Kantorowicz et al., 1989). These results were confirmed by three randomized studies that found a decrease in local recurrence from 29–39% without radiation of the breast to 10–14% with radiation of the entire breast (Table 4.**2**) (Clark et al.; 1987, Fisher et al., 1989; Kantorowicz et al., 1989). These studies indicate that radiation of the entire breast significantly decreases the risk of local recurrence. More recent publications by Fisher et al. (1995), the Early Breast Cancer Trialists Collaborative Group (1992) and the Scottish Cancer Trials Breast Group (1996) also confirm the benefit of radiation after local excision. The effectiveness of a boost to the site of primary tumor excision is less clear. Table 4.**3** shows comparative data on the risk of local recurrence in patients with breast cancer after lumpectomy and radiation of the entire breast with or without a boost to the primary tumor bed (Bedwinek et al., 1980; Chu et al., 1984; Harris et al., 1984; Nobler and Venet 1985; Romestaing et al., 1989). In conclusion, a boost of radiation marginally reduces the risk of local recurrence.

Radiobiological data indicate a moderate radiosensitivity of breast cancer. This means that a dose of about 50 Gy in 25 fractions is necessary for microscopic tumor foci. Whenever the risk of residual tumor foci is increased, a dose of 60–64 Gy in 30–32 fractions is necessary. The above-mentioned fractionated doses are within the normal tissue tolerance. The radiobiological effectiveness to tumor and normal tissue of 50 Gy in 25 fractions is approximately equivalent to 45 Gy in 18 fractions.

- *Radiation of the entire breast*: The breast is irradiated through lateral and medial tangential portals. The medial and lateral portals encompass the breast parenchyma and the chest wall. The target area begins 5 mm beneath the skin. A linear accelerator with a photon energy of 4–6 MV is appropriare. For a large breast, higher energy with skin compensation may be necessary. The radiation techniques are presented in Figure 4.**4**. Figure 4.**5** shows a film obtained with the simulator. The generally accepted radiation dose is 50 Gy in 25 fractions delivered to the isocenter.
- *Boost*: Three techniques are available for the radiation of the site of primary tumor excision (Fig. 4.**6**):
  - Wedged photon beams for a deep localized tumor in a large breast (Fig. 4.**6a**)
  - Implantation for interstitial brachytherapy, for example ^{192}Ir seeds (Fig. 4.**6b**)
  - Single electron beam (Fig. 4.**6c**)

Table 4.**2** Percentage of local recurrence in patients treated with or without radiation after breast conservation surgery

Author	Number of patients	Primary tumor volume/stage	Result	% local recurrence with radiation	% local recurrence without radiation	P-value
Fisher et al. (1995)	1450	≤ 4 cm	Recurrence after 8 years	10	39	< 0.001
Clark et al. (1987)	1504	T1–4	Recurrence after 10 years	14	29	< 0.0001
Kantorowicz et al. (1989)	237	T1–3	Recurrence not mentioned	10	30	–

Table 4.**3** Percentage of local recurrence in patients treated with or without boost radiation after breast conservation surgery

Author	Number of patients	Primary tumor volume/stage	Result	Follow-up years (median)	% local recurrence with boost	% local recurrence without boost	P-Value
Bedwinek et al. (1980)	195	≤ 5 cm	Recurrence	3.4	5	5	NS
Chu et al. (1984)	154	≤ 5 cm	Recurrence	4.2	6	19	0.010
Harris et al. (1984)	357	T1–4	Recurrence after 10 years	4.3	6	12	NS
Nobler et al. (1985)	161	T1–3	Recurrence after 6 years	3.8	6	9	NS
Romestaing et al. (1989)	384	≤ 3 cm	Recurrence	Not mentioned	1	2	NS

NS = not significant

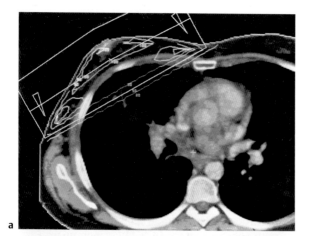

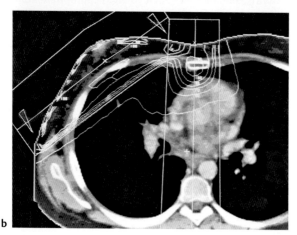

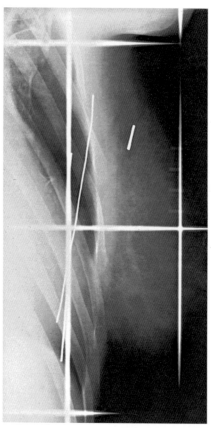

Fig. 4.5 **Example of a simulator film of tangential breast portals**. The radio-opaque clip marks the bottom of the tumor excision cavity. About 2 cm of lung tissue is invariably included in the radiation volume

Fig. 4.**4a, b Two techniques with tangential portals for radiation of the entire breast with and without internal mammary lymph nodes**
a Dose distribution of two tangential photon portals (4 MV) for radiation of the breast
b Dose distribution of the combination of two tangential photon portals (4 MV) and one anterior electron portal (13 MeV) for radiation of the breast and the internal mammary lymph nodes
Caution: subcutaneous hot spot along the junction of the portals

In our experience, radiation with electrons and interstitial brachytherapy are both well-suited for a satisfactory cosmetic result and local tumor control. Preference should be given to radiation with an electron beam in view of its relatively simple technique as well as the low patient burden. The target volume encompasses the original tumor with a margin of about 2 cm. The required dose is 14–20 Gy in 7–10 fractions for external radiation, or 15 Gy at a low dose rate for interstitial brachytherapy.
- *Radiation of regional lymph nodes:* There is no agreement regarding indications for postoperative radiation of the regional lymph nodes. Regional radiation does not significantly improve the chances of overall survival. After radiation of the supraclavicular and axillary lymph nodes the recurrence rate decreases,

but the risk of arm edema increases. Indications for radiation of the axilla and/or supraclavicular regions are limited. The axilla is radiated in cases with massive extra-nodal tumor deposits or following non-radical surgery. Indications for radiation of the supraclavicular region are four or more positive lymph nodes or positive lymph nodes in level III. Radiation is performed with the McWhirter technique to a dose of 46 Gy in 23 fractions. Radiation of the internal mammary lymph nodes is extremely controversial. A limited number of institutions apply radiation in cases with a centrally and/or medially located tumor and tumor-positive axillary lymph nodes. After scintigraphic localization, the internal mammary lymph nodes are irradiated with an anterior electron beam (9 or 13 MeV) to a dose of 46 Gy in 23 fractions (Fig. 4.4). In cases of breast conservation treatment, overlapping of the tangential and ventral beams can cause an area of high dose (hot spot) with resulting symptomatic fibrosis.

Cosmetic results and side effects:
The most important factors that determine the cosmetic results are

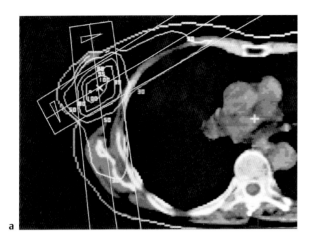

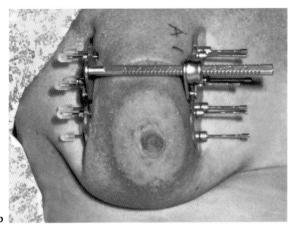

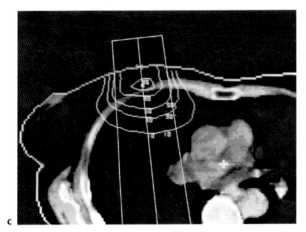

Fig. 4.6 a – c **Overview of the techniques to radiate the site of the excised primary tumor (boost)**

a Isodose pattern of two wedged photon beams (4 MV) with a low burden of lung tissue. The dose is specified in the iso-center and calculated according to the guidelines of ICRU 62

b Example of a two-level implantation. The seven hollow, stainless needles with a diameter of 1.5 mm are temporally provided with ^{192}Ir seeds. The dose is specified according to the guidelines ICRU 58

c Example of a isodose pattern of a single electron beam (9 MeV). The dose is calculated for dosis maximum according to the guidelines of ICRU 29

- Extent of tumor excision
- Method of axillary lymph node excision

The cosmetic results are also influenced by

- Total radiation dose
- Fractionation
- Homogeneity of dose distribution
- Any adjuvant chemotherapy

The major side effects after surgery and radiotherapy are local fibrosis, arm edema and telangiectasia. Pierquin et al. (1986) concluded in a large study that arm edema after axillary node dissection and radiation of the axillary region developed in 78 of 907 patients (9%). In two clinical studies with a follow-up period of five and seven years, a good to excellent result was achieved in 80 – 90% of the patients with breast conservation treatment (Olivotto et al., 1989; Rose et al., 1989)

Local recurrence after breast conservation treatment:
Recurrence after breast conservation therapy can result from the invasive component of the tumor or from incompletely excised ductal carcinoma in situ (DCIS).

Besides a recurrence, a de novo carcinoma can arise. Seventy-five percent of the recurrences appear in the immediate area of the primary tumor, 10% in other parts of the breast, and 15% in the cutis and subcutis.

As previously mentioned, the percentage of local recurrence is 8 – 10% for patients after a breast conservation procedure. However, for patients with invasive carcinoma and an extensive intraductal component (extensive intraductal carcinoma, EIC) the risk of a local recurrence increases to 28%. Extensive intraductal carcinoma is defined if more than 25% of the primary invasive tumor and/or its direct surroundings consists of intraductal carcinoma, or if one or more areas of focal invasion are present in an intraductal carcinoma (Boyages et al., 1990).

As the in situ component decreases in the periphery of the tumor, the risk of recurrence after a wide excision also declines. The need for a very wide excision is supported by the study of Holland et al. (1990). These researchers found a DCIS in 30 % of the patients with EIC at a distance of 2 cm from the primary tumor. For patients treated with a quadrantectomy, representing a wide excision, the risk of recurrence is significantly lower (Veronesi et al. 1990; Vicini et al., 1991).

The standard treatment for a local recurrence is a simple mastectomy.

Modified radical mastectomy:
For a tumor larger than 3 cm (large T2; T3) or whenever an acceptable cosmetic result with breast conservation cannot be expected, a modified radical mastectomy is the treatment of choice.

Surgical techniques:
In the modified radical mastectomy, the mammary gland together with underlying pectoral fascia is re-

moved, immediately followed by resection of the axillary lymph nodes. The major and minor pectoral muscles remain intact (modification of Madden–Auchincloss), while in the Patey variant the minor pectoral muscle is removed. The radical mastectomy according to Halsted, which removes both muscles, is considered obsolete. With tumor infiltration of the major pectoral muscle, a wide local excision of the involved muscle is sufficient.

Postoperative radiation of the chest wall:
- *Indications*: Radiation of the chest wall is advised when the resection margin is not free of tumor, when an infiltration of skin or chest wall is established (pT4), or when a large tumor (> 5 cm, pT3) is found.
- *Technique and dose*: Depending on the curvature of the chest wall and the size of the scar, an adequate radiation can be administered via a direct electron beam or via two tangential photon beams (Fig. 4.**5**). A computerized planning system is required. For microscopic disease a total dose of 46 Gy in 23 fractions is given.

Postoperative radiation of the regional lymph nodes:
- *Indications and dose*: Indications and dose for radiation of the regional lymph nodes after modified radical mastectomy are identical to those already described in the section describing breast conservation treatment (p. 45).

Results:
After modified radical mastectomy and radiotherapy, the risk of a local recurrence is 8 – 10 %. In cases of a local recurrence, clinical or subclinical distant metastases are found in 90 – 95 % of patients.

Familial or hereditary breast cancer:
 A family history of breast cancer can be found in about 30 % of patients with this disease. In almost 10 % of patients, an autosomal dominant hereditary transmission can be established. Most of those cases are linked to mutations in *BRCA1* or *BRCA2* (Hoskins et al., 1995). These mutations also increase the risk of ovarian cancers. A breast conservation procedure might lead to more local regrowths or (new) primary tumors in women with hereditary breast cancer, as compared to the general population of breast cancer patients. However, these data are not strong enough to abandon breast conservation surgery entirely. For secondary prevention, yearly mammographic examination is recommended, preferably in the early follicular phase of the menstrual cycle. MRI of the breast might be a good alternative for secondary prevention, although its role as screening procedure is not yet validated. For primary prevention a bilateral ablative procedure should be considered (Eisinger et al., 1998).

Adjuvant chemotherapy and hormonal therapy:
 With increasing local and regional extension of the primary tumor, the risk of distant metastases increases. The

Table 4.**4**   Number of tumor-positive axillary lymph nodes and the risk of distant metastases five years after treatment of breast cancer

Number of patients	Number of tumor-positive axillary lymph nodes	Risk of metastases (%)
12 299	0	19
4 192	1 – 3	37
3 442	> 3	62

Calculated from data of Nemoto et al. (1980)

Table 4.**5**   Indications for adjuvant treatment

Meno-pausal status	Axillary lymph nodes	Receptor status	
		Positive	Negative
Premeno-pausal	Positive	Chemotherapy and endocrine therapy	Chemo-therapy
Postmeno-pausal	Positive	Endocrine therapy ± chemotherapy	Chemo-therapy

Note: For premenopausal and postmenopausal patients with negative axillary lymph nodes and increased risk for metastases because of tumor volume and other prognostic factors: treatment as for lymph node-positive tumors.

number of tumor-positive lymph nodes in the homolateral axilla is a good criterion for risk of relapse. Table 4.**4** presents the relationship between the number of tumor-positive axillary lymph nodes and the risk for metastases. Curative treatment is not yet available for breast cancer with distant metastases, but results of palliative treatment are quite impressive. The ultimate treatment failure is caused by an newly developed resistance to the therapy. The risk for developing resistance increases with tumor burden. It is assumed that micrometastases have favorable cell kinetic factors compared to clinically detectable metastases and are less prone to develop resistance to treatment.

It is possible to reduce recurrence and mortality rate with adjuvant chemotherapy and/or hormonal therapy. From the results of many randomized studies, a generally accepted consensus is obtained for the indications and type of adjuvant therapy for patients treated with curative intent. These data are summarized in Table 4.**5**.

Adjuvant chemotherapy:
It is generally agreed that adjuvant chemotherapy is indicated in premenopausal patients with primary breast cancer and tumor-positive axillary lymph nodes. With a combination of cyclophosphamide, methotrexate, and 5-fluorouracil or an anthracycline-containing regimen, a relative reduction in the risks of recurrence and mortality of 35 % and 27 % is obtained during the first 10 years of treatment (Early Breast Cancer Trialists' Collaborative Group 1998 a). A chemotherapy-induced or otherwise attained cessation of ovarian function or treatment with tamoxifen in patients with a receptor-positive tumor

contributes considerably to the therapeutic effect of adjuvant chemotherapy (Beex et al., 1988; Early Breast Cancer Trialists' Collaborative Group, 1996, 1998 b). While a reduction of recurrences after treatment with adjuvant chemotherapy has been proved for node-negative tumors, overtreatment of about 80% of the patients has to be taken into account (Goldhirsch et al., 1995). For this reason, only patients with tumors of unfavorable prognostic characteristics, such as pT > 1, high proliferation rate, (lymph) vessel invasion, poor differentiation grade, and negative hormonal receptors, should be considered for this treatment. The results of adjuvant chemotherapy in postmenopausal patients, as published by the Early Breast Cancer Trialists' Collaborative Group (1998 a), indicate a minor but still significant reduction of the recurrence rate and mortality.

Adjuvant hormonal therapy:
Adjuvant hormonal therapy with tamoxifen is indicated for postmenopausal patients with primary breast cancer and tumor-positive axillary lymph nodes. In this group, the risks of recurrence and mortality during the first 10 years after treatment are reduced by about 35% and 25%, respectively (Early Breast Cancer Trialists' Collaborative Group, 1992). A positive receptor status for estradiol and/or progesterone is a favorable condition for successful treatment (Early Breast Cancer Trialists' Collaborative Group, 1998 a). Adjuvant hormonal therapy can also be considered in patients with a node-negative, receptor-positive primary tumor that have otherwise poor prognostic characteristics.

Clinical research in adjuvant therapy:
The modest results of adjuvant therapy can be seen as an affirmation of the hypothesis that micrometastases are more susceptible to treatment than clinically detectable metastases. Experimental and clinical investigations are being pursued to improve results further for different categories of patients. These investigations address (Salmon et al., 1993)

- forms of hormonal therapy other than with tamoxifen;
- the role of combined chemo-hormonal therapy;
- preoperative and perioperative chemotherapy;
- intensified chemotherapy with the help of bone marrow stimulating growth factors;
- high-dose chemotherapy and autologous bone marrow transplantation or peripheral stem cell reinfusion.

■ Palliative Therapy

Sometimes a breast cancer is too extensive for curative surgical resection. This can be caused by growth into and through the skin or chest wall (T4) or by involved and matted lymph nodes (N2). A cure cannot be expected, but a five-year survival rate of 50% is possible. The treatment aims at maximizing local/regional tumor control while minimizing disfigurement and other side effects.

Surgical treatment:
A disfiguring ablative treatment should not be performed unless this is the only measure that can correct the local problem. In this situation, a simple mastectomy is adequate, with the removal confined to the breast gland and pathological axillary lymph nodes. The hormonal receptor activity should be determined.

Radiotherapy:
- *Technique and dose:* The breast is radiated with tangential beams (Fig. 4.**5**) to a dose of 46 Gy in 23 fractions, followed by a booster dose of 24 Gy in 12 fractions to the primary tumor. The total dose to the tumor amounts to 70 Gy. In case of clinically pathological axillary lymph nodes, the axillary and supraclavicular regions will be radiated with the McWhirter technique to a dose of 46 Gy in 23 fractions, followed by a booster dose of 14–20 Gy in 7 to 10 fractions to the pathological lymph nodes. The benefit of radiating the internal mammary lymph nodes is controversial.
- *Side effects:* The necessarily high radiation dose can be expected to cause fibrosis, teleangiectasia, and edema of the arm. Radiation of the axilla has to take into account the increased risk for lymphedema of the arm, fibrosis, and damage to the brachial plexus. Chemotherapy increases the risk of these side effects.

(Neo)adjuvant therapy for patients with locally/regionally extensive breast cancer:
Studies investigating the value of adjuvant hormonal or chemotherapy for patients with stage III breast cancer have failed so far to show definite positive results. Therefore, such a therapy should be given as part of an investigational study and not be considered standard therapy. An exception is the treatment of inflammatory breast cancer (mastitis carcinomatosis). The combination of chemotherapy, surgery, and radiotherapy increases the chance of a good local/regional control of the tumor and prolongs the disease-free survival in comparison with radiotherapy alone (Rouesse et al., 1986). Furthermore, large primary tumors can be shrunk with chemotherapy and hormone therapy, making breast conservation therapy feasible.

Distant metastases:
- *Disease-free interval*: The disease-free interval is defined as the time between the primary treatment and appearance of metastases. This interval depends on
  - Growth rate of the tumor
  - Extent and size of the metastases during primary treatment
  - Effect of adjuvant therapy
  The median disease-free interval for patients who develop metastases after treatment of the primary tumor depends on the initial stage and the adjuvant

treatment, and is between 24 and 33 months, with a range of one month to more than 144 months (Koenders et al., 1991; Insa et al., 1999).

- *Dominant metastatic sites:* Metastases can be found in superficial structures, including skin, superficial regional lymph nodes and in the contralateral breast (soft-tissue metastases), in the skeleton (bone metastases), or in other organs (visceral metastases). Figure 4.7 depicts the frequency of the initial metastases in the different dominant locations in relation to the hormonal receptor status of the primary tumor. The prognosis of patients with visceral metastases is poor compared to patients with bone or soft-tissue metastases. This is evident by the fact that during the course of the disease almost all patients eventually develop visceral metastases, which ultimately lead to the patient's death.

Palliative treatment of metastases:

- *Surgical measures:* Palliative surgical treatment is especially indicated for bone metastases at risk of imminent fracture. This applies to weight-bearing

bones with involvement of the cortex by more than 50% or to the proximal femur with involvement of its medial side by more than 30%. The aim of surgical intervention is a stable fixation of the involved bone or a functional improvement of a joint. Moreover, other manifestations, such as painful or ulcerating skin lesions, peritoneal metastases with intestinal obstruction or a single brain metastasis, can be considered for surgical intervention. A simple mastectomy can be a good palliative measure for an ulcerating breast tumor.

Radiotherapy:

The classic indication for palliative radiation is an osseous metastases causing pain or at risk for fracture. A single dose of 8 Gy is sufficient for pain relief and a dose of 20 Gy in 5 fractions of 4 Gy is usually needed to treat an impending bone fracture. For spinal cord compression caused by metastases, immediate treatment with high doses of dexamethasone and radiation is indicated with a dose of 25 Gy in 5 fractions of 5 Gy. Radiotherapy is also the first choice for (multiple) brain metastases. A short but intensive treatment with a dose of 20 Gy in 5 fractions is usually sufficient. Radiotherapy is usually combined with a short course of corticosteroids. After surgical resection of a single brain metastasis, prolonged control is attainable with whole brain radiation to a dose of 20 Gy in 5 fractions followed by a boost of 15 Gy in 5 fractions of 3 Gy to the metastatic region.

Radiation can also be of great palliative value for the treatment of mediastinal or hilar lymph node metastases in cases of obstructive metastases to the trachea or bronchus, obstructive metastases in the hilar region of the liver, meningeal localizations and cutaneous metastases. The treatment of a solitary skin metastasis in the surgical scar after local excision consists of radiation to the chest wall and supraclavicular region to a dose of 46 Gy in 23 fractions and, if tumor was left behind after surgery, followed by a boost of 20 Gy in 10 fractions.

Palliative hormone therapy or chemotherapy:

Palliative hormone therapy or chemotherapy is given to stabilize or improve the quality of the patient's life (Porszolt et al., 1993). This is mainly attained through a measurable decrease in tumor tissue. Such an objective remission is accompanied by longer survival.

- *Palliative hormone therapy:* All endocrine measures have in common that they interfere with the availability of estradiol on the level of the tumor cell. Palliative hormonal therapy is only suitable for patients with receptor-positive tumors. The median chance of a first or second remission for these categories of patients is 50% and 30%, respectively. Table 4.6 shows the chance for first remission in relation to the receptor activity for estradiol and progesterone.

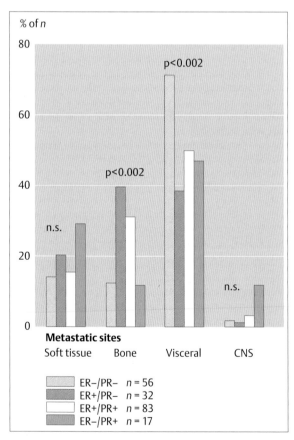

Fig. 4.7 **First localization of metastasis in relation to the receptor status of the primary tumor** (according to Koenders et al., 1991)

ER = estradiol receptor
PR = progesterone receptor
n.s. = not significant

Table 4.**6** Receptor status and chance of remission with endocrine therapy (Wittliff 1984; Harris et al. 1991)

Receptor status	Chance of objective remission (%)
ER −; PR −	< 10
ER −; PR +	45
ER +; PR −	34 (35?)
ER +; PR +	78 (70?)

ER estrogen receptor
PR progesterone receptor

The standard treatment for premenopausal patients is an ovariectomy. As an alternative treatment, a sufficient high dose of antiestrogens (tamoxifen 40 mg daily) or treatment with LHRH analogues can be considered.

The treatment for postmenopausal patients begins with tamoxifen (at least 20 mg daily). The next phase of treatment is an aromatase inhibitor or high doses of a progestin.

The median period of first and second remission is 12 and 6 months, with a variation of 3 to more than 36 months (Kimmick and Muss, 1995).

- *Palliative chemotherapy*: Palliative chemotherapy can be applied to patients with receptor-negative tumors and with metastases that are not (more) susceptible to endocrine therapy and are too widespread for surgical treatment or radiotherapy. A combination of chemotherapeutics is preferred. The decision depends upon adjuvant therapy given previously and the interval between this adjuvant therapy and the palliative treatment. Objective remissions with a median period of 9 months varying from 3 to more than 24 months are attained in 40–60% of patients with the first therapy and in 20–30% of patients treated with second-line modalities (Possinger et al., 1993; Crown, 1998).

Supplementary measures:
- *Bisphosphonates*: Morbidity caused by bone metastases can be reduced by intermittent (especially in case of tumor hypercalcemia) or continuous treatment with bisphosphonates (Müsel et al., 1992; Holten Verzandvoort et al., 1993). These drugs may also reduce the incidence of bone metastases (Diel et al., 1998).
- *Pain relief*: Adequate and careful treatment of pain is of great value to the patient. Treatment is first directed to the cause of pain, such as radiotherapy for painful bone metastases. In addition, therapy with peripherally and/or centrally acting analgesics has to be considered. It is very helpful to provide patients access to centers that offer modern techniques for intrathecal or epidural pain treatment, as well as nerve blocks.
- Other supplementary measures:
  - Treatment of arm lymphedema by means of lymph drainage or elastic bandage
  - Treatment of pleural and pericardial effusions
  - Treatment of ascites
  - Supportive measures
  - Reconstructive plastic surgery

■ Ductal Carcinoma in Situ

As a result of greater implementation of breast cancer screening programs, the diagnosis of ductal carcinoma in situ (DCIS) is more frequent today. With modern mammography, DCIS is visible as clustered microcalcifications. It is still undetermined whether all DCIS will develop into invasive breast cancer. As long as this is not known, all patients with DCIS should be treated. Two types of DCIS may be distinguished.

Subtypes of DCIS

- Comedo type (poorly differentiated)
- Non-comedo type

The comedo has the worst prognosis. The treatment of choice is a wide local excision with a margin exceeding 1 cm. For smaller margins, postoperative radiation may be beneficial (Silverstein et al., 1999). Because it is not always possible to establish the margin exactly, adjuvant radiotherapy is seen as standard treatment for any patient with DCIS.

Surgical measures:
The biopsy procedure for a nonpalpable DCIS consists of a preoperative radiographic localization, an excision guided by the localizing wire, and a radiograph of the removed specimen to determine whether the region with the calcifications has been removed. In case of extensive diffusely growing or multifocal localizations of DCIS, a simple mastectomy is indicated, without axillary node dissection. If the DCIS is poorly differentiated and laterally located, the lower axillary lymph nodes are also removed.

Radiotherapy:
If indicated, the entire breast will be radiated with tangential beams with a dose of 50 Gy in 25 fractions of 2 Gy, after biopsy. The value of a boost is still unknown.

Results:
A multivariant analysis of three studies (Fisher B et al., 1998; EORTC trial 10853; Fisher E et al., 1991) concluded that radiation therapy after lumpectomy reduced the risk of a local recurrence. In the NSABP B-17 trial (Fisher B et al., 1998), after an observation period of eight years, the cumulative incidence of recurrence was 12% after lumpectomy plus radiation therapy and 27% after lumpectomy alone. The survival rate was 95% and 94%, respectively. In the study by Sharma et al. (1997), the chance of recurrence after excision was 8–63% without

radiation therapy and 0–33% with radiation therapy. After mastectomy the chance for local control and cure is 98–100% (The Steering Committee on Clinical Practice Guidelines for the Care and Treatment of Breast Cancer, 1998).

■ Lobular Carcinoma in situ

The presence of lobular carcinoma in situ (LCIS) can be considered a risk factor for the development of an invasive carcinoma of any type of histology in both breasts. Treatment of LCIS ranges from local excision or further observation to even bilateral mastectomy, depending on additional risk factors, such as family history of breast cancer and earlier invasive breast cancer as well as the possibilities for a reliable screening procedure. In general, a contralateral mirror biopsy is not indicated for established LCIS.

■ Breast Cancer in Older Women

The treatment of primary or metastasized breast cancer in older women is in principle identical to that of younger women. Depending on the general condition and life expectancy, the standard treatment will be applied as much as possible. This means that age is not a contraindication for surgery, radiation or chemotherapy. For chemotherapy, the physiological decrease in liver and kidney function as well as the use of other medications has to be taken into account. Older patients often have hormone-responsive tumors and therefore a higher chance of a good response to hormonal therapy as compared to younger patients.

Interdisciplinary Cooperation in Diagnostic Procedures and Treatment

D.J. Dronkers

■ Team of Experts ("Breast Team")

For optimal diagnostic work-up and treatment of breast lesions, the close cooperation of radiologist, surgeon, gynecologist, cytologist, and pathologist is desirable. This cooperation is even mandatory in cases of nonpalpable lesions.

This cooperation must be based on agreements that should be laid down in a protocol. It is crucial that this team is consulted in the initial evaluation and follow-up of all cases of breast cancer.

■ Sequence of Work-up

In many cases of both clinically and mammographically detected breast lesions, routine mammographic spot views or magnification views are needed, if necessary complemented by sonography. If only MLO and CC views are obtained, it is not always possible to determine the precise location of nonpalpable lesions in the breast (Fig. 6.**36**). In these cases, an additional true lateral view (mediolateral or lateromedial) will locate the lesion.

Since women fear breast cancer, it is psychologically important to keep the time between request and performance of the examination as short as possible, and also the period between examination and definitive report.

The need for diagnostic percutaneous needle procedures should be clearly established. Needle punctures may result in a local hematoma that compromises both palpation and mammographic visualization of the lesion. A preceding cytological aspiration may also interfere with sonography since the sonographic findings after needle aspiration may resemble those of a malignant breast lesion. Therefore, punctures should be the last step in the proper sequence of diagnostic procedures.

It should be determined who performs the cytological aspiration and who prepares the slides. If the cytologist does not do both, close cooperation is necessary between the cytologist and the person performing the needle aspiration. Since cytology and histology are closely interrelated, it is advantageous for the cytologist to perform the histology as well. The terminology and classification used and guidelines for the diagnostic work-up should be defined in the protocol. When the cytology is negative, it must be established who is responsible for the histological examination that is often indispensable to exclude a false negative cytology result, depending on the level of suspicion of the mammographic and/or sonographic findings.

For nonpalpable lesions, preoperative localization with a marking system under mammographic or sonographic guidance is needed. It is generally done by the radiologist. Method, access route, and time of localization should be discussed with the surgeon. After localization, two views of the breast at right angles to each other should be taken and handed over to the surgeon. The lesion should be marked on both films.

■ Cooperation during Surgery

Surgeon and pathologist have to discuss and agree whether intraoperative frozen sections are indicated. This method is generally inappropriate for clinically nonpalpable lesions and especially for lesions presenting as microcalcifications only. Another disadvantage is the loss of substantial material when preparing the tissue.

After the excision, the specimen should be marked in at least two locations to indicate the topography of the specimen within the breast to the radiologist and pathologist. After checking the specimen radiographs, the radiologist informs the surgeon whether the lesion is included in the specimen and whether the excision was complete. If necessary, the direction needed to extend the excision must be noted. When the lesion is not found even after re-excision, the operation will generally be terminated and a new localization procedure rescheduled.

The entire specimen is handed over to the pathologist. In many cases, the specimen will be sectioned into 5 mm slices, followed by specimen radiography of the slices. Especially in nonpalpable lesions, it is possible to take the histological slices from representative tissue on the basis of the specimen radiography of the slices. The pathologist determines the type and extent of the lesion and, together with the radiologist, reports whether the biopsy is representative and complete. The pathologist is responsible for selecting and forwarding the representative tissue for the determination of steroid-hormone receptors.

The surgeon, who encounters an increasing number of breast conservation treatments, will coordinate his approach with the radiotherapy department.

■ Feedback of Histopathological Findings to the Radiologist

Know-how and experience in the interpretation of imaging of breast lesions can only be developed and extended by proper feedback of all histopathological findings to the radiologist, especially as to size, type, and differentiation of the lesion, multifocality, invasive growth, etc. These findings should be discussed by the entire team.

■ Quality Assurance and Control

Quality assurance and control should cover all aspects of diagnostic procedures and therapy:

- Preoperative localizations: measuring the distance of the tip of the localizing wire from the center of the lesion
- Positive predictive value of mammography (possibly combined with sonography)
- Positive predictive value of aspiration cytology
- Positive predictive value of core-needle biopsy
- Positive predictive value of excision biopsy

(Technical aspects of mammographic units, film – screen combinations and film processing are mentioned in chapter 5 and positioning in chapter 6.)

It is also advisable to evaluate the quality of the entire diagnostic and treatment results in each hospital or by every team, as a reflection of the joint responsibility.

Points of attention in organization:

- Is the radiologist present during all mammographic examinations?
- Is the team of technicians and radiologists specialized in breast imaging?
- Are the mammograms reviewed by the radiologist before the patient leaves the department?
- Does a protocol exist for the reporting the mammography results (findings, diagnosis, classification of tissue density)?
- Is the patient being informed immediately by the radiologist?
- Can mammography, if indicated, be immediately followed by sonographic examination and needle biopsy?
- Is the supplemental sonography performed by the radiologist who has seen the mammograms?
- Is the interdisciplinary protocol still appropriate and regularly updated?
- How effective is the feedback?

For the assessment of mammography screening, see de Wolf and Perry (1996) in "European Guidelines for Quality Assurance in Mammography Screening."

■ Patient Self-help Groups

These organizations may assist women with breast cancer and represent the patient's interests. They offer information on all aspects of breast cancer, such as treatment, breast implants, reconstruction techniques, etc. They also can act as political pressure groups. In this field several national organizations work together in the European Breast Cancer Coalition Europa Donna. In the United States these activities are executed by the National Alliance of Breast Cancer Organizations (NABCO) and by the American Cancer Society.

References

Epidemiology:

Ambrosone, C. B., J. L. Freudenheim, S. Graham, J. R. Marshall, J. E. Vena, J. R. Brasure, A. M. Michalek, R. Laughlin, T. Nemoto, K. A. Gillenwater, P. G. Shields: Cigarette smoking, N-acetyltransferase 2 genetic polymorphisms, and breast cancer risk. JAMA 276 (18) (1996) 1494–1501

American Cancer Society: Cancer Facts and Figures 1999, American Cancer Society, Atlanta 1999

Bartholomew, L. L., D. A. Grimes: The alleged association between induced abortion and risk of breast cancer: biology or bias? Obstet. Gynecol. Surv. 53 (11) (1998) 708 – 714

Baum, M., H. Schipper. In: Fast Facts-Breast Cancer (Epidemiology), Health Press Limited, Oxford, UK (1998) 6

Bleiker, E. M., H. M. van der Ploeg, J. H. Hendriks, H. J. Ader: Personality factors and breast cancer development: a prospective longitudinal study. J. Natl. Cancer Inst. 88 (20) (1996) 1478 – 1482

Boardman, L. A., S. N. Thibodeau, D. J. Schaid, N. M. Lindor, S. K. McDonnell, L. J. Burgart, D. A. Ahlquist, K. C. Podratz, M. Pittelkow, L. C. Hartmann: Increased risk for cancer in patients with the Peutz-Jeghers syndrome. Ann. Intern. Med. 128 (11) (1998) 896 – 899

Bowlin, S. J., M. C. Leske, A. Varma, P. Nasca, A. Weinstein, L. Caplan: Breast cancer risk and alcohol consumption: results from a large case-control study. Int. J. Epidemiol. 26 (5) (1997) 915 – 923

Boyd, N. F., J. W. Byng, R. A. Jong, E. K. Fishell, L. E. Little, A. B. Miller, G. A. Lockwood, D. L. Tritchler, M. J. Yaffe: Quantitative classification of mammographic densities and breast cancer risk: results from the Canadian National Breast Screening Study. J. Natl. Cancer Inst. 87 (9) (1995) 670 – 675

Brinton, L. A., J. Benichou, M. D. Gammon, D. R. Brogan, R. Coates, J. B. Schoenberg: Ethnicity and variation in breast cancer incidence. Int. J. Cancer. 73 (3) (1997) 349 – 355

Cade, J., E. Thomas, A. Vail: Case-control study of breast cancer in south east England: nutritional factors. J. Epidemiol. Community Health. 52 (2) (1998) 105 – 110

Clemmesen, J.: Carcinoma of the breast. I. Results from statistical research. Brit. J. Radiol. 21 (1948) 583 – 590

Collaborative Group on Hormonal Factors in Breast Cancer. Breast cancer and hormonal contraceptives: collaborative reanalysis of individual data on 53.297 women with breast cancer and 100.239 women without breast cancer from 54 epidemiological studies. Lancet. 347 (9017) (1996) 1713 – 1727

Collaborative Group on Hormonal Factors in Breast Cancer. Breast cancer and hormone replacement therapy: collaborative reanalysis of data from 51 epidemiological studies of 52.705 women with breast cancer and 108.411 women without breast cancer. Lancet. 350 (9084) (1997) 1047 – 1059

Coughlin, S. S., M. J. Khoury, K. K. Steinberg: BRCA1 and BRCA2 gene mutations and risk of breast cancer. Public health perspectives. Am. J. Prev. Med. 16 (2) (1999) 91 – 98

Dixon, J. M., C. McDonald, R. A. Elton, W. R. Miller: Risk of breast cancer in women with palpable breast cysts: a prospective study. Edinburgh Breast Group. Lancet. 353 (9166) (1999) 1742 – 5

Dupont, W. D., D. L. Page, F. F. Parl, C. L. Vnencak-Jones, W. D. Plummer Jr., M. S. Rados, P. A. Schuyler: Long-term risk of breast cancer in women with fibroadenoma. N. Engl. J. Med. 331 (1) (1994) 10 – 15

Feur, E. J., L. M. Wun, C. C. Boring: Probability of developing breast cancer. In: Miller BA, Gloecker-Ries LA, Hankey BF, Kosary CL, Edwards BK. National Institutes of Health Publication. Cancer Statistics Review 1973 – 1989. 92 – 2789. National cancer institute, Bethesda 1992

Furberg, H., B. Newman, P. Moorman, R. Millikan: Lactation and breast cancer risk. Int. J. Epidemiol. 28 (3) (1999) 396 – 402

Gail, M. H., L. A. Brinton, D. P. Byar, D. K. Corle, S. B. Green, C. Schairer, J. J. Mulvihill: Projecting individualized probabilities of developing breast cancer for white females who are being examined annually. J. Natl. Cancer Inst. 81 (24) (1989) 1879 – 1886

Garvican, L., P. Littlejohns: Comparison of prognostic and socioeconomic factors in screen-detected and symptomatic cases of breast cancer. Public Health. 112 (1) (1998) 15 – 20

Hakama, M., E. Pukkala, M. Heikkila, M. Kallio: Effectiveness of the public health policy for breast cancer screening in Finland: population based cohort study. BMJ. 314 (7084) (1997) 864 – 867

Hansen, J.: Breast cancer risk among relatively young women employed in solvent-using industries. Am. J. Ind. Med. 36 (1) (1999) 43 – 47

Harris, J. R., M. E. Lippman, U. Veronesi, W. Willett: Breast cancer (1). N. Engl. J. Med. 327 (5) (1992) 319 – 328

Hartmann, L. C., D. J. Schaid, J. E. Woods, T. P. Crotty, J. L. Myers, P. G. Arnold, P. M. Petty, T. A. Sellers, J. L. Johnson, S. K. McDonnell, M. H. Frost, R. B. Jenkins: Efficacy of bilateral prophylactic mastectomy in women with a family history of breast cancer. N. Engl. J. Med. 340 (2) (1999) 77 – 84

Hirayama, T.: A large scale cohort study on the effect of life styles on the risk of cancer by each site. Gan No Rinsho. (1990) Spec. No 233 – 42

Holmes, M. D., D. J. Hunter, G. A. Colditz, M. J. Stampfer, S. E. Hankinson, F. E. Speizer, B. Rosner, W. C. Willett: Association of dietary intake of fat and fatty acids with risk of breast cancer. JAMA 281 (10) (1999) 914 – 920

Howe, G. R., T. Hirohata, T. G. Hislop, J. M. Iscovich, J. M. Yuan, K. Katsouyanni, F. Lubin, E. Marubini, B. Modan, T. Rohan, et al.: Dietary factors and risk of breast cancer: combined analysis of 12 case-control studies. J. Natl. Cancer Inst. 82 (7) (1990) 561 – 569

Hoyer, A. P., P. Grandjean, T. Jorgensen, J. W. Brock, H. B. Hartvig: Organochlorine exposure and risk of breast cancer. Lancet 352 (9143) (1998) 1816 – 1820

Huang, Z., S. E. Hankinson, G. A. Colditz, M. J. Stampfer, D. J. Hunter, J. E. Manson, C. H. Hennekens, B. Rosner, F. E. Speizer, W. C. Willett: Dual effects of weight and weight gain on breast cancer risk. JAMA 278 (17) (1997) 1407 – 1411

Ingram, D., K. Sanders, M. Kolybaba, D. Lopez: Case-control study of phyto-oestrogens and breast cancer. Lancet 350 (9083) (1997) 990 – 994

Inskip, H. M., L. J. Kinlen, A. M. Taylor, C. G. Woods, C. F. Arlett: Risk of breast cancer and other cancers in heterozygotes for ataxia-telangiectasia. Br. J. Cancer 79 (7 – 8) (1999) 1304 – 1307

John, E. M., G. G. Schwartz, D. M. Dreon, J. Koo: Vitamin D and breast cancer risk: the NHANES I Epidemiologic follow-up study, 1971 – 1975 to 1992. National Health and Nutrition Examination Survey. Cancer Epidemiol. Biomarkers Prev. 8 (5) (1999) 399 – 406

Jordan, V. C.: Development of a new prevention maintenance therapy for postmenopausal women. Recent Results Cancer Res. 151 (1999) 96 – 109

Jumaan, A. O., L. Holmberg, M. Zack, A. H. Mokdad, E. M. Ohlander, A. Wolk, T. Byers: Beta-carotene intake and risk of postmenopausal breast cancer. Epidemiology 10 (1) (1999) 49 – 53

Key, T. J., G. E. Fraser, M. Thorogood, P. N. Appleby, V. Beral, G. Reeves, M. L. Burr, J. Chang-Claude, R. Frentzel-Beyme, J. W. Kuzma, J. Mann, K. McPherson: Mortality in vegetarians and nonvegetarians: detailed findings from a collaborative analysis of 5 prospective studies. Am. J. Clin. Nutr. 70 (3 Suppl) (1999) 516 – 524

Kliukiene, J., T. Tynes, J. I. Martinsen, K. G. Blaasaas, A. Andersen: Incidence of breast cancer in a Norwegian cohort of women with potential workplace exposure to 50 Hz magnetic fields. Am. J. Ind. Med. 36 (1) (1999) 147 – 154

Lancaster, J. M., M. E. Carney, P. A. Futreal: BRCA 1 and 2 - A Genetic Link to Familial Breast and Ovarian Cancer. Medscape Womens Health 2 (2) (1997) 7

London, S. J., J. L. Connolly, S. J. Schnitt, G. A. Colditz: A prospective study of benign breast disease and the risk of breast cancer. JAMA 267 (7) (1992) 941 – 944

Mann, G. B., P. I. Borgen: Breast cancer genes and the surgeon. J. Surg. Oncol. 67 (4) (1998) 267 – 274

Mettlin, C.: Global breast cancer mortality statistics. CA Cancer J. Clin. 49 (3) (1999) 138 – 144

Nordlund, L. A., J. M. Carstensen, G. Pershagen: Cancer incidence in female smokers: a 26-year follow-up. Int. J. Cancer. 73 (5) (1997) 625 – 628

Parkin, D. M., C. S. Muir: Cancer Incidence in Five Continents. Comparability and quality of data. IARC Sci. Publ. 120 (1992) 45–173

Peacock, S. L., E. White, J. R. Daling, L. F. Voigt, K. E. Malone: Relation between obesity and breast cancer in young women. Am. J. Epidemiol. 149 (4) (1999) 339–346

Roberts, F. D., P. A. Newcomb, A. Trentham-Dietz, B. E. Storer: Self-reported stress and risk of breast cancer. Cancer 77 (6) (1996) 1089–1093

Sant, M., R. Capocaccia, A. Verdecchia, J. Esteve, G. Gatta, A. Micheli, M. P. Coleman, F. Berrino: Survival of women with breast cancer in Europe: variation with age, year of diagnosis and country. The EUROCARE Working Group. Int. J. Cancer 77 (5) (1998) 679–683

Schmutzler, R. K., A. Kempe, M. Kiechle, M. W. Beckmann: Klinische Beratung und Betreuung von Frauen mit erblicher Disposition für das Mamma- und Ovarialkarzinom. Deutsche medizinische Wochenschrift. 124 (18) (1999) 563–566

Sesso, H. D., R. S. Paffenbarger Jr., I. M. Lee: Physical activity and breast cancer risk in the College Alumni Health Study (United States). Cancer Causes Control. 9 (4) (1999) 433–439

Spratt, J. S., W. L. Donegan, C. P. Sigdestad. In: J. S. Spratt, W. L. Donegan: Cancer of the Breast-Epidemiology and etiology, 4th edition, W.B. Saunders Company, Philadelphia, USA. (1995) 116–141

Stoll, B. A.: Teenage obesity in relation to breast cancer risk. Int. J. Obes. Relat. Metab. Disord. 22 (11) (1998) 1035–1040

Tseng, M., C. R. Weinberg, D. M. Umbach, M. P. Longnecker: Calculation of population attributable risk for alcohol and breast cancer (United States). Cancer Causes Control. 10 (2) (1999) 119–123

Ursin, G., L. Bernstein, M. C. Pike: Breast cancer. Cancer Surv. 19–20 (1994) 241–264

Wang, D. Y., B. L. DeStavola, D. S. Allen, I. S. Fentiman, R. D. Bulbrook, J. L. Hayward, M. J. Reed: Breast cancer risk is positively associated with height. Breast Cancer Res. Treat. 43 (2) (1997) 123–128

Welsch, C. W.: Relationship between dietary fat and experimental mammary tumorigenesis: a review and critique. Cancer Res. 52 (7 Suppl) (1992) 204–2048

Zhang, S., D. J. Hunter, S. E. Hankinson, E. L. Giovannucci, B. A. Rosner, G. A. Colditz, F. E. Speizer, W. C. Willett: A prospective study of folate intake and the risk of breast cancer. JAMA 281 (17) (1999) 1632–1637

Zhang, Y., D. P. Kiel, B. E. Kreger, L. A. Cupples, R. C. Ellison, J. F. Dorgan, A. Schatzkin, D. Levy, D. T. Felson. Bone mass and the risk of breast cancer among postmenopausal women. N. Engl. J. Med. 336 (9) (1997) 611–617

Zheng, T., T. R. Holford, S. T. Mayne, J. Tessari, P. H. Owens, S. H. Zahm, B. Zhang, R. Dubrow, B. Ward, D. Carter, P. Boyle: Environmental exposure to hexachlorobenzene (HCB) and risk of female breast cancer in Connecticut. Cancer Epidemiol. Biomarkers Prev. 8 (5) (1999) 407–411

Treatment:

Bedwinek, J. M., C. A. Perez, S. Kramer: Irradiation as the primary management of Stage I and II adenocarcinoma of the breast: Analysis of the RTOG breast registry. Cancer clin. Trials 3 (1980) 11–18

Beex, L., M. Mackenzie, J. Raemaekers u. Mitarb.: Adjuvante chemotherapy in premenopausal patients with primary breast cancer; relation to drug induced amenorrhoea, age and progesterone receptorstatus of the tumor. Europ. J. Cancer clin. Oncol. 24 (1988) 719–721

Boyages, J., A. Recht, J. L. Connelly et al.: Early breast cancer: predictors of breast recurrence for patients treated with conservative surgery and radiation therapy. Radiother. and Oncol. 19 (1990) 29–41

Chu, A. M., O. Cope, R. Russo, R. Lew: Patterns of local-regional recurrence and results in Stage I and II breast cancer treated by irradiation following limited surgery: An Update. Amer. J. clin. Oncol. 7 (1984) 221–229

Clark, R. M., R. H. Wilkinson, P. N. Miceli et al.: Breast cancer: experience with conservation therapy. Amer. J. clin. Oncol. 10 (1987) 461–468

Early Breast Cancer Trialists' Collaborative Group (EBCTCG): Systemic treatment of early breast cancer by hormonal, cytoxic or immune therapy. Lancet 339 (1992) 1–15, 71–85

Early Breast Cancer Trialists' Collaborative Group (EBCTCG): Effects of radiotherapy and surgery in early breast cancer. New Engl. J. Med. 333 (1995) 1444–1455

Early Breast Cancer Trialists' Collaborative Group (EBCTCG): Tamoxifen for early breast cancer: an overview of the randomised trials. Lancet 351 (1998a) 1451–1467

Early Breast Cancer Trialists' Collaborative Group (EBCTCG): Polychemotherapy for early breast cancer: an overview of the randomised trials. Lancet 352 (1998b) 930–942

EORTC 10853 – DCIS trial: Phase III trial of radiation therapy versus no treatment for patients with in situ ductal carcinoma of the breast. Study Coordinators: Fentiman, I. S. (London) and J. P. Julien (Rouen) in Vorbereitung

Fisher, B., M. Bauer, R. Margolese et al.: Five-year results of a randomized clinical trial comparing total mastectom and segmental mastectomy with or without radiation in the treatment of breast cancer. New Engl. J. Med. 312 (1985) 665–673

Fisher, B., C. Redmond, R. Poisson et al.: Eight-year results of a randomized clinical trial comparing total mastectomy and lumpectomy with or without irradiation in the treatment of breast cancer. New Engl. J. Med. 320 (1989) 822–828

Fisher, B., S. Anderson, C. K. Redmond, N. Wolmark, D. L. Wickerham, W. M. Cronin: Reanalysis and results after 12 years of follow-up in a randomized clinical trial comparing total mastectomy with lumpectomy with or without irradiation in the treatment of breast cancer. New. Engl. J. Med. 333 (1995) 1456–1461

Forrest, A. P., H. J. Stewart, D. Everington et al.: Randomised controlled trial of conservation therapy for breast cancer: 6-year analysis of the Scottish trial. Lancet 348 (1996) 708–713

Freeman, C. R., N. J. Belleveau, T. H. Kim et al.: Limited surgery with or without radiotherapy for early breast carcinoma. J. Canad. Ass. Radiol. 32 (1981) 125–128

Greening, W. P., A. C. V. Montgomery, A. B. Gordon et al.: Quadrantic excision and axillary node dissection without radiation therapy: the long-term results of a selective policy in the treatment of Stage I breast cancer. Europ. J. surg. Oncol. 14 (1988) 221–225

Greenwald, P., K. Sherwood, S. S. McDonald: Fat, caloric intake, and obesity: lifestyle risk factors for breast cancer. J. Amer. diet. Ass. 97, Suppl. 7 (1997) S24–30

Harris, J. R., G. F. Beadle, S. Hellman: Clinical studies on the use of radiation therapy as primary treatment of early breast cancer. Cancer 53 (1984) 705–711

Harris, J. R., S. Hellman, I. C. Henderson, D. W. Kinne: Receptors, 2nd ed. Lippincott, Philadelphia 1991

Hermaneck, P., L. H. Sobin: International Union Against Cancer: TNM Classification of Malignant Tumors, 2nd ed. Springer, Berlin 1992

Holland, R., S. H. J. Veling, M. Mravunac et al.: Histologic multifocality of Tis, T1–2 breast carcinomas: Implications for clinical trials of breast-conserving surgery. Cancer 56 (1985) 979–990

Holland, R., J. L. Connolly, R. Gelman et al.: The presence of an extensive intraductal component following a limited excision correlates with prominent residual disease in the remainder of the breast. J. clin. Oncol. 8 (1990) 113–118

Holten Verzandvoort, van A., H. M. Kroon, O. L. M. Bijvoet et al.: Palliative pamidromate treatment in patients with bone metastases from breast cancer. J. clin. Oncol. 11 (1993) 491–498

Hoskins, K. F., J. E. Stopfer, K. A. Calzone et al.: Assessment and counseling for women with a family history of breastcancer. J. Amer. med. Ass. 273 (1995) 577–585

Howe, G. R., T. Hirohata, T. G. Hislop, J. M. Iscovich et al.: Dietary factors and risk of breast cancer: combined analysis of 12 case-control studies. J. nat. Cancer Inst. 82 (1990) 561–569

Kantorowicz, D. A., C. A. Poulter, P. Rubin et al.: Treatment of breast cancer with segmental mastectomy alone or segmental mastectomy plus radiation. Radiother. and Oncol. 15 (1989) 141–150

Koenders, P. G., L. V. A. M. Beex, R. Langens et al.: Steroid hormone receptor activity of primary human breast cancer and pattern of first metastasis. Breast Cancer Res. Treatm. 18 (1991) 27–32

Lagois, M. D., V. E. Richards, M. R. Rose et al.: Segmental mastectomy without radiotherapy: Short-term follow-up. Cancer 52 (1983) 2173–2179

Montgomery, A. C. V., W. P. Greening, A. L. Levene: Clinical study of recurrence rate and survival time of patients with carcinoma of the breast treated by biopsy excision without any other therapy. J. roy. Soc. Med. 71 (1978) 339–342

Müsel, B., P. Scigalla: Pharmacology and clinical use of biphosphonates in oncology. Onkologie 15 (1992) 444–453

Nemoto, T., J. Vana, R. N. Bedwani et al.: Management and survival of female breast cancer. Results of a national survey by the American College of Surgeons. Cancer 45 (1980) 2917–2924

Nobler, M. P., L. Venet: Prognostic factors in patients undergoing curative irradiation for breast cancer. Int. J. Radiat. Oncol. Biol. Phys. 11 (1985) 1323–1331

Olivotto, I. A., M. A. Rose, R. T. Osteen et al.: Late cosmetic outcome after conservative surgery and radiotherapy: analysis of causes of cosmetic failure. Int. J. Radiat. Oncol. Biol. Phys. 17 (1989) 747–754

Pierquin, M., J. J. Mazeron, D. Glaubiger: Conservative treatment of breast cancer in Europe: report of the Groupe Europeen de Curietherapie. Radiother. and Oncol. 6 (1986) 187–198

Porszolt, F., I. Tannock: Goals of palliative cancer therapy. J. clin. Oncol. 11 (1993) 378–381

Possinger, K., W. Wilmanns: Palliative Therapieführung zur Hemmung der Tumorprogression bei Patientinnen mit metastasiertem Mammakarzinom. Internist 34 (1993) 340–350

Romestaing, P., C. Carrie, J. M. Ardiet et al.: Conservative treatment of small breast cancer. Relevance of a boost after 50 Gy on the whole breast. Preliminary results of a randomized trial. Proc. 17 th Int. Congr. Radiol., Paris 1989 (abstract 54)

Rose, M. A., I. Olivotto, B. Cady et al.: Conservative surgery and radiation therapy for early breast cancer. Arch. Surg. 124 (1989) 153–157

Rosen, P. P., A. A. Fracchia, J. A. Urban et al.: "Residual" mammary carcinoma following simulated partial mastectomy. Cancer 35 (1975) 739–747

Rouesse, J., S. Friedman, D. Sarrazin et al.: Primary chemotherapy in the treatment of inflammatory breast carcinoma: a study of 230 cases from the Institute Gustave Roussy. J. clin. Oncol. 4 (1986) 1765–1771

Salmon, S. E.: Adjuvante Therapy of Cancer. Lippincott, Philadelphia 1993 (pp. 141–257)

Sharma, S. S., A. D. K. Hill, E. W. McDermott, O'Higgins: Ductal carcinoma in situ of the breast-current management. Eur. J. Surg. Oncol. 23 (1997) 191–197

Veronesi, U., R. Saccozzi, M. Del Vecchio et al.: Comparing radical mastectomy with quadrantectomy, axillary dissection, and radiotherapy in patients with small cancers of the breast. New Engl. J. Med. 305 (1981) 6–11

Veronesi, U., A. Banfi, B. Salvadori et al.: Breast conservation is the treatment of choice in small breast cancer: longterm results of a randomized trial. Europ. J. Cancer 26 (1990) 668–670

Veronesi, U., A. Luini, M. Del Vecchio et al.: Radiotherapy after breast preserving surgery in women with localized cancer of the breast. New Engl. J. Med. 328 (1993) 1587–1591

Vicini, F. A., T. J. Eberlein, J. L. Connolly et al.: Harris: The optimal extent of resection for patients with stages I or II breast cancer treated with conservative surgery and radiotherapy. Ann. Surg. 214 (1991) 200–205

Interdisciplinary Cooperation in Diagnostic Procedures and Treatment:

Het mammacarcinoom: Richtlijn voor screening en diagnostiek. Kwaliteitsinstituut voor de Gezondheidszorg CBO (2000) ISBN 90-6910-229-3

Richtlijnen voor de kwaliteitsbewaking bij een bevolkingsonderzoek op mammacarcinoom; Screening en nadere diagnostiek. Centraal Begeleidingsorgaan voor de Intercollegiale Toetsing (CBO), Utrecht 1988

de Wolf, C. J. M., N. M. Perry: European Guidelines for Quality Assurance in Mammography Screening, 2 nd ed. Europäische Kommission, Brüssel 1996

5 Physical and Technical Aspects
of Mammography

Introduction

M. A. O. Thijssen

A radiograph of the breast, or mammogram, is obtained to gather information about the differences in type and structure of the tissues that compose this organ. This image usually constitutes the most important and often only source of information at the beginning of the diagnostic process. It is therefore of the utmost importance to optimize the *information content* of the mammogram.

Since the radiological properties of tissues, such as absorption and scattering, are known, it is possible to describe the physical mechanisms behind the generation of an image. Within the framework of these physical, technical, and radiation protection criteria, the radiologist can render a diagnostic opinion.

To understand the specific physical variables, this chapter deals with the main components of the mammographic imaging chain (see Fig. 5.**1**): generation of the radiographic image, image receptor properties and image presentation. Radiation protection and quality control complete the chain of mammographic imaging.

■ The Imaging Chain

Following the pathway from the production of X-rays in the X-ray tube to the interpretation of the image by the radiologist, several steps can be identified where information is added or modified:

Step 1: Generation of the X-rays. X-rays are produced in the X-ray tube whenever high voltage is applied between cathode and anode. Tube voltage and anode material as well as type and thickness of the added filter determine the *transparency* of the breast tissue in the displayed image. Shape and size of the focal spot and the geometrical configuration of the radiographic device de-termine the maximum *attainable resolution* of the imaging system as a whole.

Step 2: Generation of the radiation image. The display of tissue as an image is achieved by the relative absorption of X-rays in tissue. The *radiation image* represents the distribution of X-ray intensities at the plane of the image receptor. It is produced by X-rays emanating from the tube and traveling through breast tissue, thereby being modulated by absorption and scattering according to the properties of the different tissue components. *The radiation leaving the breast carries the information extracted from the tissue as the distribution of intensity and direction of the X-rays. No new information can be added on the pathway to the image display. Information can only be selectively emphasized or suppressed, or even deliberately eliminated.*

Step 3: Image improvement through the antiscatter grid. The radiation leaving the breast consists of *primary radiation*, which contains the entire image information, and *scattered radiation*. The intensity differences in the primary radiation (primary contrast) caused by attenuation (absorption and scattering) are diminished by simultaneous scattering of radiation. The grid modifies the radiation beam before it reaches the image receptor by absorbing the scattered radiation to a greater degree than the primary radiation. This improves the image contrast, since only the modified radiation image with less scattered radiation is recorded by the image receptor.

Step 4: Absorption of the radiation in the image receptor. The image receptor partly absorbs the X-ray quanta and transfers the image information to other informa-

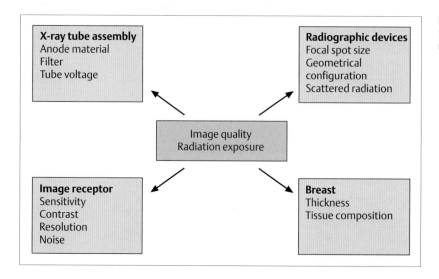

Fig. 5.**1** **Physical characteristics that affect image quality and radiation exposure**

tion carriers: an intensifying screen emits *light quanta* by luminescence that can be detected by a film or CCD chip, whereas some direct digital detectors release *electrons*. The better the absorption of the X-ray quanta in the image receptor, the better will be the transmission of the image information that is contained in the spatial distribution to the subsequent imaging chain. The more light quanta (in the intensifying screens) or the more free electrons (in the direct digital detectors) that are generated, the more sensitive the total imaging system becomes.

The physical quantity introduced to describe the effectiveness of this signal transformation is the detective quantum efficiency (DQE). The DQE determines the exposure needed to obtain an image of a defined quality.

Step 5: Transformation of the image information in the detector. The light quanta or the electrons generated in the detector cannot be used directly for image display; the information has to be transferred to another suitable information carrier. Several steps might be needed before a latent image can be passed on for further processing. The *latent image* in film – screen mammography is the distribution of activated grains in the emulsion of the film. The *latent image* ("*raw image*") in digital imaging is the distribution of the numerical values for each pixel in the memory of the image data processor. The numerical values correspond to the X-ray energy absorbed in the pixel or the corresponding computed signal value.

Step 6: Film processing/image processing. The latent image on the film can be taken to the darkroom, where it will be manipulated by the film processing before it can be viewed on the viewbox. The same holds for the digital raw image, which is stored in the memory of the computer but still needs further processing before it can be displayed on a monitor. Processing of the film or digital data does not add new information to the image, but it renders the information contained into a form that the radiologist can interpret.

Step 7: Image presentation. After development, a film image is viewed on the viewbox, while a digital image is viewed after transformation of the numerical values/pixel into grey levels/pixel on a viewing monitor (or on

the viewbox as hard copy as well). At this point, the information is presented to the examining physician. The result (i.e., the diagnosis) depends—as well as on the skill of the observer—on the information content that is left after all image transformations, on the working conditions in the reading area, and on the ambient light level.

■ Definitions

To evaluate the quality of the imaging chain for a given exposure technique, it is sufficient to limit the number of variables to the three most important characteristics: sharpness, contrast, and noise. All other variables contribute directly to the values of these.

Sharpness. The ability of an image receptor to display small details is defined by the sharpness in the image. What is subjectively called sharpness can be quantitatively described by the concept of resolution at very high contrast.

It is difficult to distinguish between two small objects (details) that are close to each other. The better the *resolution*, the smaller the individual objects that can be recognized separately in the image. The object size defined in this way can be taken as a criterion for the visual resolution limit. This limit will be achieved for high contrasts and can be measured by imaging a lead bar pattern (contrast lead/air, see Fig. 5.**2**). The contrast between two lines (a "line pair") can be quantified by their difference in optical density on the film or intensity on the monitor. The thinner the lines are, the more difficult it is to visualize the lines separated from each other, and therefor the higher the resolution has to be. Measurements obtained with a lead bar pattern show reproducible results. Further details are described on p. 64.

Along with the *geometrical configuration* of the radiographic device, the *size of the focal spot* and *the intensity distribution of the radiation in the focal spot* determine the resolution of the entire imaging system. In addition, the resolving power of the image receptor has to be considered. This is determined by the design of the intensifying screen and/or the pixel size of the digital detector. The highest number of line pairs per mm (lp/mm) displayed separated from each other is called the *visual resolution limit of the entire imaging device*.

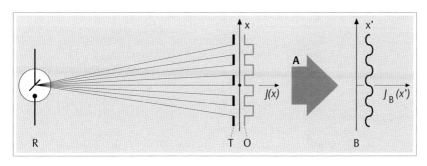

Fig. 5.**2 Imaging of a test pattern made from thin lead strips** (Morneburg, 1995) **for the evaluation of the visual resolution**
A   Image system
B   Image plane
J, J$_B$ Intensities
O   Object plane
R   X-ray tube
T   Test grid

Contrast. The ability to convert subtle density differences in the tissue into visible information is called *contrast resolution*. Contrast is generated by differences in attenuation of X-rays in the breast tissue (i.e., adipose relative to glandular tissue), or breast areas of different thickness (i.e., the superficial region close to the skin relative to the thicker region near the chest wall). Furthermore, the contrast in the image is affected by the *X-ray spectrum*, which is determined by tube voltage, anode material, and total added filtration. The contrast in the radiation image (*radiation contrast*) contains all information on composition and thickness of the breast obtainable with the selected X-ray spectrum. The image receptor and the subsequent processing transform the *radiation contrast* into *image contrast*: different optical densities on the radiographic film or different levels of brightness on the monitor (see Table 5.**1**). The *image contrast* is influenced by the *gradation* of the film–screen system and by the setting of the window level and -width in the digital image. The higher the contrast, the more conspicuous the bright and dark image areas will be. Alhough this effect creates the subjective impression of a sharper image, it delivers no additional information.

Noise. Noise is the component in the optical density or brightness of the image that contains no useful information. It permeates the image information. Noise can be recognized within homogeneous tissue areas by statistical fluctuations in optical density or brightness.

In an X-ray image the tissues are not presented as a smooth distribution of their corresponding optical densities, but noise is superimposed on that density. The distribution of the number of absorbed X-ray quanta over the film area builds up the image, with the contribution of each individual X-ray quantum adding to the picture. The more X-ray quanta are represented per image area, the better the density will be defined statistically, resulting in lower noise. The number of X-ray quanta absorbed by the image receptor from the radiation image therefore determines the contribution of the quantum noise.

Moreover, the number of absorbed X-ray quanta (see Step 4) and the efficiency of transforming the absorbed energy into visible light or electrons contribute to the noise, since both processes limit the number of light quanta available for building up the visible image (see Step 7). In addition, the total noise is affected and increased by the system noise, i.e., the statistical fluctuations within the imaging system, whether it is a film–screen system (graininess) or a digital system (e.g., electrical noise) (see Table. 5.**2**).

■ Image Quality

The information content of an image is determined by the visibility of details of the imaged tissues that are important to the diagnostic process. In mammography, these are *small details*, such as microcalcifications, and *larger details*, such as masses.

- Small high-contrast details like microcalcifications need to appear as small bright spots on the background to become visible. This is only possible when the imaging system is able to resolve those small calcifications as separate structures, implying a sufficient sharpness of the system.
- Low-contrast details like masses require a minimum contrast relative to the background to become visible. This threshold contrast depends on the size of the lesion and the noise in the imaging system. This implies the need for an optimal contrast transfer of the system.
- The observation that small details need high contrast and large details are adequately seen at lower contrast is expressed to by the formula proposed by Rose (1973):

$$C \times D = k \tag{5.1}$$

Table 5.1 Contrast definition

Definition	Linear contrast	Logarithmic contrast
Radiation contrast	$C_r = (X_o - X_b)/X_b$	$C_r = \log X_o - \log X_b$
Modulation	$C_m = (X_o - X_b)/(X_o + X_b)$	$C_m = \log X_0 - \log X_b$
Image contrast (monitor)	$C_L = (L_o - L_b)/L_b$	$C_L = \log L_o - \log L_b$
Image contrast (film)	–	$C_D = D_o - D_b$

o object
b background

Table 5.2 The influence of individual steps on image quality

step property	X-ray image	Screen	Film	Digital
Resolution	Focal spot Geometry	Graininess	(Graininess)	Screen grain Pixel size
Contrast	Tube voltage Anode material Filter	–	Gradient Processing	Window level
Noise	Dose	Absorption Efficiency	Sensitivity	Bits/pixel Electronic

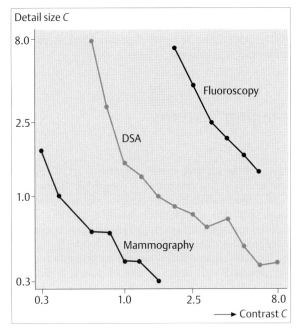

Fig. 5.**3**   **Examples of contrast – detail curves** (Thijssen et al., 1989)
•–• Mammography
•–• Digital subtraction angiography (DSA)
•–• Fluoroscopy

Equation (5.1) means that the product of contrast C and detail size D is constant at the visibility threshold (Fig. 5.**3**). The constant k is important in quantifying the image parameters: when image quality improves, smaller details and/or lower contrasts are visualized. Consequently, the lower the value of k, the better the imaging system. The limits are determined by the system properties and dose constraints (Thijssen et al., 1989). Optimizing physical parameters can change this constant. Improvement of information content will result in a better (lower) k.

The visualization of low-contrast objects has not been defined or standardized so far. Since there is no universal physical measure for visibility at the moment, evaluation of visibility has to be restricted to physical quantities with measurable parameters (Table 5.**2**).

Medical Quality Criteria of X-ray Mammography

M. Säbel

In Europe the medical standard for X-ray investigation of the female breast is documented in the "European Guidelines on Quality Criteria for Diagnostic Radiographic Images," published in 1996 by the European Commission (EC). This document establishes medical quality criteria for basic investigations with X-rays—and therefore includes mammography—as well as guidelines for radiographic techniques. These guidelines are discussed in the following sections.

The diagnostic requirements comprise image criteria, crucial image details, and critical structures (Table 5.**3**).

- The image criteria specify the anatomical structures that should be visible on a mammogram for accurate diagnosis. These criteria depend in part on correct positioning and patient cooperation and in part on the technical performance of the imaging system.
- Crucial image details provide quantitative information on the minimum size of important anatomical details that should be discernible on a mammogram.
- Critical structures are findings that are relevant for the diagnostic statement and for the quality of the image.

Stating the minimum size (0.2 mm) of mammographically visible microcalcifications provides important

guidance for the development of quality-assurance programs. Moreover, it is very helpful for solving optimization problems that arise in the process of developing

Table 5.**3**   European Guidelines on Quality Criteria for Diagnostic Radiographic Images: Breast, craniocaudal (CC) projection

Image criteria related to positioning
- Visually sharp reproduction of pectoral muscle at image margin
- Visually sharp reproduction of retroglandular fat tissue
- Visually sharp reproduction of medial breast tissue
- Visually sharp reproduction of lateral glandular tissue
- No skin folds seen
- Symmetrical images of left and right breast

Image criteria related to exposure parameters
- Visualization of skin outline with bright light (but barely without it)
- Reproduction of vascular structures seen through most dense parenchyma
- Visually sharp reproduction of all vessels and fibrous strands and pectoral muscle margin (absence of movement)
- Visually sharp reproduction of skin structure (rosettes from pores) along the pectoralis muscle

Important image details
- Microcalcifications of 0.2 mm

mammography units. Unfortunately, the EC document does not specify under what conditions these small microcalcifications are adequately delineated to become recognizable. The present state of knowledge makes it sensible to assume that these requirements refer to an average-sized breast (about 5 cm compressed breast thickness) with its tissue equally composed of glandular and adipose tissue and with exposure parameters typical for this size of breast.

Resulting Demands on Radiological Imaging Systems

H. Aichinger

The special demands on imaging systems used in mammography can be found in the recommendations shown in Table 5.**3**. Image quality and radiation exposure cannot be evaluated independently from each other. Figure 5.**1** demonstrates the different components and technical parameters that influence absorbed dose and image quality of the mammographic imaging system. The physical characteristics of the X-ray tube assembly and the imaging device must be adapted to the medical requirements in such a way that the image receptor, e.g., the film–screen combination, can generally produce an optimal X-ray image that displays the finest microcalcifications and tissue structures of the breast at the lowest possible exposure. Since the X-ray image contains the entire image information (see p. 60, Step 2), it is useful to optimize this image primarily with respect to the medical question—assuming an ideal image receptor—and only then to consider the actual image receptor used (see pp. 60 and 61, Steps 4–6, and see p. 62, Table 5.**2**).

The most important characteristics of the radiographic device presented in the Introduction will be discussed here in detail, and subsequently the demands on the imaging system.

■ Sharpness

In mammography, the image must display very fine structures (see p. 63, Table 5.**3**). The theoretical description of X-ray imaging often expresses the detail size as "spatial frequency ν" (see Fig. 5.**4**), which equals the reciprocal value of twice the detail size, i.e., $\nu = 1/(2 \cdot \text{detail size})$. Microcalcifications 0.2 mm in diameter correspond to a spatial frequency of 2.5 lp/mm. To display such tiny microcalcifications, the resolution of the imaging system has to be at least ≥ 2.5 lp/mm. Since sharpness requires a high contrast not achievable with microcalcifications of 0.2 mm diameter, the resolution of the whole radiographic system, including focal spot, geometric setup, and image receptor, must be substantially better. In Germany, a resolution of at least 8 lp/mm is therefore demanded; in other countries (e.g., The Netherlands, The United States), as high as 10–13 lp/mm. Microcalcifications can only be successfully displayed by an imaging system if its so-called modulation transfer function MTF(ν) shows a high-contrast transfer in the spatial frequency range from 2 to 5 lp/mm. The modulation transfer function indicates the contrast be-

havior of the imaging system relative to detail size and spatial frequency, respectively. Figure 5.**5** illustrates a typical modulation transfer function with respect to a focal spot size of 0.4 (according IEC 60336), a SID (source-to-image distance) of 60 cm and the film–screen system Kodak OM1/MinR.

From its original definition, the modulation transfer function MTF(ν) is based on the sinusoidal modulation of the radiation intensity by a bar pattern inserted into the path of the X-ray beam (Morneburg, 1995). This is hard to implement in a radiographic system, and the MTF is instead most often measured by a lead grid made of lead bars and spaces of equal width (see Fig. 5.**4**). The rectangular radiation intensity distribution produced by this test pattern in the object plane is displayed in the image plane more or less smoothed, depending on the quality of the imaging system (see Fig. 5.**2**). Coltman (1954) has given a correction formula that allows the determination of the correct MTF(ν). This represents the line pairs/mm (lp/mm) as units on the x-axis of the MTF diagrams rather than periods/mm (per/mm).

■ Contrast

Since the difference of the attenuation coefficients of parenchyma, infiltrating ductal carcinoma and adipose tissue is small and decreases rapidly with increasing X-ray energy (see Fig. 5.**6**) (Yaffe, 1992), mammography requires low-energy ("soft") radiation and steep film–

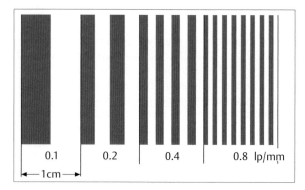

Fig. 5.**4** **Principle outline of a test grid** One line pair consists of one dark and one light stripe. In mammography, lead bar patterns with a line pair number up to 20 lp/mm are used

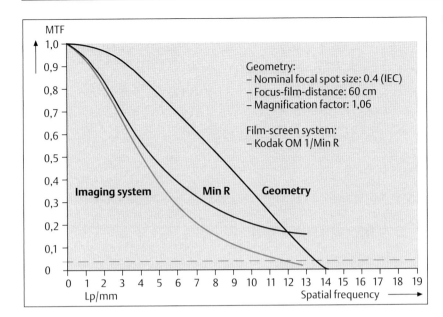

Fig. 5.**5** **Modulation transfer function of imaging geometry, film–screen system, and the complete imaging system**

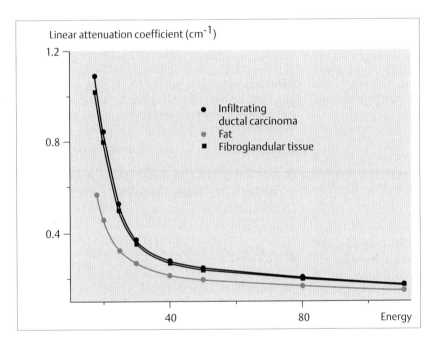

Fig. 5.**6** **Linear attenuation coefficients of fibroglandular tissue, infiltrating ductal carcinoma, and adipose breast tissue as function of the X-ray energy** (Yaffe, 1992)

screen systems for adequate image contrast. The *soft radiation* results in higher radiation exposure, making patient dosimetry an important issue in mammography.

■ Noise

The image signal in mammography is created by the "important image details" listed in Table 5.**3**, e.g., by microcalcifications or circular structures that are diagnostically discernible against the background of the normal breast tissue. Perceptibility is compromised by noise due to statistical fluctuations of the X-ray photons that make

up the mammographic image. The difference between signal and noise must therefore be as high as possible. On theoretical grounds, the eye needs a *signal-to-noise ratio* (SNR) of at least 3–5 to recognize image detail with sufficient reliability (Rose 1973). Selecting the appropriate image receptor is therefore of great importance. Film–screen systems of very high sensitivity absorb fewer X-ray photons to acquire an image and cause the mammogram to show quantum mottle, which might interfere with the perceptibility of fine details.

The model shown in Figure 5.**7** indicates that the SNR is proportional to the product of the thickness (t) of the detail (e.g., a microcalcification) times the difference

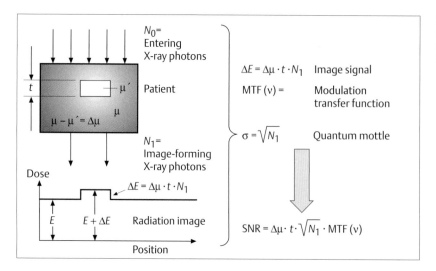

Fig. 5.7 **Determination of the signal-to-noise ratio (S/N) for small image details ($\Delta\mu \cdot t \ll 1$); monoenergetic model**

($\Delta\mu$) of the absorption coefficients of the detail (μ') and its surrounding medium (μ), in addition to being proportional to the square root ($\sqrt{N_1}$) of the number of the image-forming X-ray photons (N_1). The image signal (ΔE) is proportional to the number of X-ray photons N_1 exiting from the breast and the quantum mottle (σ) proportional to the square root of N_1. Thus, the SNR is also proportional to the square root of the number of photons ($\sqrt{N_1}$):

$$\text{SNR} \propto \Delta\mu \times t \times \sqrt{N_1} \qquad (5.2)$$

The SNR in the X-ray image (assuming an ideal focal spot) has to be multiplied by the modulation transfer function MTF(v) of the film–screen system:

$$\text{SNR} \propto (\Delta\mu \times t \times \sqrt{N_1}) \cdot \text{MTF}(v) \qquad (5.3)$$

Sharpness, contrast, and noise, as defined in the Introduction, are the physical quantities that determine the SNR, which is a derived physical characteristic for describing the image quality (5.3). Optimizing the SNR of the "radiation image" means optimizing the imaging geometry (i.e. MTF) and the radiation quality as determined by the thickness of the breast (i.e. $\Delta\mu$) and, concomitantly, minimizing the dose absorbed in the breast with consideration of the quantum mottle of the recorded image.

■ Image Quality Figure

The image quality, which incorporates the aspect of minimizing radiation exposure, can be assessed with the help of the concept of the image quality figure (Aichinger et al., 1994). The image quality figure (IQF), also referred to as figure of merit (FOM), is defined as the quotient of the square of the signal-to-noise ratio, $(\text{SNR})^2$, and the average glandular dose (AGD).

■ Dose

To calculate the image quality figure (IQF), e.g., for the display of microcalcifications, it is most sensible to take the average glandular dose (AGD) as reference (see p. 92), since this dose is most relevant for estimating the risk of carcinogenesis. With the introduction of the SNR and IQF, whereby $\text{IQF} = (\text{SNR})^2/(\text{AGD})$, the tools are available for describing further the quantities that determine sharpness, contrast, and noise (see Fig. 5.1).

■ The Effect of the Radiographic Imaging System on Dose, Contrast, Resolution, and Noise

H. Aichinger

■ Contrast

The contrast of a mammogram is fundamentally determined by the radiation quality (Step 1 of the imaging chain, p. 60), i.e., by the physical properties of the X-ray tube listed in Figure 5.1, such as anode material, filtration, and tube voltage, but also by the characteristics of the imaging system (antiscatter grid, compression device) and by the constitution of the breast itself (compression thickness, tissue composition).

In addition to the Mo-anode/Mo-filter system, which has been the most frequently used system for more than 20 years, other systems are available (Aichinger et al., 1994): the Mo-anode/Rh-filter system, the W-anode/Mo-filter system, the W-anode/Rh-filter system, and the Rh-anode/Rh-filter system (Mo = molybdenum, Rh = rhodium, W = tungsten). Figures 5.8 and 5.9 show the X-ray spectra generated by the Mo/Mo, W/Mo, and W/Rh systems at tube voltages of 25 kV and 30 kV, respectively.

The radiation quality optimal for mammography can be determined by calculating the figure of merit

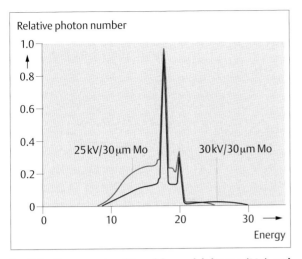

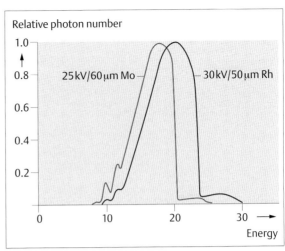

Fig. 5.**8** **X-ray spectra filtered by molybdenum (Mo) and produced by a molybdenum anode at tube voltages of 25 kV and 30 kV**

Fig. 5.**9** **X-ray-spectra filtered by molybdenum (Mo) and by rhodium (Rh) and produced by a tungsten anode at tube voltages of 25 kV and 30 kV, respectively**

under the theoretical assumption of ideal mono-energetic X-radiation. As indicated in Figure 5.**7**, this method first calculates the SNR for the microcalcifica-tion (e.g., simulated by $CaPO_4$) and then determines the average glandular dose (AGD) (see p. 92), with both values used to arrive at the image quality figure $IQF = (SNR)^2/(AGD)$.

Figure 5.**10** shows the energy dependence of the re-sult for various phantom thicknesses. For each object thickness, the most favorable X-ray energy can be read from the x-axis where the image quality figure reaches its maximum. It begins at about 17 keV for an object thickness of 3 cm and reaches 22 keV for an object thick-ness of 8 cm. From the radiological point of view, these

energies are the most favorable compromise between SNR and radiation exposure of the patient.

When using X-rays from a molybdenum or tungsten tube (or a dual-track tube with two focal spots and the anode made of Mo/Rh or Mo/W), it should be attempted to approximate the ideal monoenergetic radiation as closely as possible by varying tube voltage, filter mate-rial, and filter thickness. An approximation can be real-ized by a simulation calculation with data of measured X-ray spectra and using the model of a standard breast phantom introduced by Dance (Dance, 1990). Figure 5.**11** shows a representatively calculated SNR of an optimized combination of tube voltage and filter as a function of the object thickness for a molybdenum anode, and

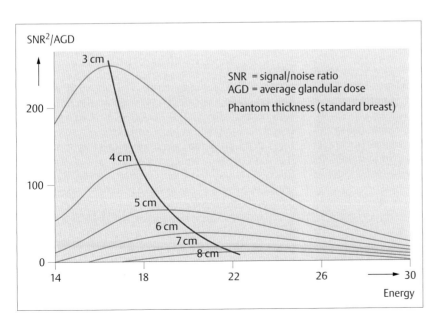

Fig. 5.**10** **Image quality figure (IQF) as function of the X-ray energy for various phantom thicknesses**

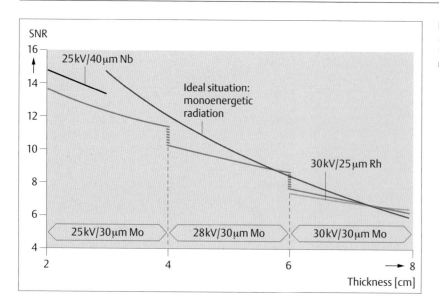

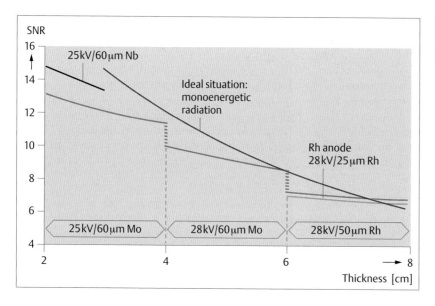

Figure 5.**12** the corresponding dependence for a tungsten anode. Both anodes can produce mammograms of high quality with either material (Mo or W).

It also might be of interest to use niobium (Nb) as filter material together with Mo and W anodes (Aichinger et al., 1994). In clinical practice, Mo/Nb systems and W/Nb systems are not used, since they are only suitable for very thin breasts.

■ Dose

In contrast to the SNR, the resulting average glandular dose (AGD) is strongly dependent on the anode material. Figures 5.**13** and 5.**14** show the dependence of the average glandular dose on the object thickness for the same

anode–filter combinations as in Figures 5.**11** and 5.**12**. The simulation calculation is based on the film–screen system Kodak MinR/SO177 or OM1/MinR. At a given system dose, a detailed comparison of these results reveals that the tungsten tube offers advantages with respect to the molybdenum anode, above all within the object thickness range of 6–8 cm. Compared to the Mo/Mo system, a reduction of the average glandular dose to about 50% can be achieved (p. 92).

The *system dose* designates the dose reaching the image receptor and producing a mean optical density in the range of 1.2–1.6 above base and fog. The system dose of the film–screen system OM1/MinR amounts to 70μGy, meeting the dose requirements in Germany. The system dose is mainly determined by the number of X-ray quanta absorbed by the film–screen system, the amplifi-

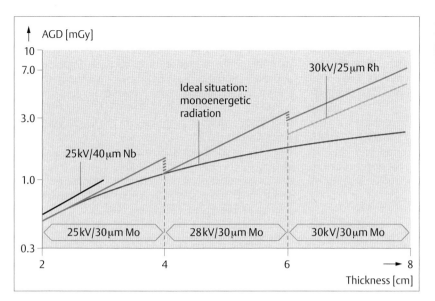

Fig. 5.**13** **Average glandular dose (AGD) as function of the phantom thickness: Mo anode in combination with K-edge filter**

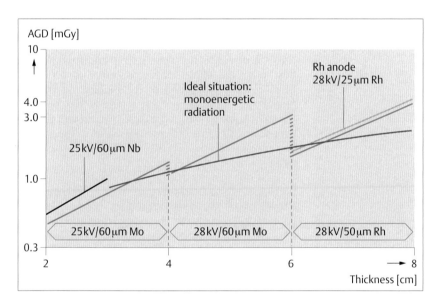

Fig. 5.**14** **Average glandular dose (AGD) as function of the phantom thickness: W anode in combination with K-edge filter**

cation factor (i.e., the number of light quanta produced for every X-ray quantum absorbed in the screen), and the sensitivity of the film. The number of absorbed X-ray quanta determines the noise on the radiographic film.

Quantum noise, i.e., the fluctuations of the optical density in a mammogram in relation to the average of absorbed X-ray quanta, is proportional to

$$1/\sqrt{N_1} \tag{5.4}$$

Expression (5.4) also demonstrates the interrelation of image quality and dose (see Fig. 5.**1**). An ideal image receptor would absorb 100% of the impinging X-ray-quanta without deteriorating the image resolution. These interrelations will be discussed in detail on p. 80.

■ Compression

Contrast is also affected by the compression device (see Fig. 5.**1**), which insures the immobilization of the breast (minimizing of motion artifacts) and changes its conical form into a largely flat form. The compression is of great importance for image quality (lower scatter fraction, less beam hardening of the imaging radiation) and reducing patient exposure (smaller object thickness).

■ Antiscatter Grid

Like any other radiographic system, mammography can improve its image contrast most effectively by employing antiscatter grids. These are made of an alternating arrangement of very thin lead strips and low-absorption medium (see Fig. 5.**15**). The effectiveness of antiscatter grids can be described by the physical properties of selectivity Σ, contrast improvement factor C, and Bucky factor B (Morneburg, 1995). The *selectivity* Σ is the ratio of the primary radiation transmission T_p and the scattered radiation transmission T_s of the grid. The *contrast improvement factor C* is the ratio of the contrast with the grid to that without it (see Fig. 5.**16**). The *Bucky factor B* gives the factor by which the entrance dose with the grid must be increased to compensate for the dose reduction at the image receptor caused by the lower amount of

scattered and primary radiation. The higher the transmission for primary radiation, the lower (better) the Bucky factor. When antiscatter grids are employed in mammography, a compromise between image quality and dose increase must be found. Investigations have shown that in mammography it serves no purpose to increase the grid ratio above $r = 4$ to 5 (Friedrich, 1975). The grid ratio r is defined as the ratio of the height of the lead strips to the thickness of the interspace medium (see Fig. 5.**15**). At compressed breast thickness values smaller than 4 cm, the use of grids should be abandoned in favor of a lower radiation exposure for the patient. Everything being equal, the radiation exposure will be increased by a factor of 2 at a breast thickness of 4 cm.

■ Sharpness

Resolution of an imaging system characterizes its ability to display fine details faithfully and with good sharpness (p. 64). The influence of the detail size on the perceptibility of small details has not yet been considered in the discussion about contrast. Only the so-called "high-contrast resolution" has been discussed so far. For the analysis of the display of fine details, the modulation transfer function of the whole imaging system must be known (see Fig. 5.**5**). Application of the modulation transfer function to the focal spot must consider not only the geometric dimensions of the focal spot but also the distribution of the radiation intensity within it. The product of contrast times the MTF also determines the resulting signal-to-noise ratio (see equation 5.3).

As a rule, quality assurance checks only the resolution limit. As discussed above (see p. 64), the recommendations of the "Bundesärztekammer" (General Medical Council) in Germany require a visual resolution > 2.4 lp/mm. According to the German "Röntgenverordnung", (Regulation for the Use of X-rays) the acceptance test must measure a resolution limit of at least 8 lp/mm. The "European Protocol for the Quality Control of Technical Aspects of Mammography Screening" requires 13 lp/mm. The lead bar pattern used for these measurements is placed close to the chest wall at a defined distance from the cassette holder. The requirements in the United States are very similar. These various specifications reflect the general uncertainty about the effect of the resolution limit on the image quality. From the medical point of view, the detail contrast is important in the spatial frequency range 2–5 lp/mm. This range of the spatial frequency falls into the detail sizes of microcalcifications that are visible under optimal exposure conditions.

A high resolution limit does not inevitably imply a good contrast reproduction at low spatial frequencies, since the composite modulation transfer function is also determined by the radiation intensity distribution within the focal spot. In particular, extrafocal radiation is undesirable arising around the focal spot. A focal spot that has a high contrast transfer predominantly around 2–5 lp/mm will deliver mammograms of better quality

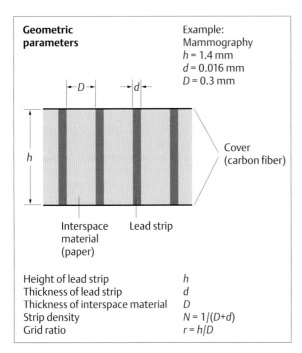

| Geometric parameters | Example: Mammography h = 1.4 mm d = 0.016 mm D = 0.3 mm |

Height of lead strip	h
Thickness of lead strip	d
Thickness of interspace material	D
Strip density	$N = 1/(D+d)$
Grid ratio	$r = h/D$

Fig. 5.15   Geometrical characteristics of an antiscatter grid in mammography

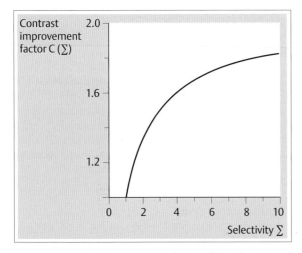

Fig. 5.16   Contrast improvement factor $C(\Sigma)$ as function of selectivity Σ at a scatter fraction of 50 %

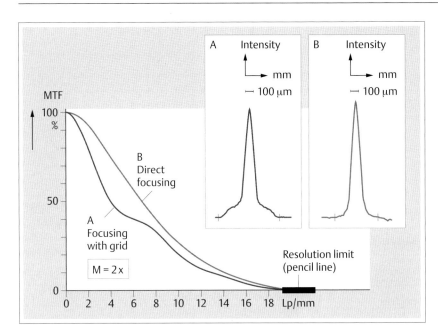

than a focal spot that shows an extremely high resolution limit but low detail contrast in the spatial frequency range of particular interest to diagnostic imaging.

The Effect of the Image Receptor on Dose, Contrast, Resolution, and Noise

T. von Volkmann

In most cases, the radiographic image is recorded using a film–screen system as an image receptor. Integral components of this film–screen system include the cassette and film processing.

All four components (film, screen, cassette, and processing) affect dose and image quality of the mammogram.

A single intensifying screen (as the back screen) in conjunction with a single-emulsion film is used almost exclusively for mammography to reduce screen blur, albeit at the cost of speed.

Description of physical image quality by four parameters

- Optical density
- Contrast
- Blur
- Noise

Composition of Mammography Films

Unlike films used for general radiography, mammography films are usually coated with a light-sensitive emul-

sion on one side only. The emulsion contains the light-sensitive silver halides embedded in gelatin. The base is usually made of polyester. A coating is applied to protect the emulsion from damage, which also helps reduce electrostatic discharge through the inclusion of special additives.

Structure of Intensifying Screens

Intensifying screens consist of a phosphor layer coated on a support (usually polyester). At present, mammography screens from almost all manufacturers have gadolinium oxisulfide ($Gd_2O_2S:Tb$) as phosphor, in contrast to the wide variety of phosphors found in the intensifying screens used for general radiography. The phosphor layer is coated with a protective layer.

Characteristic Curve

The characteristic curve describes the relation between exposure, including processing, and the resultant optical density (previously called blackening and referred to as "density" in the following text). Important film properties, such as film contrast and maximum density, can be derived from the characteristic curve (Fig. 5.**18**).

Speed of the Film–Screen System

The speed of the film–screen system determines to a large extent the dose of a mammogram.

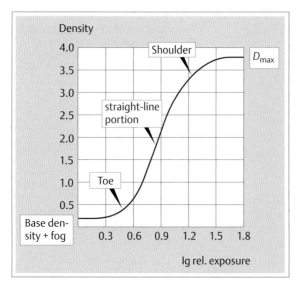

Fig. 5.**18**   **Characteristic curve of an X-ray film**

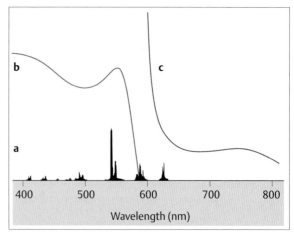

Fig. 5.**19**a–c   **Spectral curves**
a Emission spectrum of intensifying screen (Gd_2O_2S)
b Spectral sensitivity of an orthochromatic film
c Spectral transmission of a safelight

Parameters of speed

- Intensifying factor of the intensifying screen
- Speed and spectral sensitivity of the film
- Processing
- Beam quality used (kVp value, anode material, filter material)

The speed also determines the exposure time for the radiographic films and, consequently, the extent of the possible motion blur.

Intensifying Factor of Screens

Because the sensitivity of photographic film is considerably less for X-rays than for visible light, the X-rays are converted through phosphors (luminescence) into visible light, which in turn exposes the film. This substantially reduces the dose required to expose the radiographic film.

The intensification is determined by the degree of absorption of X-rays by the intensifying screen and by the degree of conversion of the absorbed X-rays into visible light (conversion efficiency). Both parameters can be influenced by the selected phosphor material and by the structure of the intensifying screen.

Depending on the type of phosphor used, intensifying screens emit light of various colors (wavelengths). With screens using gadolinium oxisulfide as phosphor, the greatest percentage of light is in the green range (Fig. 5.**19**a).

Speed and Spectral Sensitivity of the Film

Just like photographic film, the speed of X-ray film is inversely proportional to the amount of light needed to

blacken the film. The spectral sensitivity of the film defines the range of the light spectrum to which the film is sensitive.

The speed of a film is not a constant parameter, but depends also on the condition of the film (age, storage conditions, fog) and on the length of the exposure time (reciprocity failure). Film speed decreases as exposure time increases.

Factors for long exposure times

- Low-speed film–screen systems
- Large and/or dense breast
- Magnification technique
- Low power high voltage generator
- Low output X-ray tubes
- Low kVp values

For the essentially green emission of gadolinium oxisulfide screens, it is necessary to use so-called orthochromatic films with a spectral sensitivity in the blue and green region (Fig. 5.**19**b).

The spectral sensitivity of the film also determines the color of the suitable safelight. Orthochromatic film, for example, may only be exposed to red light (Fig. 5.**19**c). Improper safelight increases fog and reduces the contrast of the radiograph.

Processing

The effect of processing (especially developing) on dose and image quality is frequently underestimated. The various factors that affect film development are well known, but often are not adequately taken into consideration.

Factors that influence processing

- Developer temperature
- Developing time
- Motion (transport rollers, film throughput, chemical recirculation)
- Type of processor
- Activity of developer:
  - composition and mixture
  - concentration
  - replenishment rate
  - age of developer
  - oxidation
  - impurities
  - type and quantity of other films being processed

The values specified by the manufacturer for speed and contrast of the film–screen system are valid only when the processing conditions recommended by the manufacturer are followed. It is important to note that different types of film can respond differently to processing variations.

Figure 5.**20** illustrates the influence of developer temperature and developing time on speed, contrast and fog of a film. This behavior is exhibited by essentially all types of film, differing only in extent and temperature range, both of which depend on the other developing parameters.

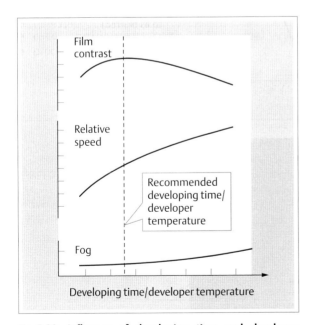

Fig. 5.**20 Influence of developing time and developer temperature on relative speed, contrast, and fog (representative diagram).** The speed S published by the manufacturer is achieved when the recommended developer is used at the recommended combination of developing time and developer temperature

Speed S of a Film–Screen System

The speed S of a film–screen system is inversely proportional to the dose at the image receptor that yields the density $D = 1$ on the film above fog and density of the base (ISO 9236 – 1 and ISO 9236 – 3).

The speed of modern mammography film–screen systems is usually between 10 and 30.

The often used term "(nominal) speed class" defines only a broad speed category in a given scheme,where the speed is doubled or halved on going from one class to the next (…,12, 25, 50, 100, 200,…). Sometimes the speed is also given in values relative to an arbitrary standard.

Only the speed S, however, can be used for calculating the radiation dose to the patient.

◼ Density of the Mammogram

The density of the radiograph has a major influence on image quality, especially on the radiographic contrast.

The European guidelines recommend that, for diagnostically relevant parts, the range of density shall lie between 0.6 and 2.2 with a mean density of the mammogram between 1.3 and 1.8. This mean density is somewhat higher than the value for general diagnostic radiography ($D = 1.0 – 1.4$). The difference reflects the unique anatomy of the breast. Densities above 2.2 must be viewed with a bright light.

These values are basically in accordance with the ACR recommendations, which refer especially to the correct exposure of the glandular tissue: the optical density of the glandular tissue is optimal in the range 1.4 – 2.0 and shall not be below 1.0 or above 3.0.

A higher mean density enhances the exposure latitude of the film, which is of special advantage with modern high-contrast films, but more frequently requires the use of the bright light (Fig. 5.**21**).

Detail visibility at densities below 0.6 and above 2.2 is limited since the film contrast becomes lower at the toe of the characteristic curve (Fig. 5.**22**) and contrast perception of the human eye decreases at higher density levels (greater than 2.2) (Fig. 5.**36**). Regions with higher density levels can, however, be evaluated with a bright light.

These density values result from the physiology of the human eye, the brightness of the viewbox and the shape of the characteristic curve (see p. 72).

Cutis and subcutis as well as other regions frequently have a density level above 2.2 as a consequence of the recommended higher mean density for mammograms, and must, as recommended in the guidelines, be viewed with a bright light.

Microcalcifications require a special consideration: Since microcalcifications must be imaged in their "size, shape, and arrangement," but not in their inner structure, the density level for a microcalcification may be lower than $D = 0.6$, as long as it stands out against the

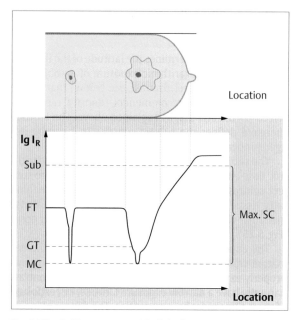

Fig. 5.**25**   **Subject contrast SC of the breast**
lg I_R   Radiation dose behind the breast
Sub   Subcutis
FT   Fatty tissue
GT   Glandular tissue
MC   Microcalcification
Max. SC Maximum subject contrast

High film contrast

- Structures are conspicuous
- Pleasant, brilliant radiographs
- Subjectively less blurred (contrast is perceived as sharpness)
- Narrow film latitude, i.e., the subject contrast to be properly imaged is confined
- Reduced exposure latitude
- Film contrast too high: loss of information ("black and white" radiographs)

Low film contrast

- Wider film latitude, i.e., greater range of subject contrast can be properly imaged
- Structures are less conspicuous
- Less pleasant, low-contrast radiographs
- Subjectively more blurred
- Wider exposure latitude
- Film contrast too low: unnecessary loss of conspicuity

Selection of film contrast should be based on the subject contrast and clinical context, not on subjective preferences (see below).

Film contrast is not a constant parameter. Even the same film type can change its contrast, especially as a re-

sult of processing and exposure of the radiograph. Improperly processed and underexposed or overexposed radiographs have less contrast.

If the radiographic contrast is too high ($\Delta D > 1.6$), important structures are not imaged well or not at all on the radiograph, which results in loss of information. If the radiographic contrast is too low ($\Delta D < 1.6$) structures become less conspicuous and may be missed or overlooked.

Because of the stored mental image ("engram") acquired by the radiologist over many years, any change in contrast, even when improving the image quality, will require some time to get accustomed to.

Correct contrast of a mammogram. A mammogram has the required contrast when subject contrast (p. 75) and film contrast have been matched in such a way that all diagnostically relevant regions have a density between 0.6 and 2.2, except for cutis/subcutis and microcalcifications (Fig. 5.**23**). The cutis and subcutis may be imaged darker, but must then be reviewed using the bright light. Microcalcifications can be imaged somewhat lighter, as long as they stand out against the surrounding tissue.

High film contrast has the advantage that structures within the recommended density range (0.6–2.2) are imaged conspicuously, but requires that the subject contrast is matched to the narrow film latitude. This is possible using modern X-ray equipment that offers not only adjustable tube voltage (kVp value) but also a choice of several anode and filter materials, to be adapted to different breasts. This is especially important for detecting focal densities and microcalcifications, particularly if located in dense glandular tissue. An additional advantage is the lower radiation dose, making this technique very recommendable. A mammogram has the correct radiographic contrast when subject contrast and film contrast have been matched in such a way that the subject contrast coincides with the correct exposure range determined by the film latitude. (Fig. 5.**26**).

For a large and dense breast and inadequate radiation quality (e.g. 28 kV Mo/Mo), the subject contrast may exceed the subject contrast recordable on the film, resulting in regions of the radiograph being too dark or too light (Fig. 5.**27 a**). In this case, either a harder radiation quality (e.g. 30 kV, Mo/Rh, Fig. 5.**26**) or a film with a lower contrast (Fig. 5.**27 b**) must be selected to achieve the correct contrast.

If the radiation quality selected for the given object is too hard (e.g. 32 kV, Rh/Rh), the resulting subject contrast falls short of the subject contrast that the film can properly image and the radiograph is low in contrast (Fig. 5.**28 a**). In this case, a softer beam quality or a film with higher contrast must be used (Fig. 5.**28 b**) to achieve the desired radiographic contrast.

■ Image Blur

Diffusion of the light in the screen and in the film results in image blur in addition to the blur caused by the

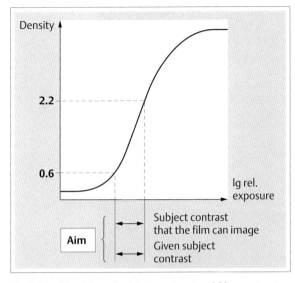

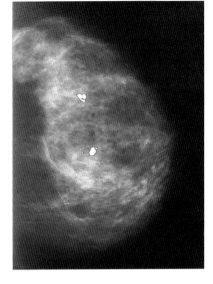

Fig. 5.**26**   **Matching of subject contrast and film contrast**

geometric conditions (focal spot size, focus–film distance, object–film distance) and by motion (exposure time).

These three components of image blur—geometric, motion, and screen blur—are interrelated by the uniformity rule. This states that the individual contributions to the blur must be as low and as equal as possible. If one particular blur is considerably greater than the others, it will determine the blurring of the radiograph. For example, the large geometric blur of a large focal spot cannot be eliminated by a screen that may have the highest resolution possible.

Poor film–screen contact caused by defective cassettes or entrapped air may lead to unnecessary additional blur (see below).

Mammography film–screen systems consist almost universally of only one intensifying screen combined with a single-emulsion film. The intensifying screen is used as a back screen because the X-rays are absorbed preferentially at the tube side. This reduces light diffusion in the screen, resulting in less blur (Fig. 5.**29**).

The objective measure for the image blur of an image receptor is the modulation transfer function (MTF). The resolution is frequently stated as the 4% value of the MTF. Expressed as the 4% value of the MTF, the resolution of modern mammography film–screen systems is higher than 15 lp/mm.

Visual resolution determined by a lead bar test pattern is very subjective and also depends on the film contrast. Exclusive use of this assessment of the image quality of film–screen systems can be misleading since an essential criterion, the latitude of the film–screen system, is not taken into account.

A detail size of ≤ 0.2 mm formally corresponds to a structure of ≥ 2.5 lp/mm (p. 64). However, this value cannot be compared to a resolution determined with a lead bar test pattern because periodic structures of high contrast detail (lead) are easier to recognize than a single detail with a low subject contrast (microcalcification). Therefore, a considerably higher modulation transfer function (MTF) is needed.

According to the European Guidelines, a spatial resolution > 10 lp/m is acceptable and > 13 lp/mm is desirable, measured with a lead bar test pattern on top of a 45 mm PMMA plate.

To mimimize radiation absorption by the cassette, mammography cassettes are not made of metal, as are most cassettes used for general radiography, but of plastic, which absorbs less radiation. However, plastics are less stable than metal. Furthermore, any air entrapped after closing the plastic cassettes may not escape as quickly as from metal cassettes.

The distance between the film and the screen created by air trapped in the cassette causes avoidable blur on the mammogram. Depending on the type of cassette that is used, a waiting period from 5 to 15 minutes should be observed for mammography cassettes between loading and exposing. The required waiting time should be stated in the instructions for the cassette.

■ Noise

The ability to recognize details is also influenced by the noise ("graininess") of the radiograph. However, the same level of objective noise is perceived as being more or less bothersome by different viewers.

Noise refers to the "grainy" appearance of the radiographic film—the statistically distributed density fluctuations that are not caused by the object being imaged. The noise in film–screen systems is to a large degree quantum mottle and less film grain or screen structure.

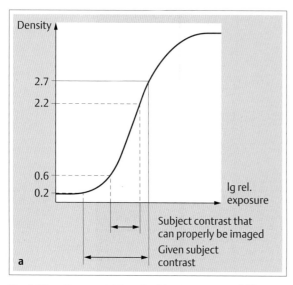
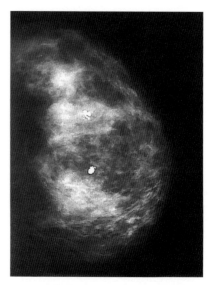

Fig. 5.27 a **Poor matching of subject contrast and film contrast**. Given subject contrast is too high for given film contrast

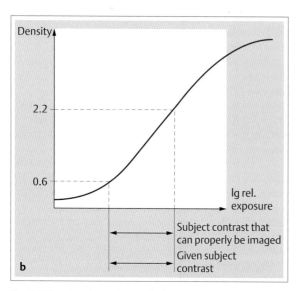
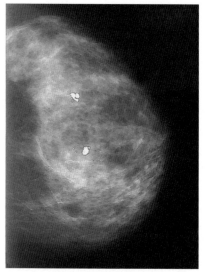

Fig. 5.27 b **Good matching of subject contrast and film contrast**. High subject contrast with low film contrast

In contrast to a widely held opinion, noise is not a function of the speed of the film–screen system or entrance dose, but rather of the number of photons that are absorbed by the screen to expose the film.

If the speed of the film–screen system is increased by selecting a highly absorbing phosphor or a thicker phosphor layer, the quantum noise does not increase because the number of absorbed X-ray photons remains the same. If, however, the speed of the film–screen system is increased by using a film with higher speed or by more aggressive processing, the noise level will rise because the number of required X-ray quanta decreases.

In addition to the level of quantum mottle, conspicuousness is also relevant. As for the representation of small details in general, conspicuousness depends on screen blur, the contrast of the film and the density of the radiograph. This means that a film with a higher contrast will bring out noise more conspicuously than a film with a lower contrast. The same applies to a high-resolution screen.

■ Summary

Density. The European guidelines recommend that the mean density for mammograms should lie between D = 1.3 and 1.8. The ACR mainly refers to the optical density for imaging the glandular tissue, with the optical

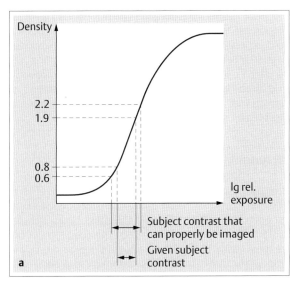

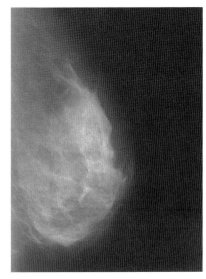

Fig. 5.**28 a**   **Poor matching of subject contrast and film contrast**. Film contrast is too low for given subject contrast

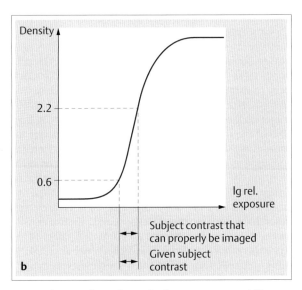

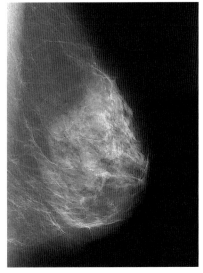

Fig. 5.**28 b**   **Good matching of subject contrast and film contrast**. Low subject contrast with high film contrast

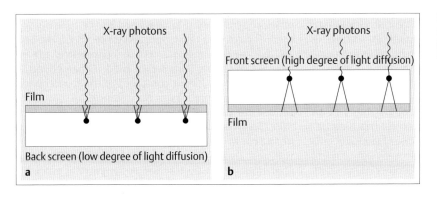

Fig. 5.**29 a, b   Screen blur, use of intensifying screen** as
a Back screen: low blur
b Front screen: high blur

density best in the range of 1.4 – 2.0, but not below 1.0 or above 3.0. Densities above 2.2 must be viewed with the bright light.

Contrast. Subject and film contrast should be matched to each other in such a way that all diagnostically significant details are imaged with a density between 0.6 and 2.2, except for subcutis and microcalcifications.

A higher film contrast will increase the conspicuousness of the details in the recommended density range. At the same time, this has the risk of other diagnostically significant structures to be less or not at all recognizable when they fall outside this density range. This can be prevented by appropriate selection of tube voltage (kVp value), anode and filter material with respect to the object.

Blur and noise. Blur and noise correlate only under certain circumstances with the speed of the film–screen system. The systems can be optimized with respect to blur or noise by selecting the appropriate film and screen.

For single-emulsion mammogram film–screen systems, the following simplified rules apply:

- As the intensifying factor of the screen increases, the blur (modulation transfer function) usually decreases while quantum noise remains the same, since usually only the screen thickness is changed.
- As the speed of the film increases, the level of quantum noise also increases but the blur (MTF) remains the same.

Evaluation. Evaluation of film–screen systems with a lead bar test pattern alone is misleading. Contrast detail diagrams are better suited.

■ The Importance of Constancy and Reproducibility of the Entire Imaging System

H. Aichinger

Optimizing the quality of mammograms requires correct exposure of every radiographic image. All exposure parameters must be kept constant and reproducible within narrow limits. This especially applies to "screening mammography" since retakes are undesirable for medical reasons (additional radiation exposure, induced anxiety) and financial reasons (additional film costs and labor).

When judging constancy and reproducibility of an imaging system, the tolerance of the contributing parameters must be considered. It is quite obvious and immediately noticed if the automatic exposure control (AEC) does not work, but a change of other parameters, such as the tube voltage, may not be noticed right away. This illustrates why quality-control programs are especially important in mammography.

Since the X-ray generators (high-frequency generators) used today in mammography units have such a high reproducibility, the constancy of mammograms is primarily determined by correct patient positioning (see chapter 7), suitable film material, stable film processing, and careful adaptation of the AEC to the film–screen system, as well as by correct sensor placement in relation to the breast.

■ Automatic Exposure Control

The purpose of the automatic exposure control is to achieve a constant mean optical density of each mammogram independent of breast thickness, breast density, and selected exposure parameters. This requirement can be most easily fulfilled by placing the sensor directly in front of the film cassette, as is customary in general radiology. This arrangement has not become established in mammography, however, because a sensor in this location would increase the distance between object and image receptor and reduce the achievable resolution. For reasons of achieving optimal image quality and keeping the absorption of the imaging radiation through intermediate layers as low as possible, the sensor is generally placed behind the film cassette. Consequently, the sensor is not recording the imaging radiation, but the radiation transmitted through the film–screen system and the cassette. As the film–screen system absorbs the major fraction of the imaging radiation, only a small fraction of the radiation hitting the cassette is available for measuring the exposure. This fraction depends on the radiation quality (tube voltage, anode-filter combination), on the thickness and the composition of the breast tissue, and, finally, on the film–screen system and the cassette. As a result, the optical density decreases considerably with increasing thickness and physical density of the breast, unless special measures are taken to reduce this effect (see Fig. 5.**30**) (Aichinger et al., 1990). In clinical practice, therefore, the technologist has to use a phototimer technique chart (La France et al., 1988) according to the compressed breast thickness.

In Germany, the "Guidelines of the Bundesärztekammer" (General Medical Council) require that the automatic exposure control be adapted to the thickness and physical density of the breast and to the tube voltage used. The goal is a mean optical density (including base and fog) in the range 1.2 – 1.6, independent of the individual exposure parameters used. Other countries demand an even higher constancy of the mean optical density. In the United States, for instance, the mean optical density will not be allowed to deviate more than ±0.15 from the mean value in the object thickness range from 2 cm to 6 cm Plexiglas for the corresponding tube voltages. This will be in effect in October 2002. The gradation γ of the film–screen system used is crucial in meeting this requirement.

Different automatic exposure control systems are employed today to achieve the required constancy of the

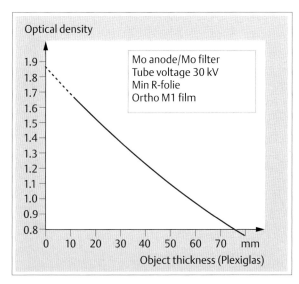

Fig. 5.**30** **Optical density as function of the object thickness when using automatic exposure control (conventional system without transparency compensation)**

mean optical density of mammograms. Determining the correct exposure based on the compression thickness is very limited, since the tube current time product (mAs) required for maintaining a constant optical density can vary by a factor of 5 to 6 for the identical thickness of compressed breast (Klein et al., 1997). A preexposure "test shot" might determine the right cut-off dose more accurately. This method has the additional advantage (if a dual-track tube is employed) that anode and filter material, together with the tube voltage, can be automatically adapted to the X-ray transparency of the breast. Only a short interruption of the exposure must be accepted.

An automatic exposure control system produces a signal that is directly proportional to the transparency of the breast. To meet the requirements of constancy with respect to the mean optical density as discussed above, a double sensor with two semicircular semiconductor detectors is used (Aichinger et al., 1990). An additional brass filter is arranged between these detectors (see Fig. 5.**31**). While the signal of the upper detector switches off the tube voltage as in conventional exposure control systems, the detector element located below the additional filter serves to determine a correction factor for the cut-off dose. The correction factor is determined by the processor system of the AEC after obtaining a quotient of the two detector signals S_1 and S_2. For a given anode-filter combination and film–screen system and a particular tube voltage, the "transparency correction" is an unambiguous function of the object transparency. Figure 5.**32** shows the results of phantom measurements with and without automatic transparency compensation. Over the whole object thickness range from 10 mm to 70 mm Plexiglas, a constancy of the mean optical density better than 1.3 ± 0.1 relative to 40 mm Plexiglas is obtained.

The efficacy of the automatic transparency compensation can also be demonstrated with radiographs of a phantom made of materials simulating different tissue compositions (see Fig. 5.**33**), with Plexiglas used for glandular and styrene for adipose tissue. Different breast compositions can be "realized" by combining various numbers of Plexiglas and styrene layers and placing them in the area measured by the AEC.

Figure 5.**34** shows four different representative "tissue compositions" at a "breast thickness" of 50 mm

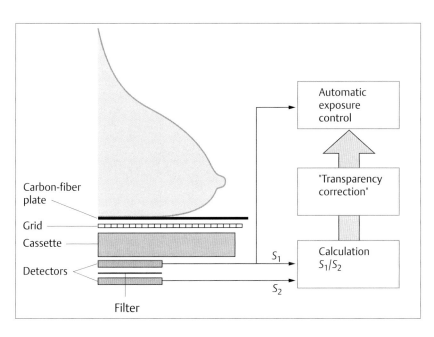

Fig. 5.**31** **Diagram of the principle of an automatic exposure control system (AEC) with automatic transparency correction**

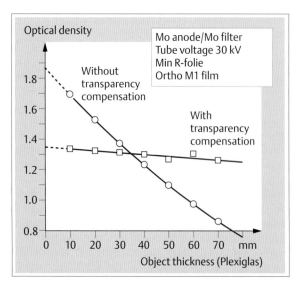

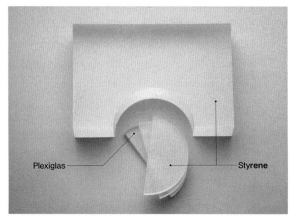

Fig. 5.32 Optical density as function of the object thickness when using automatic exposure control in mammography (with and without automatic transparency compensation)

Fig. 5.33 Test phantom for the simulation of different tissue combinations:
Glandular tissue = Plexiglas, adipose tissue = styrene

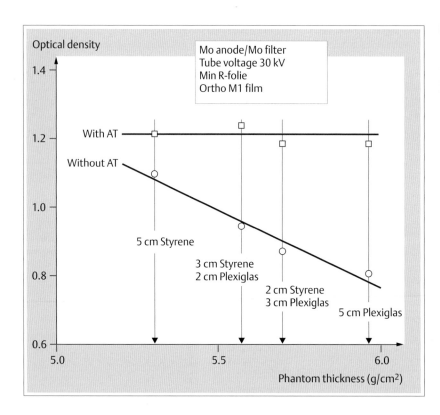

Fig. 5.34 Optical density as function of the tissue combination with automatic exposure control (with and without automatic transparency compensation)
AT = automatic transparency compensation

with and without automatic transparency compensation. This method of maintaining mean optical density is possible because the double detector scores the radiation quality of the imaging radiation behind the breast, which is—at a given object thickness—dependent on the tissue composition (see Fig. 5.35).

To guarantee constant and reproducible exposure of mammograms, the following factors have to be taken into consideration for calculating the exposure correction factors ("transparency correction")

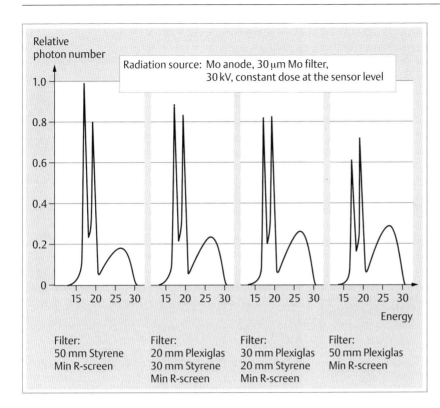

Fig. 5.**35**   X-ray spectra in the detector plane: beam hardening is dependent on the tissue composition in the area of the measuring field of the automatic exposure control (Aichinger et al., 1990)

Factors determining the exposure

- Anode material
- Filter thickness and filter material
- Tube voltage
- Antiscatter grid
- Characteristics of the cassette
- Characteristics of the screen
- Characteristics of the film
- Reciprocity law failure
- Tissue thickness
- Tissue composition
- Characteristics of the AEC detector

To obtain an optimal exposure of mammograms at all times, the automatic exposure control system must be carefully adjusted to the routine work in the clinical practice. Because of complex interrelationships, all factors, especially the constancy of the film processing, have to be checked regularly.

■ The Role of the Viewbox and Viewing Conditions

T. von Volkmann, M. A. O. Thijssen and A. Stargardt

The process of viewing radiographic images has so far been given less attention than the performance of imaging systems. Optimal viewing conditions, however, are very important, particularly in mammography.

A relatively bright viewbox (at least 3000 cd/m^2) with masking possibility and a sufficiently low ambient light level (below 50 lux) is required for viewing mammograms. In addition, a bright light and a magnifying lens with 2 × to 4× magnification must also be available. The visibility of details depends on three prerequisites:

- The quality of their representation on the radiograph (pp. 60 – 83)
- The capacity of human vision
- The viewing conditions

Viewbox and viewing conditions must consider the characteristics of human vision. Acuity and contrast resolution depend on the level of luminance, and are reduced by low luminance since the receptors responsible for acuity (cones) have a threshold around 20 cd/m^2, with an increasing reaction above this level. The maximum acuity and contrast resolution lies between 100 and 300 cd/m^2 (Fig. 5.**36**).

The general requirements for the viewbox and the viewing conditions are derived from these correlations.

■ European Quality Assurance Guidelines for Mammography Screening

- The luminance should be in the range from 3000 to 6000 cd/m^2.

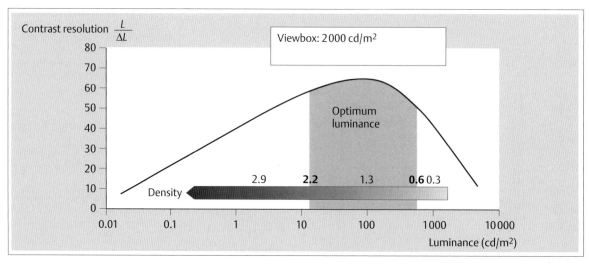

Fig. 5.**36**   **Contrast resolution of human vision as a function of the luminance behind the radiograph for various densities using a viewbox with a luminance of 2000 cd/m² (König-** Brodhun/Wucherer). A density of $D = 1.3$ corresponds to attenuation by a factor of 20

- The luminance across a single viewbox should be within ± 30% in the area 5 cm from the edge of the pane.
- The intensity of the different viewboxes in the department should be within 15% of the average (measured in the center of the viewing area).
- To prevent color deviation, all lamps shall be of the same brand, type, and age.
- All lamps shall be replaced once a year.
- Regular cleaning of the viewbox is essential.
- The ambient (extraneous) light level shall be below 50 lux.

■ Luminance of the Viewbox

To achieve good vision and contrast resolution, the luminance behind the mammogram shall be at least 100 cd/m², preferably 300 cd/m².

The optimal luminance of the viewbox can be calculated from the mean density of the mammogram. As density is a logarithmic quantity, a mean density of $D = 1.5$ means that light is attenuated by a factor of $10^{1.5} = 32$. The luminance of the viewbox is calculated according to the following relationship:

Luminance behind the mammogram (viewers side)	×	Attenuation factor of the light by the mammogram	=	Luminance of the viewbox

Optimum conditions mean:

$$100 \, cd/m^2 \times 32 = 3200 \, cd/m^2 \qquad (5.5)$$

In actual practice, mammograms are, unfortunately, often underexposed with resultant low contrast, and viewboxes often lack adequate luminance. Both of these factors are detrimental to diagnostic quality.

Brandt (1991, 1994) and others demonstrated for chest radiographs how the density of the radiograph and the luminance of the viewbox influence the diagnostic quality. Since the critical structures (small or low-contrast lesions) are comparable, these results can be transfered to the reading of mammograms. Furthermore, it must be taken into account that the cones, which are responsible for acuity, require a longer adaptation time than the rods. The eyes need at least 10 minutes to adapt from bright sunlight to a darkened room.

■ Illuminance of Ambient Light

The state of adaptation of the eyes is also influenced by the ambient light. Its illuminance should be matched to the luminance behind the darkest regions of the radiograph relevant for interpretation. Any deviation compromises detail recognition.

Consequently, the illuminance of the ambient light should not exceed 50 lux for reading properly exposed mammograms and adequate luminance of the viewbox. Paper documents can still be read at illuminance levels slightly less than 50 lux.

The viewbox must be installed in such a way that extraneous light (sunlight and artificial lighting) is not reflected by the viewbox or the mammograms.

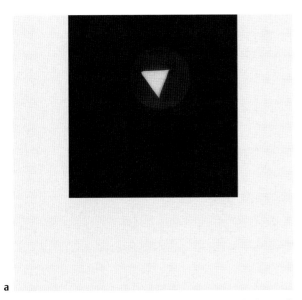

a

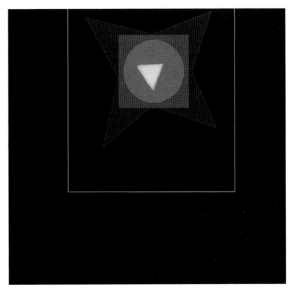

b

Fig. 5.37 a, b   Influence of masking and ambient light on the contrast resolution of the human vision
a Poor masking   **b** Correct masking

■ Masking

Good masking is very important when viewing mammograms, in particular with high-luminance viewboxes and high-density mammograms. Without masking, the adaptation of the eye to the luminance of the mammogram on the viewbox is adversely affected (Fig. 5.**37**); this is especially the case at the edge of the mammograms. Viewboxes with automatic masking are now available.

The physician reading mammograms must not only be aware of the physiological processes of vision (such as adaptation times), the relationship between density of the radiograph and the.luminance of the viewbox, the influence of ambient light, the use of bright lights and magnifying glasses or masking, but must also keep in mind that both the contrast resolution and the accommodation capacity of the human eye deteriorate rapidly after the age of 30 years (Wucherer, 1995).

■ A New Digital Film-Reading Modality

D. J. Dronkers and G. Rosenbusch

A new digital film viewer has recently been introduced (Smartlight). This system uses optronic technologies, which optimize film reading.

This film viewer fully eliminates glare by providing automated seamless masking. The light intensity emanating from the film is optimized electronically. By the use of micro-optic beam forming that produces coned light, film scatter (Callier effect) is suppressed, which improves contrast significantly.

Othe important characteristic are the facility of a local spotlight and mammography reading features such as automated masking for comparing small areas of left and right breast simultaneously. This technique is also used in motorized viewers.

■ Possible Digital Image Receptors

H. Aichinger

Film–screen mammography is still the most important examination method for detecting and diagnosing breast cancer, but it has limitations that may be overcome by direct digital acquisition of the image. The most salient limitation is the narrow dynamic range of about 1 : 25 or less for steep film–screen combinations. A desirable latitude would be about 1 : 100 (Yaffe, 1992; Yaffe and Rowlands, 1997). Especially in young women, it is very hard to detect microcalcifications and small masses in very dense breasts. This is expected to improve with digital imaging because of its wider dynamic range. Figure 5.**38 a, b** illustrates this point by comparing a conventional and a digital mammogram of the same patient (Thijssen, 2000). Furthermore—depending on the ability of post-acquisition processing of the image—a higher-contrast resolution can be achieved.

Film–screen combinations provide an excellent spatial resolution of high-contrast details not yet achievable with digital image receptors. This display of high spatial frequencies is crucial for faithful visualization of microcalcifications since their shape and arrangement often provide information decisive for diagnosis and therapy. The answer to the question of the resolving power really needed for the diagnosis at optimal contrast transfer has great impact on the concept and success of digital mammography.

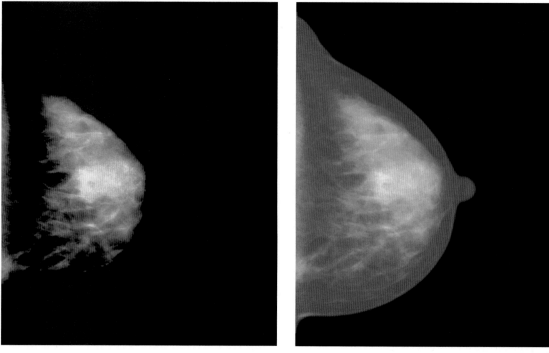

a   b

Fig. 5.**38 a, b**   Comparison of an conventional mammogram and a digital mammogram of the same patient. The dynamic range in the digital image is considerable improved.

■ Digital Detectors (Full-field Mammography)

Digital image receptors for mammography can be realized as line and area detector systems (Yaffe, 1992; Yaffe and Rowlands, 1997).

   CCD (charge-coupled device) detector arrays, coupled with a fiberoptic taper or a demagnification camera system to a scintillator material, such as Gd_2O_2S:Tb or CsI, are primarily suitable for the first cate-

gory because of their mechanical dimensions. CCD detectors consist of photosensitive semiconductor elements arranged as a matrix (see Fig. 5.**39**). The signal of the image matrix elements (pixels) is read out serially for each pixel line by line. The literature reports a line detector consisting of 4096×64 detector elements, which was assembled by connecting a strip of photostimulable phosphor with two CCD sensors (Yaffe, 1992). Combined with a mammographic imaging unit based on the scan-

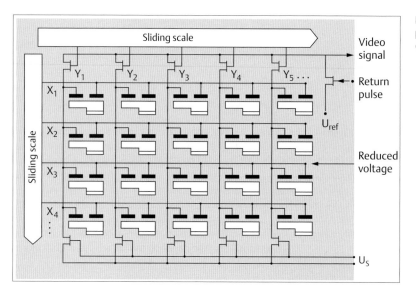

Fig. 5.**39   Diagram showing the principle of a CCD (charge-coupled device) detector**

ning slit technique, an image matrix size of 4096 × 4096 pixels, corresponding to a resolution limit of 10 lp/mm (i.e., detail size of 50 μm diameter), can be obtained. The slit technique collimates the X-ray beam close to the tube and image receptor to form a fan beam, which is guided over the breast with the focal spot as pivot (see Fig. 5.**40**). A critical aspect of the scanning slit technique is the extreme heat loading of the X-ray tube. Compared to conventional full-field mammography, the tube loading increases approximately by a factor equal to the ratio of the field length to the slit width. It is possible to improve the efficiency of such a system by scanning with a multiple-slit assembly. Besides the high tube load, the increased mechanical complexity is another disadvantage of such a scanning system.

Storage phosphor screens, detectors made of amorphous silicon or selenium or large-area CCD arrays (e.g., 3 × 4 single CCD chips joined together), belong to the second category of digital full-field detectors.

Storage phosphor screens (also called photostimulable phosphors) are very similar to normal intensifying screens, but the photostimulable phosphor has the ability to storing the image information for a long time. This latent image can be read out by scanning with a focused laser beam. During the line-by-line scanning process analogous to the intensifying screen, visible light is emitted and measured, e.g., by a photomultiplier tube. After analog–digital conversion, the resulting electrical signal is sent to a digital storage device. The quality of the

laser beam essentially determines the resolution obtainable.

As a rule, a CsI scintillator layer is used as input screen for image receptors based on CCD and amorphous silicon technology to convert the absorbed X-ray energy to visible light. In the large-area CCD arrays, the light coupling is again made by fiberoptic tapers; in the so-called flat-panel detector (FD detector), the light is detected directly by the photodiodes deposited on the amorphous silicon layer. In image receptors based on the amorphous selenium technology, the X-ray energy is directly converted to a electrical signal. Amorphous selenium can be produced for large areas by evaporation and vapor deposition on an array of thin-film transistors (TFT technology). Since the signal is no longer generated through emitted visible light, this system offers the potential for increased spatial resolution (Yaffe and Rowlands, 1997).

Plates of amorphous selenium are well-known from xeromammography, but when they are used in digital imaging the latent electrostatic image is no longer made visible with a powdered toner. The image information is read line by line with microelectrodes or, in the same manner as FD detectors, with a transistor-matrix in thin-film transistor technology (TFT-matrix; Yaffe and Rowlands, 1997).

Full-field detectors have the advantage that they can be operated with the exposure technique well-established for film–screen mammography. The question of the image matrix size is still open. Current investigations of digital imaging that address the limiting resolution still use digital mammograms generally obtained by digitizing conventional film images. This conversion achieves a pixel size of 50 μm, corresponding to a resolution limit of 10 lp/mm. For a film size of 18 cm × 24 cm, this results in an image matrix size of 3600 × 4800 pixels.

The only digital image receptor already available so far in routine mammography (i.e., the storage phosphor screen) has a pixel size of 100 μm, corresponding to a resolution limit of 5 lp/mm for the grid technique. Various investigators have shown a detectability of microcalcifications that is comparable to that of conventional mammograms (Karssemeijer et al., 1993). This could be documented with the contrast-detail phantom shown in Figure 5.**41**.

The measured contrast–detail curves for a disk-shaped object published by Karssemeijer are shown in Figure 5.**42**. The graph illustrates the threshold contrast as function of the detail size for the original film and the digitized film image. The digital imaging performs better for larger-detail diameters. The detection threshold for small objects does not differ notably, with about 130 μm being the lowest-diameter detail perceptible with either modality.

An investigation by Thijssen (Thijssen 2000) confirms the expected improvement of the contrast resolution of digital images mentioned above. Figures 5.**43** and 5.**44** reproduce radiographs of the contrast detail phantom (see Fig. 5.**41**) made with a full-field amorphous sil-

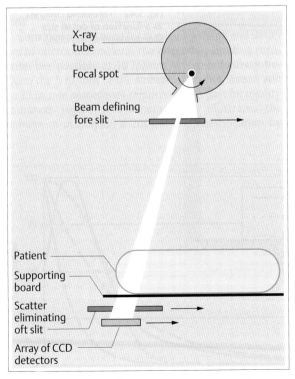

Fig. 5.40   Principle of the scanning mammographic slit assembly

Radiation Exposure

M. Säbel

The radiation dose delivered to the breast through mammography has found renewed interest in connection with quality assurance and the introduction of breast cancer screening. Radiation exposure mainly depends on the X-ray beam quality, breast thickness, and breast composition, but also on the particular components of the imaging system (Fig. 5.1). The numerical dose value is also determined by the dose quantity used for describing the radiation exposure.

For situations requiring a simple comparison only (e.g., in connection with technical quality assurance), it is often sufficient to state the air kerma (**k**inetic **e**nergy **r**eleased in **ma**tter) or entrance surface dose. For example, in the revised document of the European Commission mentioned on p. 63, a dose reference value of 10 mGy is given for the entrance surface dose of a standard-sized breast (5 cm compressed breast thickness, with antiscatter grid).

These dose quantities are less suited for estimating the radiation risk. Presently, it is generally assumed that the glandular tissue of the breast is most vulnerable to the induction of cancer by ionizing radiation. Therefore, the average glandular dose is increasingly used as the risk–relevant dose. Average glandular dose cannot be measured directly. As a rule, it is calculated under certain assumptions from the relation

$$AGD = ESAK \cdot g \tag{5.6}$$

where ESAK is the measured **e**ntrance **s**urface **a**ir **k**erma and g a conversion factor. This conversion factor can be calculated from measured depth–dose distributions or by Monte Carlo methods directly from the X-ray beam energy spectrum. It depends mainly on radiation quality, compressed breast thickness, and breast tissue composition (Klein et al., 1997).

The influence of the image receptor and the other components of the X-ray imaging system on image quality was presented on p. 60. As a rule, these technical parameters also influence radiation exposure (Fig. 5.1). This will be demonstrated with some examples important for clinical practice.

A reduction of radiation exposure can be achieved by adapting radiation quality (by the use of an optimized combination of tube voltage, anode material, and filtration) to breast thickness and tissue composition, especially for large breasts (p. 68). In comparison to the conventional Mo/Mo anode/filter combination, the following approximate dose reductions are possible:

- 25% with Mo/Rh
- 35% with Mo/Pd
- 50% with W/Rh and Rh/Rh, respectively

The thickness of the compressed breast represents a factor strongly affecting radiation exposure. At average tissue composition and with typical radiographic parameters (tube voltage 28 kVp, Mo anode, 30 µm Mo added filtration), an increase of breast thickness by 1 cm results in a 25% higher average glandular dose. At constant breast thickness, the average glandular dose varies by a factor of about 5 to 6, indicating the differences between the radiation absorption in breasts with a large fraction of adipose tissue and in those essentially consisting of glandular and fibrous tissue.

Radiation exposure is increased by use of an antiscatter grid. This increase can be expressed with the Bucky factor B (p. 70). In general, values of B are in the range of 2 to 3 for moving grids. Due to the aluminum interspace of the grid, values up to 3.5 were determined for stationary grids.

Average glandular dose is directly proportional to the dose that switches off the automatic exposure control unit. The reciprocal value of this so-called "system dose" is proportional to the sensitivity of the film–screen system. For instance, changing the film speed from 12 to 25 reduces average glandular dose to 50% of the initial value.

Mainly in conjunction with the intended introduction of mammography as a screening method, risk/benefit analyses of this breast imaging technique have repeatedly been carried out over the last few years. Present knowledge about the risk of radiation-induced breast cancer originates essentially from data taken from three series of irradiated women:

- Women who were treated with pneumothorax for tuberculosis and underwent frequent fluoroscopy of the thorax region to monitor the pneumothorax therapy. Some women had more than 200 fluoroscopies.
- Women who were irradiated as treatment for pathological alterations of the breast (especially postpartum mastitis).
- Females who were exposed to radiation as survivors of the Hiroshima and Nagasaki atomic bomb detonations.

The data resulting from these investigations on radiation-induced breast cancer are consistent with the following generalizations:

- The development of a radiation-induced breast carcinoma is clearly dependent on the hormonal status of the woman.
- Radiation-induced breast cancers are similar in age distribution and histopathological types to breast cancers resulting from other or unknown causes.
- Women who are irradiated at less than 20 years of age are at a higher relative risk for breast cancer induction than those who are irradiated later in life.
- The incidence of radiation-induced breast cancer shows little or no decrease when the total radiation dose is received in multiple exposures rather than in a single short exposure.

The risk/benefit analyses carried out during the last few years mostly demonstrate that the benefit of mammography (i.e., lowering of breast cancer mortality) significantly exceeds the radiation risk in women at age 40 or even at age 35. It should be pointed out, however, that the reduction of breast cancer mortality due to mammographic screening may vary between screening programs and may be restricted to women of age 50 years and over. With the present state of knowledge, routine screening cannot be recommended for young women.

Quality Assurance

H. Aichinger, M. Säbel, and M. A. O. Thijssen

Quality-assurance measures in diagnostic radiology are an essential component of the efforts to improve diagnostic validity and avoid unnecessary examinations. This statement is valid also for X-ray mammography and especially for mammography screening programs, where the demand for comprehensive quality assurance is a central theme. All steps of preventive medical care, i.e., the invitation of the participants, the mammographic examination itself, and, if necessary, additional diagnostic examination, as well as therapy and follow-up, must be considered.

This section deals only with the physical and technical aspects of quality assurance (QA), i.e., the quality control (QC) in mammography. In the United States, the basis of QA is the "Mammography Quality Standards Act (MQSA)," which was passed on 27 October 1992 to establish a national quality standards for mammography. For provision of mammography services legally after 1 October 1994, the MQSA required that all facilities, except facilities of the Department of Veterans Affairs, must be accredited by an approved accreditation body and certified by the Secretary of Health and Human Services. The authority to approve accreditation bodies and to certify facilities was delegated to the Food and Drug Administration (FDA). On 28 October 1997, the FDA published the final regulations of the MQSA in the *Federal Register*. The final regulations became effective on 28 April 1999 and replace the interim regulations that previously regulated mammography facilities under MQSA.

The European Union promotes quality assurance in diagnostic radiology as well. In this context, the section "Medical quality criteria of X-ray mammography" of the document "European Guidelines on Quality Criteria for Diagnostic Radiographic Images" has already been mentioned. The European Union especially supports mammography screening. As early as 1993 the "European Guidelines for Quality Assurance in Mammography Screening" were published. These guidelines, revised in 1996, contain the "European Protocol for the Quality Control of the Physical and Technical Aspects of Mammography Screening (EPMS)."

The aim of quality control, according to the European Protocol EPMS, is to ensure the following.

- The radiologist is provided with images that have the best possible diagnostic information obtainable when the appropriate radiographic technique is employed.

- The image quality is stable with respect to information content and mean optical density.
- The breast dose is "as low as reasonably achievable (ALARA)" for the diagnostic information required.

The basis for this approach is to assure every single woman who undergoes a mammographic examination that every reasonable action is undertaken to avoid a misdiagnosis for technical reasons: "Each Screening Unit should perform Technical Quality Control on their equipment, to assure the appropriate image quality for every single woman attending the screening project."

The protocol is meant to be a basic guideline, leaving local or national authorities to prescribe a protocol that might be more strict. The actions in this protocol are basically comparable with those of MQSA. Some of the actions that are part of such a QC program can be performed by the local staff on a daily basis. More elaborate measurements should be performed less frequently by medical physicists who are trained and experienced in diagnostic radiology and specifically trained in mammography quality control.

Both the MQSA (or the ACR Quality Control Manual) and the European Protocol for the Quality Control of the Physical and Technical Aspects of Mammography Screening aim to provide assurance of an adequate level of quality of the images used for diagnosing the presence or— which is even more difficult—the absence of tumors in the breast.

■ Quality Control Regarding ACR and EPMS

The success of mammography, whether for screening or diagnosis, depends on delivering high-quality, low-dose images. To reach this goal, quality control (QC) begins with the specification and purchase of mammography equipment that meets the accepted standards of performance. Before the system is put into clinical use, it must undergo acceptance testing to ensure that its performance meets these standards. This applies to the X-ray tube, image receptor, film processor, and QC equipment. After acceptance, the performance of all equipment components must be maintained at the highest level possible, at least above the minimum level.

In the United States, QC addressing these physical and technical aspects is generally carried out according to the protocol developed by the American College of Radiology (ACR: Quality Control Manual 1999), which is in agreement with the requirements of the MQSA. In Europe, national protocols have been applied for mammography equipment to date; e.g., the DIN 6868 standard is the basis for quality control in Germany. In the future, the "European Protocol for the Quality Control of the Physical and Technical Aspects of Mammography Screening" will gain more importance for mammography in general. Both protocols—MQSA/ACR and EPMS—are very similar, except for the following points:

- Accuracy and the reproducibility of the tube voltage.
- Object thickness compensation (after 28 October 2002, the requirements will be the same).
- According to the EPMS, the entrance surface air kerma (ESAK) shall be < 15 mGy (< 14 mGy, desirable) with respect to a 4.5 cm PMMA phantom and for a net film density of 1.4 OD; according to the MQSA/ACR, the average glandular dose for a 4.2 cm compressed breast shall be ≤ 3 mGy.
- In comparison with the EPMS, the ACR protocols are less rigorous with respect to the cassette sensitivity. The cassettes have to be grouped by size and sensitivity. Within one group, the density difference between the lightest and the darkest film shall not exceed 0.3. The film–screen contact shall be tested with a 40 mesh copper screen only in the ACR protocol.
- In the EPMS, no specific test phantom is recommended for the evaluation of the physical and technical characteristics of the mammographic X-ray equipment. In contrast, the ACR protocol prescribes a particular mammographic phantom for the assessment of image quality (Radiation Measurement Inc. RMI-156 or Nuclear Associates 18–220). This phantom is equivalent to a 4.2 cm thick compressed breast consisting of 50% glandular and 50% adipose tissue, containing appropriate test objects (fibers, specks, and masses) that range from visible to invisible on the mammographic image.

References

Aichinger, H., J. Dierker, M. Säbel, S. Joite-Barfuß: Bildqualität und Dosis in der Mammographie. Electromedica 62 (1994) 7–11

Aichinger, H., S. Joite-Barfuß, P. Marhoff: Die Belichtungsautomatik in der Mammographie. Electromedica 58 (1990) 68–69

Blanks, R. G., M. G. Wallis, S. M. Moss: A comparison of cancer detection rates achieved by breast cancer screening programmes by number of readers, for one- and two-view mammography: results from the UK National Health Breast Screening Programme. J. Med. Screen. 5 (1998) 195–201

Bollen, R., J. Vranckx: Influence of ambient light on the visual sensitometric properties of, and detail perception on, a radiograph. Proc. SPIE 273 (1981) 57–62

Brandt, G.-A.: Der Einfluß objektiver Parameter der Röntgenbilderzeugung auf die Sicherheit bei der diagnostischen Entscheidungsfindung. In Moderne Röntgenfotografie 4/83. VEB, Berlin 1983 (S. 27–40)

Brandt, G.-A.: Einfluß technischer Parameter auf die Diagnosequalität. Akt. Radiol. 1 (1991) 16–22

Brandt, G.-A.: Bedeutung der optischen Dichte für die Röntgenbildbetrachtungsbedingungen. Akt. Radiol. 4 (1994) 75–78

Brandt, G.-A., F. Boitz, L. Mansfeld, K.-H. Rotte: Zum Stellenwert der Röntgenfilmbetrachtungsbedingungen für die Diagnosequalität bei Thoraxaufnahmen. Radiol. diagn. 24 (1983) 85–90

Chan, H. P., K. Doi, C. J. Vyborny et al.: Improvement in radiologist's detection of clustered microcalcifications on mammograms. Invest. Radiol. 25 (1990) 1102–1110

Chan, H. P., B. Sahiner, M. A. Helvie, et al.: Improvement of radiologists' characterization of mammographic masses by using computer-aided diagnosis: An ROC study. Radiology 212 (1999) 817–827

Coltman, J. W.: The specification of imaging properties by response to sine wave input. J. opt. Soc. Amer. 44 (1954) 468–471

Curry III, Th. S., J. E. Dowdey, R. C. Murry: Christensens's Physics of Diagnostic Radiology. Lea & Febiger, Philadelphia 1990

Dance, D. R.: Monte Carlo calculation of conversion factors for the estimation of mean glandular dose. Phys. Med. Biol. 35 (1990) 1211–1219

van Dijck, J. A. M., L. M. Verbeek, J. H. C. L. Hendriks, R. Holland: The current detectability of breast cancer in a mammographic screening program. Cancer 72 (1993) (1933–1938

DIN 6856–1: Betrachtungsgeräte und -bedingungen, Anforderungen für die Herstellung und den Betrieb von Betrachtungsgeräten zur Befundung von Durchsichtsbildern in der medizinischen Diagnostik. Beuth, Berlin 1994

DIN 6856–2: Betrachtungsgeräte und -bedingungen; qualitätssichernde Maßnahmen; Prüfverfahren, Meßgeräte. Beuth, Berlin 1994

DIN 6867–1: Sensitometrie an Film-Folien-Systemen für die medizinische Radiographie. Teil 1: Verfahren zur Ermittlung des Verlaufs der sensitometrischen Kurve, der Empfindlichkeit und des mittleren Gradienten. Beuth, Berlin 1997

European Guidelines on Quality Criteria for Diagnostic Radiographic Images. EUR 16260. Februar 1996

European Guidelines for Quality Assurance in Mammography Screening, 2nd ed. European Commission. Juni 1996

Friedrich, M.: Der Einfluß der Streustrahlung auf die Abbildungsqualität bei der Mammographie. Fortschr. Röntgenstr. 123 (1975) 556–566

Haus, A. G.: Technologic improvements in screen–film mammography. Radiology 174 (1990) 628–637

Haus, A. G., J. E. Gray, T. R. Daly: Evaluation of mammographic viewbox luminance, illuminance, and color. Med. Phys. 20 (1993) 819–821

Hoeschen, D.: Bildqualitätsparameter von Folien-Film-Kombinationen. Röntgen-Bl. 40 (1978) 193–199

Jiang, Y. L., R. M. Nishikawa, D. E. Wolverton, et al.: Malignant and benign clustered microcalcifications: Automated feature analysis and classification. Radiology 198 (1996) 671–678

Karssemeijer, N., J. H. C. L. Hendriks: (1997) Computer-assisted reading of mammograms. Europ. Radiol. 7 (1997) 743–748

Karssemeijer, N., J. T. M. Frieling, H. C. L. Hendriks: Spatial resolution in digital mammography. Invest. Radiol. 28 (1993) 413–419

Kassenärztliche Bundesvereinigung: Qualifikationsvoraussetzungen gemäß § 135 Abs. 2 SGB V zur Durchführung von Untersuchungen in der diagnostischen Radiologie und Nuklearmedizin und von Strahlentherapie (Vereinbarung zur Strahlendiagnostik und -therapie). Dtsch. Ärztebl. 90 (1993) 292–302

Kegelmeyer Jr., W. P., J. M. Pruneda, P. D. Bourland, A. Hillis, M. W. Riggs, M. L. Nipper: Computer-aided mammographic screening for spiculated lesions. Radiology 191 (1994) 331–337

Klein, R., H. Aichinger, J. Dierker et al.: Determination of average glandular dose with modern mammography units for two large groups of patients. Phys. Med. Biol. 42 (1997) 641–671

Kirchner, J., J. Kollath: Qualitätssicherungsmaßnahmen im Rahmen der DIN 6856: Anpassung der Filmbetrachtungsgeräte und -bedingungen der Röntgenabteilung einer Universitätsklinik. Fortschr. Röntgenstr. 164 (1996) 146 – 149

Leitlinien der Bundesärztekammer zur Qualitätssicherung in der Röntgendiagnostik. Dtsch. Ärztebl. 92 (1995) C 1515 – 1527

Morneburg, H.: Bildgebende Systeme für die medizinische Diagnostik. Publicis MCD, Erlangen 1995

Pizzutiello Jr., R. J., J. E. Cullinan: Introduction to Medical Radiographic Imaging, Health Science Division. Eastman Kodak Company, Rochester 1993

Richtlinien zur Durchführung von Prüfungen zur Qualitätssicherung in der Röntgendiagnostik nach § 16 der Röntgenverordnung.

Rose, A.: Vision: Human and Electronic. Plenum, New York 1973

Säbel, M., H. Aichinger: Recent developments in breast imaging. Phys.Med.Biol. 41 (1996) 315 – 368

Schmidt, T., H. Kaselowsky, G.-A. Brandt, H.-S. Stender: Qualitätskontrollen an Filmbetrachtungskästen. Akt. Radiol. 1 (1991) 223 – 225

Schober, H.: Allgemeine physiologische Grundregeln für die Detailwahrnehmung im Röntgenbild. In Stieve, F. E.: Bildgüte in der Radiologie. Fischer, Stuttgart 1966

te Brake, G. M., N. Karssemeijer: Automated detection of breast carcinomas that were not detected in a screening program. Radiology 207 (1998) 465 – 47

Thijssen, M. A. O., H. O. M. Thijssen, J. L. Merx, J. M. Lindeijer, K. R. Bijkerk: A definition of image quality: the image quality figure. BIR REPORT 20 (1989) 29 – 34

von Volkmann, T.: Film-Folien-Systeme. In Ewen, K.: Moderne Bildgebung. Thieme, Stuttgart 1998 (S. 98 – 114)

Vyborny, C. J.: Can computers help radiologists read mammograms? Radiology 191 (1994) 315 – 317

Warren Burhenne, L. J., S. A. Wood, C. J. D‹Orsi, et al.: The potential contribution of computer-aided detection to the sensitivity of screening mammography. Radiology 000 (2000) 000 – 000

Wucherer, M.: Filmbetrachtungsgeräte – aktueller Stand. Was wird heute gefordert? Akt. Radiol. 5 (1995) 335

Yaffe, M. J.: (1992) Digital mammography. In Syllabus: A Categorical Course in Physics: Technical Aspects of Breast Imaging. RSNA, Oak Brook 1992 (pp. 245 – 256)

Yaffe, M. J., J. A. Rowlands: X-ray detectors for digital radiography. Phys.Med.Biol. 42 (1997) 1 – 39

6 Positioning in Mammography

Henny Rijken

Technical Aspects

■ Equipment

The X-ray unit, processor, and film–screen combination must be tested and found to be in compliance with the criteria of the quality assurance program to maintain a high technical quality.

Quality control tests of mammographic systems used for screening

- Acceptance test
- Semiannual constancy test
- Daily quality control

The technical specifications are stated in the "European Protocol for the Quality Control of the Physical and Technical Aspects of Mammography Screening" (part of the "European Guidelines for Quality Assurance in Mammography Screening"). (See chapter 9). The same quality requirements apply to clinical mammography.

In the United States the ACR (American College of Radiology) Committee on Quality Assurance in Mammography established practices and standards for quality control in film – screen mammography. Since the original publication in 1990, it has been updated and revised several times. The 1999 edition reflects changes mandated as a result of the implementation of the Food and Drug Administration's Final Rules for the Mammography Quality Standards Act (MQSA).

■ Ergonomics

The ergonomics of the mammography unit are important for positioning. The technologist should find the equipment easy to operate, with knobs and buttons within easy reach. The space around the mammography unit should be adequate for working with the equipment.

The mammography unit should be equipped with a compression paddle that is operated by a foot pedal to keep the hands of the technologist free for positioning the breast.

The design of the mammography unit should not intimidate the women and should be free of any sharp edges that might cause discomfort during positioning. Color, size, and arrangement of the mammography unit are important to create a calm and confidence-promoting ambience in the mammography room. Ideally, the room should be exclusively used for breast imaging.

■ Film processing

A dedicated processor is strongly recommended. To maintain processor stability, sufficient throughput of films (a minimum of 20 mammograms a day) is advisable. The instructions of the manufacturer should be followed concerning developer temperature, replenishment rates, processor cycle time, and processor maintenance.

Tasks of the Radiologic Technologist (Radiographer) within the Breast Imaging Team

It is recognized that producing optimal mammograms requires good teamwork. The team responsible for obtaining optimal mammograms consists of the radiologist, the physicist, and the technologist.

The technologist's responsibilities within the team are as follows:

- To produce an optimum image with respect to positioning and technical aspects
- To produce the image in a manner tolerated by the woman
- To carry out quality control checks on the equipment.

To ensure good quality images, it is desirable to have a specialized, motivated group of technologists with special training and interest in mammography.

■ Technical Quality Control

Quality control is the basis for technically optimal mammograms. Image quality standards must be established to guarantee a high level of technical quality. It is the technologist's duty to carry out quality control checks, to monitor and evaluate these standards and to take corrective action if necessary. In the quality control program, the technologist must be involved in

- equipment specification and selection;
- commissioning and acceptance tests;
- in-service consistency testing;
- image quality assessment using a recognized phantom.

Several measurements can be performed by the local staff. Medical physicists trained and experienced in diagnostic radiology and with additional training in mammography quality control programs should undertake the more elaborate measurements.

Social Skills

The communication between technologist and woman is one of the most important aspects of the examination. In screening programs, the technologist is frequently the only healthcare professional the woman may encounter. Even when seeing a large number of women on any single day, the technologist should be friendly and caring and do her best to generate comfort and confidence in each woman.

In a pleasant, calm and informative atmosphere, the woman is more likely to relax. The technologist should answer inquiries, explain the procedure thoroughly, and emphasize the importance of proper compression to obtain understanding and cooperation from the woman. The woman should feel at ease and have the impression of being treated as important individual. The technologist should treat the woman the same way she would like to be treated.

Introduction to the Examination

The technologist welcomes the woman, introduces herself, and establishes eye contact. Wearing a name badge may contribute to a more personal relationship. Before performing the examination, the technologist must ask the woman several questions:

- Have there been breast problems in the past or are there any current breast problems?
- How long have they existed?
- In case of a known lump, since when was it palpable and where is it located?
- Was a mammogram performed previously and what was the woman's experience of it?
- Is there a history of previous biopsy?

The technologist must inspect the breasts:

- Are there any specific anatomical characteristics that need to be taken into consideration (for instance, thoracic kyphosis or scoliosis, see p. 121, caudocranial view)?
- Does the patient have a pacemaker (in which case it should be explained that the radiation does not affect its functioning or discharge the batteries)?

The inspection of the breasts is best performed immediately before positioning. The technologist should look for any changes in the breast: scars, skin lesions such as moles or warts, eczema of the nipple, nipple secretion or retraction (especially if it is of recent onset), local skin retraction, or any other information relevant for the radiologist, and record this on the appropriate worksheet (Fig. 6.1).

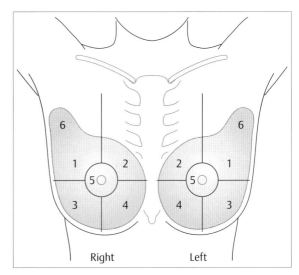

Fig. 6.**1** **Classification of the breast in quadrants**. Chart to record the radiographer's findings
1 Upper outer quadrant
2 Upper inner quadrant
3 Lower outer quadrant
4 Lower inner quadrant
5 Central area
6 Axillary tail ("tail of Spence")

If the technologist feels an additional lump, observes a skin-retraction, or notes any abnormal sign during the examination, the radiologist should be informed about it. It is not the technologist's task to palpate the breast routinely, but in case of a palpable mass, the technologist has to ensure that the lesion will be included on the mammogram. In case of a surgical scar, the reason for it should be noted (biopsy, breast augmentation, trauma, mastitis). Any nipple secretion during compression of the breast should be recorded by the technologist, especially when the secretion is brownish or bloody.

The technologist has to be aware of the anxiety and apprehension of many women induced by the fear of a breast carcinoma.

During the introductory talk explaining the examination, the technologist should cover the following points:
- The procedure, including the number of views and an outline of the positioning
- The importance of good compression
- The process of notification of the results
- The possibility of additional views, such as magnification views, and supplemental examinations, such as sonography

Good cooperation between technologist and woman will lead to satisfactory results.

The technologist should review any previous mammogram, if available, to determine the proper positioning of the automatic exposure control (AEC) detector.

Positioning

■ Compression

The technologist should understand the need for compression in mammography. A good quality mammogram can only be achieved with an adequately compressed breast. Compression makes the breast substantially thinner, distributing the thickness more equally over its entire surface. Compression is used for the following reasons:

- Less scattered radiation, which improves the contrast of the images
- Less radiation to the tissue
- Less blurring due to improved geometry and immobilization
- Separation of the various structures and less overlapping of tissue shadows, providing better visualization of the breast tissue
- More homogeneous film density
- Improved visualization of distortions (abnormal tissue structures)

The importance of proper compression should be explained to the woman before the breast is compressed. Most women experience the compression as unpleasant, some even find it painful. Women generally tolerate compression better after its purpose has been explained to them. It is helpful to mention that the compression will only last a few seconds.

The breast should be compressed adequately but not more than necessary. When the breast tissue has been maximally spread out, any attempt at further compression is useless since image quality will not improve further and the risk of pain increases rapidly.

The usual range of the compression force to be applied to the breast varies between 100 and 180 newtons. The degree of compression tolerated by women varies. Women with sensitive breasts in the premenstrual phase should have their mammograms performed one week after the beginning of menstruation.

During the compression, the technologist should observe the woman to note any early pain reaction. Compression is better tolerated when the woman is asked to indicate when compression becomes uncomfortable.

■ Placement of Automatic Exposure Control (AEC) Detector

Prerequisites for proper exposure

- Accurate automatic exposure control device
- Proper tube voltage
- Sufficient tube current
- Correct focal spot

Correct positioning of the AEC detector is crucial. The AEC detector must be movable so that it may be shifted underneath the most dense area of the breast, which is usually in the retroareolar area. With the central region of the breast placed over the center of the cassette holder, the proper position of the detector is in the anterior one-third of the breast behind the nipple, regardless of the degree of parenchymal involution. For very small breasts, positioning of the detector can be difficult and manual exposure may then be preferable. Underexposure may lead to loss of information and thereby to false negative diagnoses. While an underexposed film is unacceptable, an overexposed film may still reveal satisfactory information with the use of a bright light.

Reviewing previous films, if available, may be helpful to determine the correct position of the detector. Modern mammography units automatically select not only the correct dose before the exposure but also the lowest possible tube voltage.

■ Anatomical Basis for Mammographic Projections

The following anatomical conditions complicate imaging in different views:

- Considerable individual difference in size and shape of the breast
- The disklike shape of the fibroglandular body and its axillary tail
- The complicated shape of the underlying structures constituting the oblique course of the pectoralis muscle and the vertically and horizontally curved chest wall formed by the ribs

Imaging must use the anatomy as basis for the standard views, especially incorporating the following anatomical facts:

- The natural mobility of the breast, with good mobility of the inferior and lateral portion of the breast against the thoracic wall and restricted mobility of the medial and superior portion (Fig. 6.2). This is important for positioning and compression. Before compression, as much breast tissue as possible should be placed toward the less-mobile portions of the breast, the medial and the superior borders.
- The longitudinal axis of the fibroglandular body, including axillary tail, forms an angle of about 45° with the horizontal and vertical planes. The lower edge of the pectoralis muscle also runs from the upperlateral aspect to the lower-medial aspect, more or less parallel to the longitudinal axis of the fibroglandular body. Consequently, the view perpendicular to this axis provides a complete image of the entire glandular body (Fig. 6.3). This projection is the mediolateral oblique (MLO) view. When the glandular

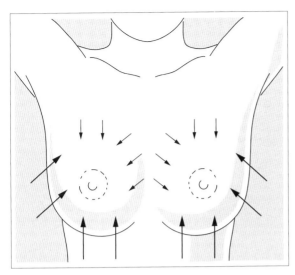

Fig. 6.**2**   **Mobility of the breast**. Lateral and inferior parts are mobile (long arrows), while the superior and medial parts are relatively immobile

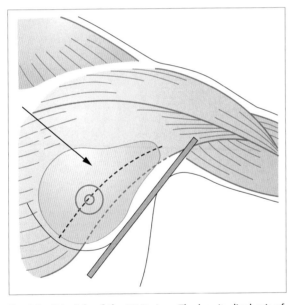

Fig. 6.**3**   **Principle of the MLO view**. The longitudinal axis of the fibroglandular body and lateral lower edge of the pectoralis muscle are parallel to the film

body is gently pulled away from the chest wall, the posterior border of the fibroglandular body and the retroglandular fat tissue as well as the frontal border of the pectoralis muscle can be imaged.
• The convergence of the lactiferous ducts toward the nipple requires that the nipple is imaged in profile in all views. In this way, the diagnostically important retroareolar area can be optimally visualized with compression. An additional advantage is that the nipple is well-recognizable on the film and does not resemble a round breast lesion.

■ Positioning

Proper positioning of the breast for mammography is an art. Inadequate positioning is the most frequent problem encountered when reading mammograms. Therefore, high standards should be set to achieve optimal positioning in mammography.

■ Standard Projections

• Craniocaudal (CC) view
• Mediolateral oblique (MLO) view

■ Craniocaudal (CC) View

The CC view can be performed with the woman seated or standing (Fig. 6.**4**). The sitting position of the woman is easier for the technologist if the technologist is short. The examination chair should be adjustable and easily moved and locked when in the desired position. The tube-arm should be vertically oriented with the central ray in the craniocaudal direction.

Although this projection cannot always encompass the medial and lateral aspects of the gland close to the chest wall in one view, it succeeds in imaging the entire fibroglandular body, including its axillary extension, in most patients due to the natural mobility of the lateral portion of the breast (Fig. 6.**5**).

A single view will fail whenever the axillary tail extends dorsomedially beyond the border of the pectoralis muscle (the so-called "tail of Spence"). An exaggerated craniocaudal view (the so-called "Cleopatra" view) is required in these cases (see p. 120).

The criteria for positioning are the same for sitting and standing women.

The woman should be erect (with the back straightened), about 5–10 cm away from the unit (Fig. 6.**6**). Both arms rest on the woman's lap. The side of the breast to be examined is anteriorly rotated about 10° and the woman's head turned away from it. The technologist stands on the medial side of the breast to be examined. The correct height of the cassette holder can be best determined and adjusted considering the different mobility of the upper and lower part of the breast. The breast should be positioned horizontally on the cassette holder. Lifting the breast moves the inframammary fold upward (Fig. 6.**7**) and the cassette holder is raised to the level of the inframammary angle (Fig. 6.**8**). (When compression is afterwards applied in this position, extreme traction on the skin and upper part of the breast, which is uncomfortable for the woman, is avoided.) The technologist now lifts the breast with both hands and pulls it forward over the cassette holder to image as much breast tissue as possible (Fig. 6.**9**). The technologist holds the breast in the proper position with one hand and supports the woman's back with the other arm to prevent

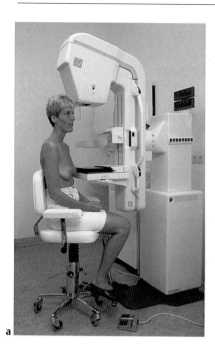

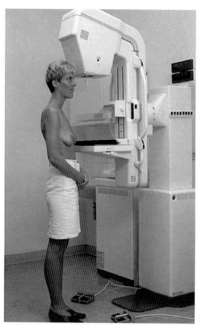

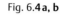
Fig. 6.**4a, b**

a

b

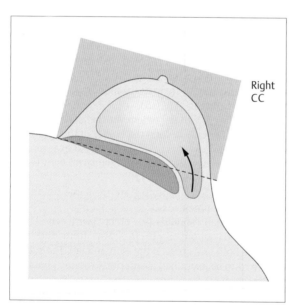

Right
CC

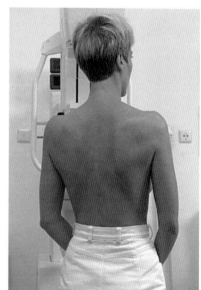

Fig. 6.**5 Diagram for the CC view of the right breast**. The axillary tail is situated outside the exposure area. The axillary tail consists of glandular tissue and reaches upward laterally, partly along the lateral edge of the pectoralis muscle. Part of the posterolateral tissue can be pulled onto the exposure field immediately before compression (arrow). The medial part of the breast tissue must be imaged completely. The retroglandular fat tissue should be visualized, if possible also the pectoralis muscle

Fig. 6.**6**

her from leaning backward (Fig. 6.**10**), placing the hand on the shoulder on the side to be examined and applying gentle downward pressure. The breast is compressed slowly and evenly and the breast tissue is smoothed forward, while the hand of the technologist gradually moves toward the nipple (Fig. 6.**11**).

Specific criteria for assessing the CC view:
The medial portion of the breast must be imaged completely and the lateral portion as much as possible. The nipple should be in neutral position, i.e., in the center of the image (Fig. 6.**12**).

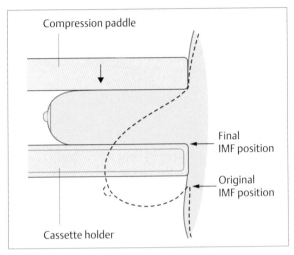

Fig. 6.7 Adjustment of the cassette holder with respect to the inframammary fold. Lifting the breast is possible because of its mobility. The inframammary fold (IMF) then moves upward, which is important for determining the correct height of the cassette holder

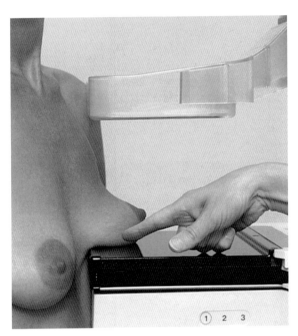

Fig. 6.**8**

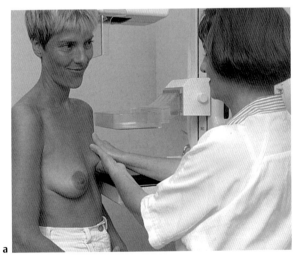

a

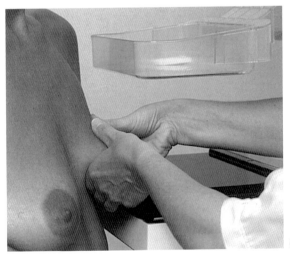

b

Fig. 6.**9 a, b**

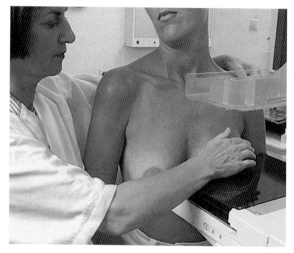

Fig. 6.**10**

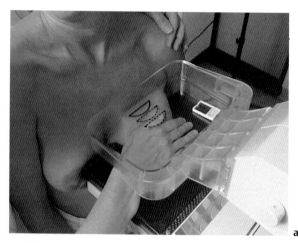

a

Fig. 6.**11 a – c**

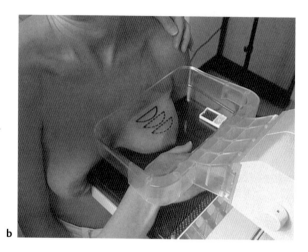

b

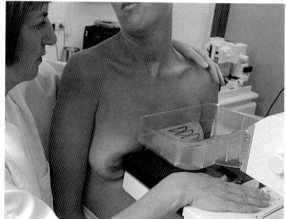

c

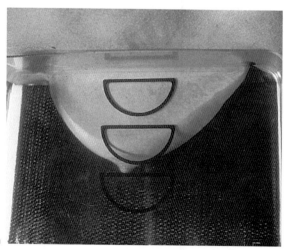

a

Fig. 6.**12 a, b**

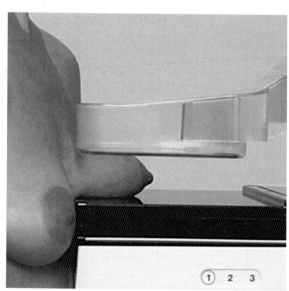

b

Visualization of the pectoralis muscle on the CC view is desirable, but not achievable in many cases, and its nonvisualization is not necessarily a sign of incorrect positioning. When the pectoralis muscle is not visible, a line can be drawn directly posterior from the nipple to the edge of the film, to have an indication of the amount of posterior tissue imaged on the CC view. In general this line should be within 1 cm of its length on the properly positioned MLO view. Usually the length of this posterior nipple line is greater on the MLO than on the CC view.

Exaggerated imaging of the medial tissue leads to loss of visualization of the lateral tissue, and vice versa.

On the CC view an ill-defined triangularly shaped density, a continuation of the chest wall, can occasionally be seen on the medial side. This density, which may give the impression of an invasive cancer, can be attributed to the insertion of the pectoralis muscle (Britton et al., 1989).

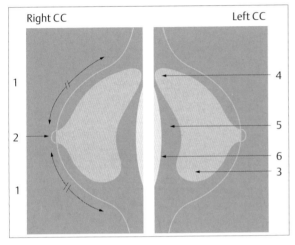

Fig. 6.**13 a**   **Diagram of CC views with radiological – anatomical features for optimal positioning** (see text)

Criteria for assessing the CC view (Fig. 6.**13**)

- Nipple in the center and in profile (1 + 2)
- The medial border of the breast is imaged (3)
- As much of the lateral aspect of the breast as possible is imaged (4)
- Central part of retroglandular fat tissue should be imaged (5)
- If possible, the pectoralis muscle shadow is displayed on the posterior edge of the breast (6)

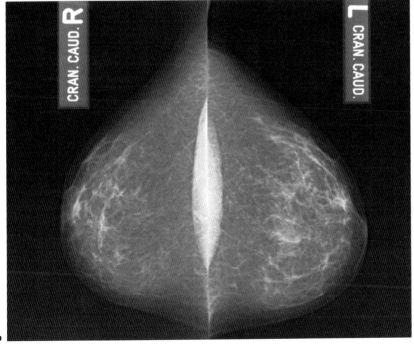

Fig. 6.**13 b, c**   **CC views right and left**

Common errors

- Inadequate height of the cassette holder. Compression might be more painful and the nipple is not visualized in profile. Cassette holder too high (Fig. 6.**14**). Cassette holder too low (Fig. 6.**15**).
- The breast is insufficiently pulled forward: the posterior portion of the fibroglandular tissue is not visualized (Fig. 6.**16 a**); the same breast well-positioned (Fig. 6.**16 b**). Posteriorly located cancers in front of the pectoralis muscle may remain undetected when the breast is not sufficiently pulled forward (Fig. 6.**17**).
- Skin folds in the lateral part due to incorrect positioning and insufficient smoothing of the skin during compression (Fig. 6.**18**).
- Incorrectly placed AEC detector, e.g., posterior to the fibroglandular tissue, resulting in unterexposure of the fibroglandular tissue (Fig. 6.**19**).

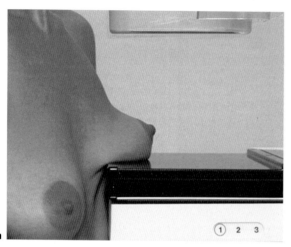
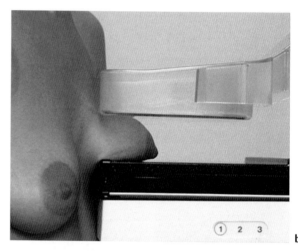

a   b

Fig. 6.**14 a, b**

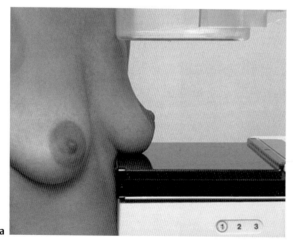
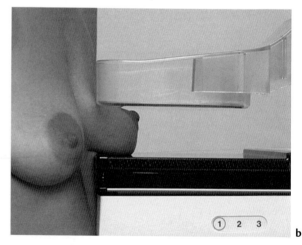

a   b

Fig. 6.**15 a, b**

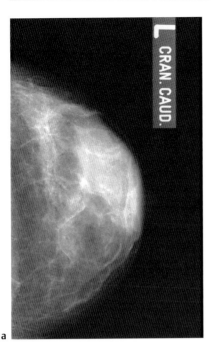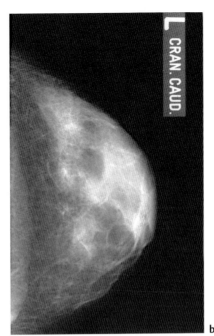

Fig. 6.**16 a, b**

a

b

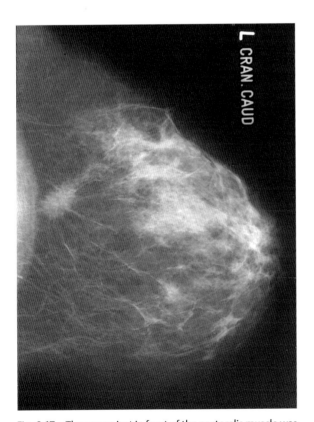

Fig. 6.**17**   The cancer just in front of the pectoralis muscle was detected only by pulling the breast sufficiently forward

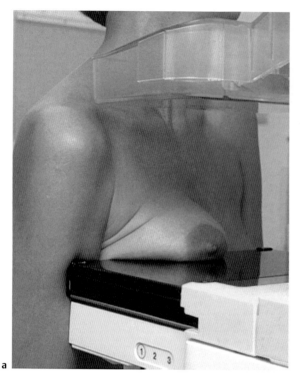

a

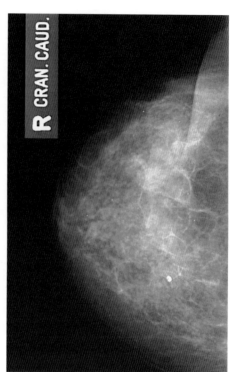

b

Fig. 6.**18 a, b**

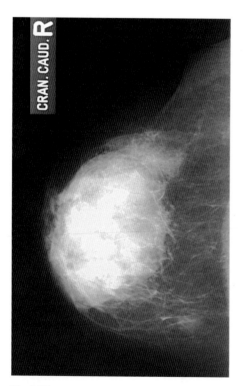

Fig. 6.**19**

■ Mediolateral Oblique (MLO) View

The MLO view is performed with the woman standing (Fig. 6.**20**). The X-ray beam passes from the superomedial to the inferolateral aspect of the breast with a 45° angle. Sometimes the angle must be adjusted to place the cassette holder parallel to the pectoralis muscle (Fig. 6.**3**). In tall, slender women the angle from the vertical may be slightly smaller (cassette holder in steeper position); in smaller, more corpulent women the angle from the vertical may be slightly greater (cassette holder in flatter position). The woman is standing upright, rotated 45–50°, with the breast to be examined facing the unit (Fig. 6.**20**). The woman's hand on the side being examined should be resting on the handle bar of the tube arm. The height of the cassette holder is adjusted. The cassette holder lies immediately anterior to the posterior axillary fold (Fig. 6.**21**). After compression, the upper outer corner of the compression plate should be positioned just below the clavicle (Fig. 6.**22**). Stand-

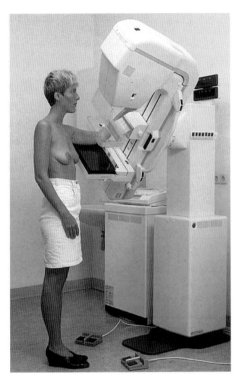

Fig. 6.**20**

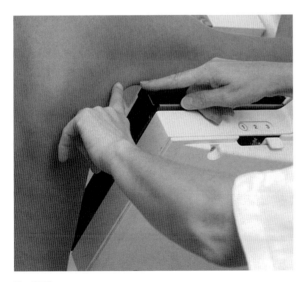

Fig. 6.**21**

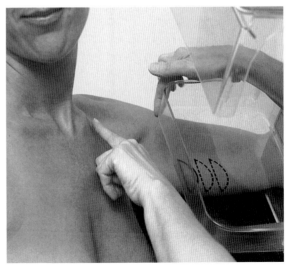

Fig. 6.**22**

ing at the opposite side of the woman, the technologist takes hold of the woman's upper arm with one hand and of the woman's entire breast with the other hand (the sternum of the technologist is placed against the hanging arm of the woman) (Fig. 6.**23**). Both the technologist and the woman lean slightly forward into the mammography unit. The cassette holder is positioned immediately anterior to the posterior axillary fold to ensure inclusion of the axillary tail, which is partially located behind the pectoralis muscle. The lateral lower portion of the breast is placed on the cassette holder (Fig. 6.**24**). The technologist finds the clavicle with her fingers to ensure that the upper outer corner of the compression plate will be positioned exactly under the middle of the clavicle (Fig. 6.**25**). The fingers of the hand holding the breast rotate out from underneath the breast (the thumb remains in contact with the breast) (Fig. 6.**26**). The breast is pushed up and forward, away from the chest wall. When compression is applied, the breast tissue is smoothed out (Fig. 6.**27**). The edge of the compression plate should touch the sternum. The upper corner of the compression plate will now lie just below the clavicle. The central beam runs from the upper medial quadrant to the lower lateral quadrant, i.e., slightly above the nipple level, and reaches the cassette perpendicularly.

It is desirable to show the nipple in profile. Any possible skin folds at the inframammary angle are to be

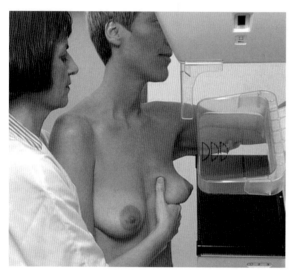

Fig. 6.**23**

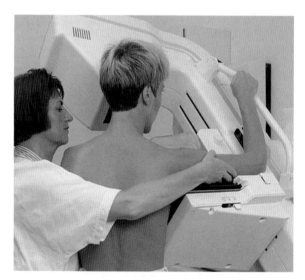

Fig. 6.**24**

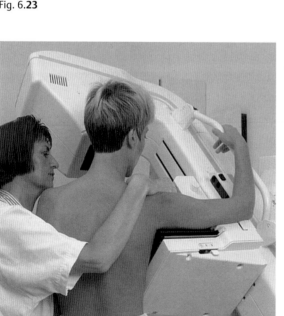

a

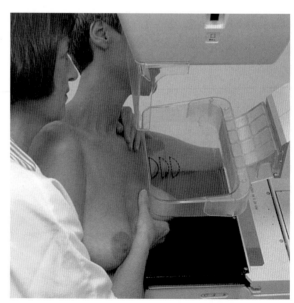

b

Fig. 6.**25 a, b**

smoothed out. If necessary, the woman should hold her opposite breast out of the way. (Fig. 6.**28**).

In the MLO view, the longitudinal axis of the fibroglandular body is positioned parallel to the film to display the entire gland (Fig. 6.**29**). Therefore, this view is the most important standard view. Only this view enables imaging of the deeper structures of the upper outer quadrant of the breast.

Specific criteria for assessing the mediolateral oblique view:

The soft tissues density of the pectoralis muscle must be seen as low as or even lower than the posterior nipple line. The posterior nipple line extends from the nipple posteriorly and is perpendicular to the anterior outline of the pectoralis muscle. A gently convex anterior outline indicates that the muscle is relaxed for the compres-

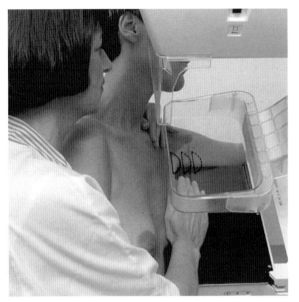

Fig. 6.**26**

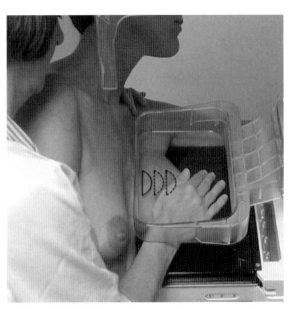

Fig. 6.**27**

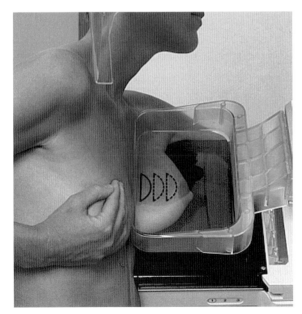

Fig. 6.**28**

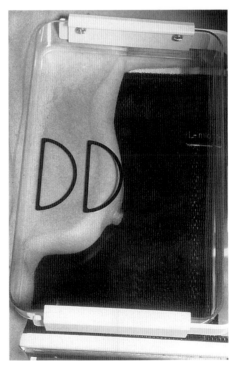

Fig. 6.**29**

sion and adequately displaced medially together with the fibroglandular tissue. The retroglandular fat tissue must be seen posterior to the fibroglandular tissue.

The fibroglandular tissue must be elevated from the chest wall and should not sag, causing the linear structures in the lower aspect of the view to be stretched, radiating toward the chest wall.

The skin of the inframammary fold must be stretched without any overlapping skin folds.

Criteria for assessing the MLO view (Fig. 6.**30**)

- The entire breast tissue is clearly shown (1)
- The pectoralis muscle is shown and extends to or below the nipple line (2)
- Nipple in profile (3)
- Inframammary angle clearly demonstrated (4)

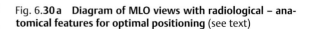

Fig. 6.**30 a**   **Diagram of MLO views with radiological – anatomical features for optimal positioning** (see text)

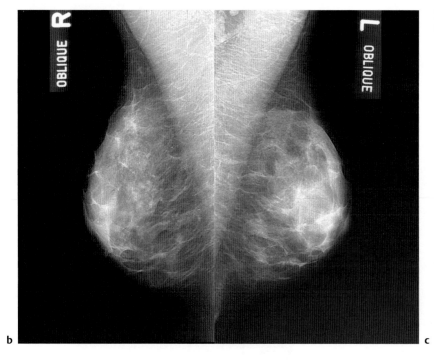

Fig. 6.**30 b, c**   **MLO views right and left**

Common errors

- Cassette holder too high: too much of the pectoralis muscle is under the compression plate, resulting in inadequate compression of the breast (Fig. 6.**31 a,b**); the same breast well positioned (Fig. 6.**31 c**). The cassette holder too low: the upper part of the breast is not imaged. Incorrect placement of the detector (Fig. 6.**32**).
- The shoulder and the pectoralis muscle are not relaxed and the woman is leaning backward, leading to no or incomplete visualization of the muscle (Fig. 6.**33**).
- No contact between the chest wall of the woman and the cassette holder, so that the lower posterior portion of the breast is not visualized (Fig. 6.**34 a,b**); the same breast after proper positioning (Fig. 6.**34 c**).
- Insufficient rotation of the woman, preventing imaging of the medial part of the breast (Fig. 6.**35 a,b**); the same breast after proper positioning (Fig. **6.35 c**).

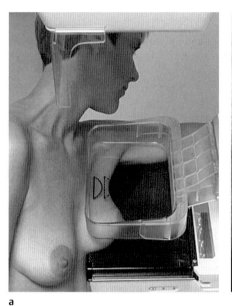
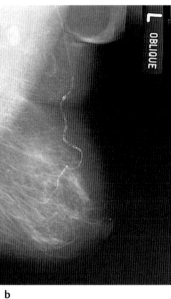
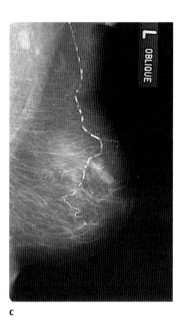

a   b   c

Fig. 6.**31 a – c**

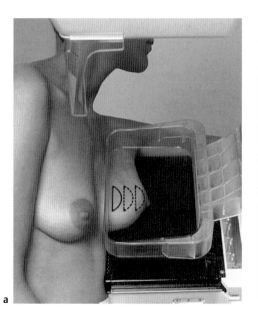
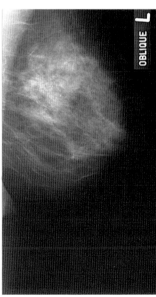

Fig. 6.**32 a, b**

a   b

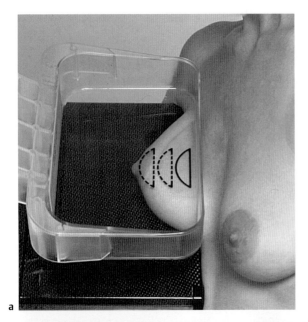

a

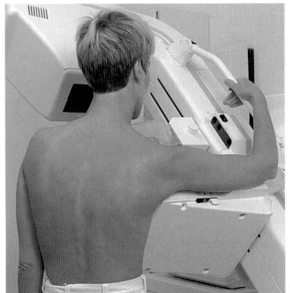

b

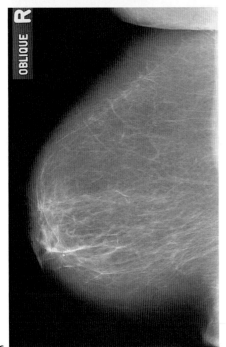

c

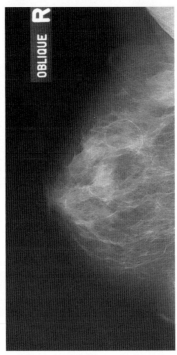

d

Fig. 6.**33a–d**

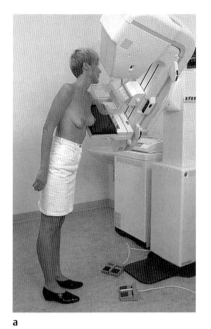

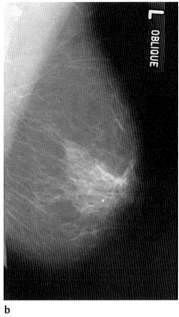

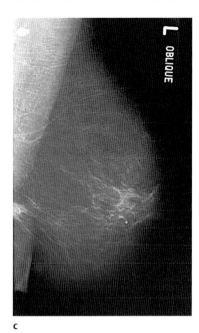

a

b

c

Fig. 6.**34** a – c

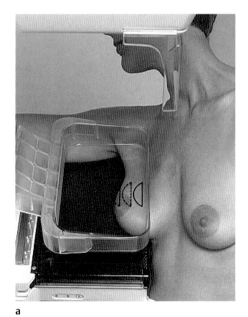

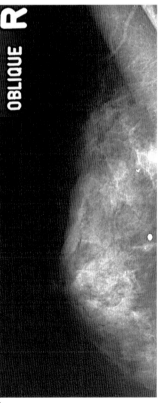

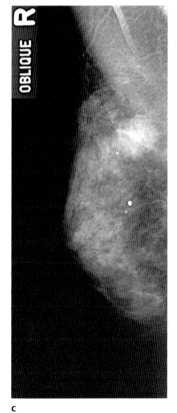

a

Fig. 6.**35** a – c

b

c

■ Most Important Additional Projections

■ Lateral Projections (Mediolateral, Lateromedial)

MLO and CC views cannot always determine the exact location of a breast lesion (Fig. 6.**36**). In these cases, a true lateral projection is needed. A lateral projection is also obtained for a lesion visible on either MLO or CC view only. The lateromedial view is obtained for medially located lesions and the mediolateral view for laterally located lesions. These supplementary views can confirm or exclude a summation density due to superimposed structures.

Both mediolateral and lateromedial views are obtained with a horizontal beam after 90° rotation of the tube-arm. The woman is seated or standing.

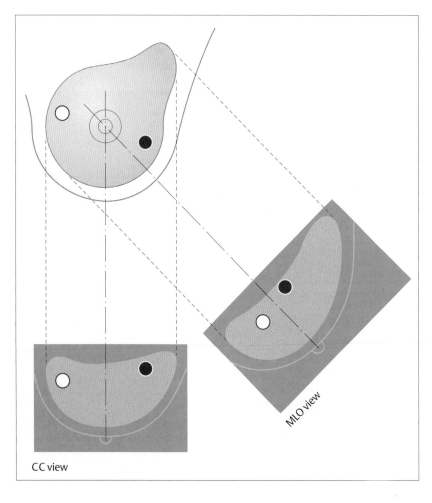

CC view

MLO view

Fig. 6.**36**   Schematic illustration of the two major projections (MLO and CC views of the left breast). Lesions in the upper part of the lower outer quadrant are projected in the upper half of the breast on the MLO view; lesions in the lower part of the medial upper quadrant are projected in the lower half on the MLO view

Mediolateral view. The woman stands or sits facing the unit, slightly rotated. with the breast to be examined forward. The technologist takes hold of the woman's ipsilateral upper arm with one hand and lifts the breast with the other hand. The woman is encouraged to lean forward into the unit. The technologist pushes the breast up with the flat hand, away from the chest wall. The woman's upper arm should rest on top of the cassette holder. The corner of the cassette holder is in the axilla. Compression is applied and the breast tissue is smoothed out. The compression paddle should skim the sternum. The nipple is in profile. The woman should hold the opposite breast back, away from the breast being radiographed. The convexity of the chest wall usually precludes the display of the entire axillary tail (Fig. 6.**37**).

Laterally located lesions in this projection will be imaged most distinctly.

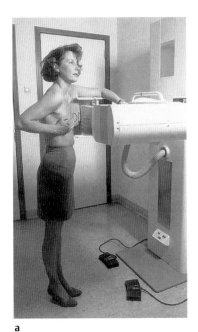
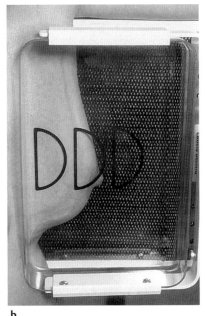
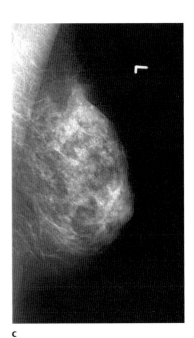

a   b   c

Fig. 6.**37 a – c**

Lateromedial view. The woman faces the unit, slightly rotated medially and leaning forward. Her sternum is placed against the cassette holder. The woman's arm on the side of the breast examined is placed on top of the cassette holder. The breast is pushed up and away from the chest wall, and during compression the glandular tissue is smoothed in an upward direction. The nipple is in profile.

■ Spot and Magnification Views

Spot views are used to obtain more information about a possible lesion. Often, spot views (focal spot view, coned-down spot view, spot compression view) are combined with magnification, and are then called spot magnification views (synonym: paddle magnification view), to gain further information. Magnification views

Fig. 6.**38 a – d**

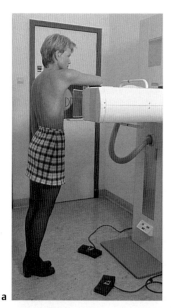

a

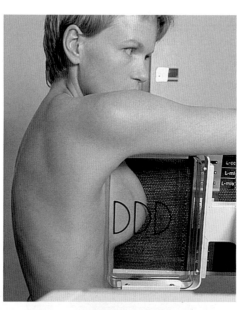

b

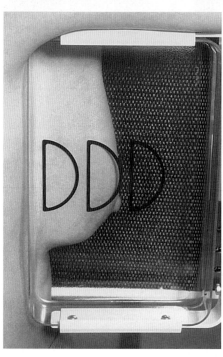

c

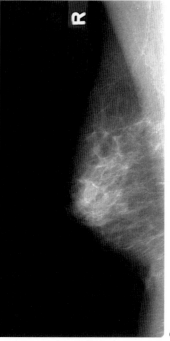

d

require an X-ray tube with a microfocal spot to compensate for the geometric unsharpness from the magnification. It also requires a special magnification table (see also chapter 7, p. 126).

Spot (magnification) views are always performed in two different projections. A dedicated spot-compression device applies localized compression more effectively (Fig. 6.**39**). Lesions are better visualized by spreading overlying structures (Fig. 6.**40**). The collimation of the X-ray beam reduces the scattered radiation, resulting in better image contrast. A palpable lesion in the breast is positioned under the center of the compression cone. For a nonpalpable lesion, the area of interest is determined on the original mammogram. On the films of the preceding mammogram, the technologist measures

- The depth of the lesion by drawing a line from the nipple back toward the chest wall;
- the distance of the lesion above or below that line (or medial or lateral to that line);
- the distance from the lesion to the skin surface.

The measurements are transferred to the breast and the location of the lesion is marked on the skin. This mark is then positioned under the center of the spot-compression device.

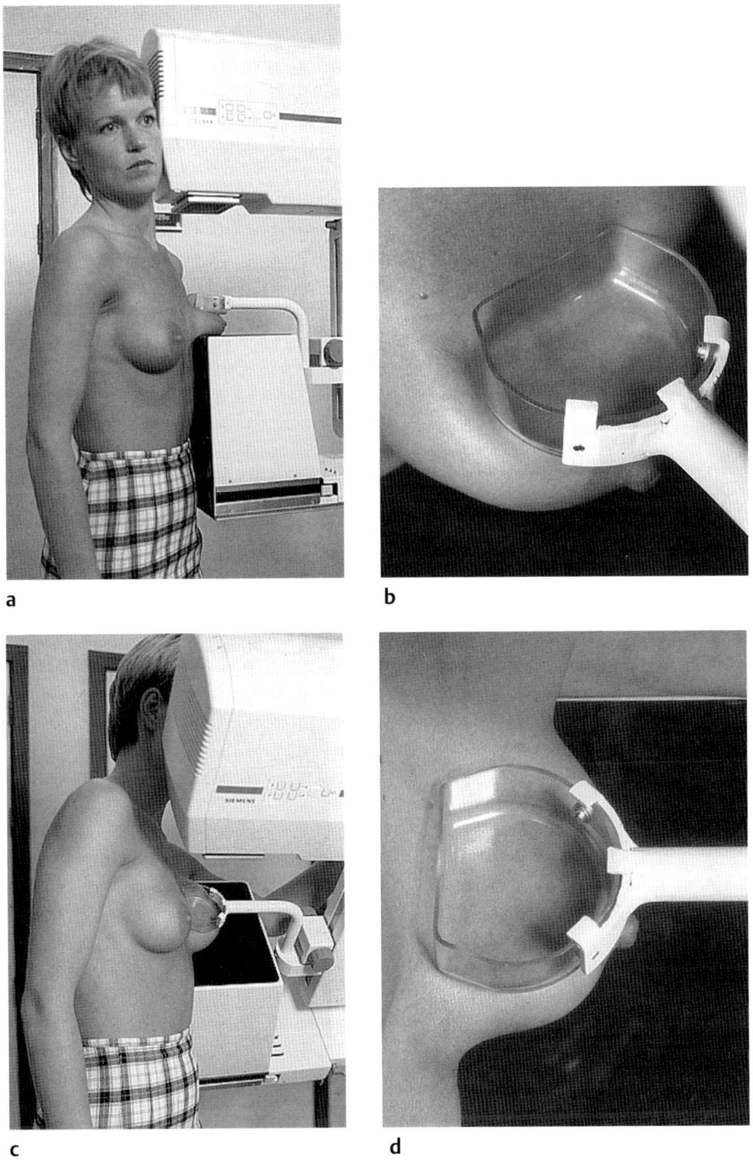

Fig. 6.**40a, b   Good visualization of microcalcifications on spot magnification views**. Histology: DCIS, poorly differentiated
a CC view
b MLO view

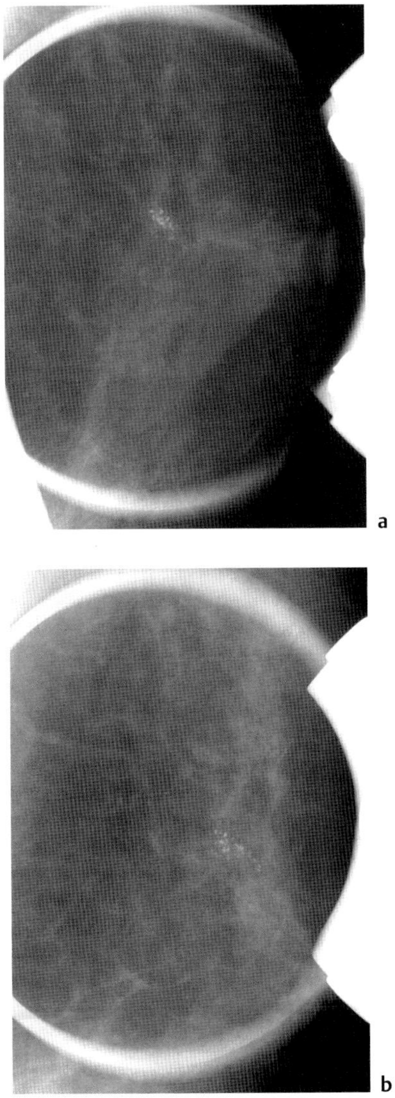

Fig. 6.**39a–d**

7 Supplemental and Advanced Examinations

Magnification Mammography

J .H. C. L. Hendriks and G. Rosenbusch

Technique

Requirements:

Molybdenum anode tube with an 0.1 mm focal spot (0.15 mm as upper limit), often with dual focal spots (0.1 mm and 0.3 mm).

- *X-ray generator*: The X-ray generator must have sufficient capacity and support the power rating of the tube. The exposure time should be less than one second, which requires a 12-pulse or high-frequency generator. Automatic exposure control with compensation for transparency, object thickness, and beam quality.
- *Screen–film combination*: Normal mammography film, i.e., single emulsion film with high contrast, mean gradient ±3, faster intensifying screens. Because of geometric consideration determined by the X-ray unit, a faster intensifying screen may be used to prevent motion blurring.
- Always spot compression of the area of interest. The compression paddles should be transparent (usually Plexiglas) to facilitate correct positioning. The compression cone must be made of material generating little scattered radiation. A collimator, 3 cm × 4.5 cm or 4 cm×6 cm, should always be used.

- The distance between breast and film determines the degree of magnification.
- *Radiographic magnification*: The image quality depends on the effective focal spot size: 0.1 mm focal spots allow magnification factors of 1.5 – 1.8. Smaller focal spots have a low photon flux and require long exposure times, increasing the risk of motion unsharpness.
- No antiscatter grid. Scatter is reduced by the air gap.
- *Exact collimation*: The X-ray beam should not exceed the size of film or cone.
- Always two views perpendicular to each other: craniocaudal and mediolateral or lateromedial projections. Important for analyzing microcalcifications (teacup phenomenon).

Goals:
- Adding information of a mammographically suspicious area (Figs. 7.**1** and 7.**2**).
- Eliminating causes of poor definition and relatively low contrast of conventional mammographic views.

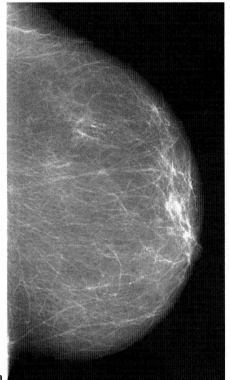

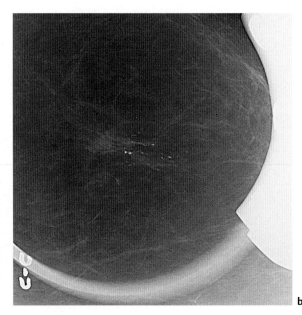

b

Fig. 7.**1 a, b Magnification mammogram for improved differentiation of clustered microcalcifications**
a Mammogram
b Magnification mammogram. Histology: Poorly differentiated DCIS

a

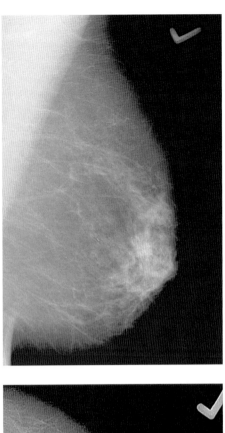

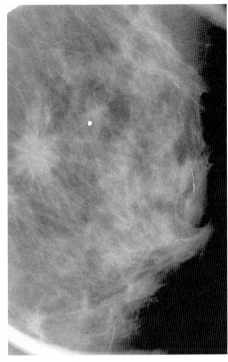

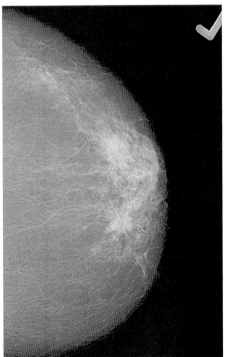

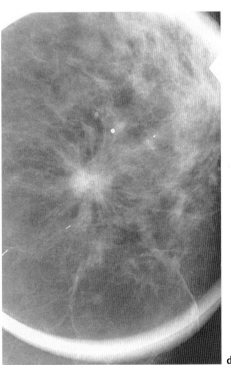

Fig. 7.**2 a – d**   **IDC with extensive intraductal components of carcinoma in situ**. The magnification mammogram shows the extent of the carcinoma in situ, indicating that the lesion is not suitable for breast-conservation treatment
a MLO view
b Magnification view, ML projection
c CC view
d Magnification view, CC projection

Advantages:
- Less noise due to a higher effective photon flux.
- Less scattered radiation reaches the film due to the air gap between breast and film–screen combination, leading to higher contrast with more conspicuous delineation of the structures.

- Better definition of the lesion by simultaneous spot compression, which displaces surrounding tissue, decreases the tissue volume to be radiated and achieves better immobilization of the breast.
- Better analysis and classification of the calcifications due to improved contrast.

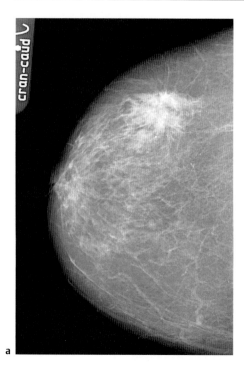

a

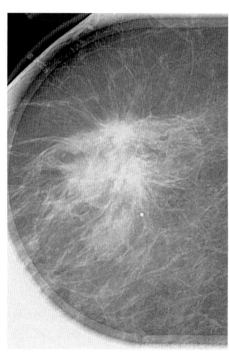

b

Fig. 7.**3 a, b Palpable asymmetric density**. Magnification mammography offers more detailed information
a CC view
b Magnification view, CC projection
Histology: ILC with 15 mm diameter, axillary lymph nodes negative

- Increase in the number of correct interpretations:
  - in a selected group, a definite diagnosis could be made in 70% of uncertain mammographic findings (Sickles 1980),
  - in a screening program, the mammographic specificity could be increased.

Remark: Radiographic magnification hardly achieves any better spatial resolution.

Any apparent gain in spatial resolution can be ascribed to increased contrast and enlarged display. The mentioned advantages cannot be achieved with video magnification (electronic) or with a magnifying glass (optical) since both methods increase the noise level at the same time.

Disadvantages:
- Careful positioning of the region of interest is required.
- Since the breast is only partly imaged, getting oriented may be difficult.
- The radiation dose increases with the additional exposures; no higher skin dose in comparison with the conventional mammographic view since faster intensifying screens are used, antiscatter grids are removed, and smaller radiation fields are selected.
- The longer exposure time may lead to blurring due to patient motion, which in most cases can be limited or eliminated by compression. Breath holding is necessary. Motion unsharpness caused by transmitted cardiac or vascular pulsation may be unavoidable with long exposure times!

- Lesions near the thoracic wall are less accessible due to mechanical constraints of the compression device and X-ray tube!
- Magnification mammography should be used as secondary method added to regular mammography, not as primary method.

Indications

- Microcalcifications:
  - Not clearly discernible.
  - Further clarification regarding form, density, number, distribution (diffuse or aggregated), and improved differentiation between malignant and benign.
  - Can a biopsy be avoided? Increasing the mammographic specificity!
- Asymmetric densities:
  - Internal structure: homogeneous or heterogeneous, e.g., radiolucency in the center of a stellate lesion
  - Margins: circumscribed or spiculated. Increase in mammographic sensitivity!
- Differentiation of uncertain or questionable lesions, also palpable lesions, especially in dense breasts.
- "Lesions" that are only visible in one projection and requiring clarification to determine whether they are true lesions or pseudo-lesions caused by superimposed structures.
- Establishing possible multifocality of an already known cancer. Detecting calcifications near the tumor is very important:

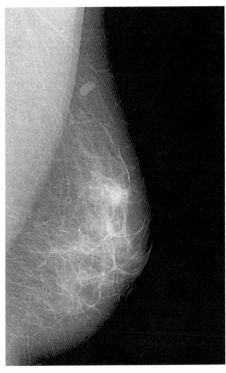

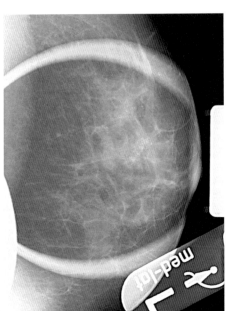

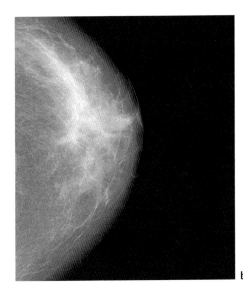

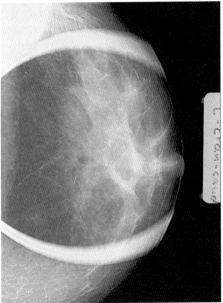

Fig. 7.**4a–d** Assessment of an uncertain finding by magnification mammography

a, b MLO and CC view with a pseudotumor due to superimposed glandular structures

c, d The magnification mammogram no longer shows a suspicious lesion

– decisive for planning of excision, especially in breast-conservation surgery; cases with satellite clusters of microcalcifications (extensive intraductal component) need a more extensive excision or even a total mastectomy.

• Gaining additional information on lesion detected by MRI and not seen on standard mammographic views.

• Gaining additional information on palpable or sonographically detected lesions that are not seen on standard mammographic views.

• Evaluating sites of earlier excision or other surgical procedures.

• Specimen: Locating the lesion for histopathological examination.

Concluding Remark

Magnification mammography should be seen as a supplementary method. In uncertain findings, it often leads to a higher diagnostic confidence (Fig. 7.**4**).

Percutaneous Diagnostic Procedures, Preoperative Localization, and Specimen Radiography

D. J. Dronkers

The increasing use of mammography, especially for screening, has increased the number of mammographically detected breast lesions, most of which are not palpable.

Unless the lesions can be ranked as probably benign, at least after additional spot-compression and/or magnification views, further evaluation is needed by cytology and/or histology. The image-guided percutaneous needle biopsy has become important in these cases. Furthermore, image-guided localization procedures are needed for preoperative localization of mammographically detected lesions that are not palpable. Finally, specimen radiography is an integral part of the localization procedure and indispensable for quality control of the entire diagnostic process.

Percutaneous diagnostic procedures

- Diagnostic puncture of cysts
- Fine-needle aspiration cytology (FNA)
- Core-needle biopsy

For nonpalpable lesions, needle guidance sonography or stereotactic mammography are required.

■ Percutaneous Diagnostic Procedures

■ Diagnostic Puncture of Cysts

When sonography cannot differentiate between cyst and solid tumor, diagnostic puncture is indicated. For nonpalpable lesions, this is done under sonographic guidance.

Technique

Sterile gloves and sterilization of the skin with antiseptic solution are necessary. Local anesthesia is rarely needed. When the lesion is located behind the mamilla, the sensitive areolar region should be avoided by pulling the areola aside and obliquely inserting the needle through the skin outside the areola. Because using very thin needles entails the risk that viscous fluid will not spontaneously drain from the cyst, at least an 18-gauge needle must be used.

Table 7.1 shows the relation between cyst volume and diameter.

For a cyst under 25 mm in diameter, a 10 ml syringe is adequate. For larger cysts, at least a 20 ml syringe is needed.

When a cyst is punctured, as much fluid as possible should be aspirated. For puncture under sonographic guidance, images before and after aspiration should be obtained for documentation.

Fluid under pressure will drain spontaneously or even squirt when the cyst is punctured. The color of the fluid can vary from light yellow to black, depending on the age of the cyst. The darker the color, the older the cyst.

Leakage of fluid from a cyst (due to puncture, seatbelt injury, vigorous compression during mammography) may cause an aseptic (chemical) inflammation in the surrounding breast tissue.

Clinical Contribution

When the aspirated fluid is clear, cytological analysis is superfluous.

Sanguine fluid may be caused by perforation of a small vessel near the cyst but may indicate an intracystic lesion, and cytological examination of the fluid is mandatory. If an infection is suspected, a specimen for bacterial culture should also be obtained. By replacing the fluid with air, a pneumocystogram is seen on subsequently obtained mammographic films (p. 149).

In addition to the possibility of detecting intracystic lesions, pneumocystography provides a window in the dense breast tissue, permitting inspection of tissue that earlier was superimposed by the fluid-filled cyst. If fluid cannot be aspirated, a solid lesion must be assumed and FNA should be performed next. If material for cytological analysis cannot be aspirated, a core biopsy or surgical excision is indicated. If pus is found in large inflamed cysts or an abscess is encountered, insertion of a drain is advisable after consultation with the referring physician.

■ Fine-Needle Aspiration (FNA) for Cytology

FNA cytology is often the first step in evaluating mammographically or clinically detected suspicious breast lesions. Only familiarity and experience with FNA cy-

Table 7.1   Content of cysts of different diameters

Diameter (mm)	Content (ml)
10	0.5
15	1.8
20	4
25	8
30	14
35	22
40	33
45	48
50	65

tology assure acceptable diagnostic results. This applies not only to aspiration of the lesion and preparation of the aspirated material but also to the interpretation of the specimen.

If a cytopathologist cannot be present for instant review of the aspirated material and experience with this method is limited, the percentage of nondiagnostic results can be 30% or higher.

Material inadequate for cytological analysis and false negative results are encountered more often with benign breast lesions, probably related to the large proportion of connective tissue in benign lesions and the relative scarcity of cells (fibroadenoma).

As these nondiagnostic findings are not always entered in published studies, the results of FNA cytology found in the literature are not always comparable. Experienced cytopathologists achieve quite reliable results for both palpable and nonpalpable lesions and, as systematically applied complementary examination, FNA cytology will increase the potential of mammography to detect malignant lesions early.

Furthermore, FNA cytology can decrease the ratio of benign to malignant excisional biopsies.

False negative findings, however, are unavoidable and negative findings can never exclude a malignancy entirely. In contrast, false positive findings are rare. This means a not always impressive sensitivity of FNA cytology, but a high specificity. Most patients tolerate the FNA well and the risk of severe complications is negligible. For all practical purposes, there are no contraindications.

A major shortcoming of FNA cytology is the lack of any information about the invasiveness of positive cell samples. This calls for additional histological examination whenever malignant cells are found. Moreover, FNA cytology cannot determine the degree of differentiation. It does allow receptor analysis.

Technique

For cytological smears, many aspirated tissue fragments about equal in thickness to the cell diameter should be spread on the slide next to each other. The necessary fragmentation of the biopsy material can be accomplished by using thin needles (21, 22, or 23 gauge) and by creating a sufficient vacuum (negative pressure). The negative pressure required for aspiration during puncture can be reached with a specially designed syringe holder. Both 20 ml and 10 ml syringes are used. (Fig. 7. **5**).

Positioning the needle into palpable lesions generally does not create a problem. Sonographic guidance is used for nonpalpable lesions. For microcalcifications, which are barely, if at all, visible sonographically, mammographic guidance by means of a two-dimensional coordination system or stereotactic device is indicated to aspirate material from different parts of the site in question.

Local anesthesia of the skin is hardly ever required when using the thin needles used for aspiration. After

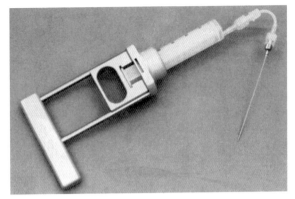

Fig. 7.5 Syringe holder used to attain a negative pressure for fine-needle aspiration (FNA)

disinfection of the skin, the needle is inserted and advanced to the lesion. As slanted needle tips may deviate the needle during insertion, accurate positioning can be improved by rotating the needle during insertion. With a negative pressure created in the syringe, the needle is repeatedly entered into the lesion in a fanlike fashion (Fig. 7.**6**). The negative pressure is released before withdrawal of the needle. This keeps the cell material in the needle from being sucked into the syringe. Finally, the air in the syringe is used to push the material in the

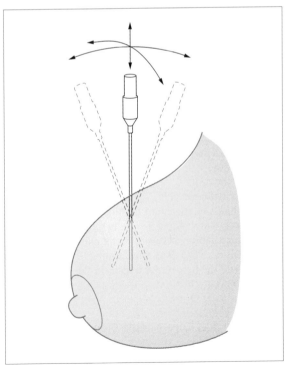

Fig. 7.6 Technique of FNA for cytology (up-and-down movement and swiveling of the needle in a small angle around the puncture axis (Philips Medical Systems, Hamburg, Germany)

needle onto a slide, where it is smeared and fixed. As long as sterile slides are used, re-puncturing with the same needle is permitted.

Add-on stereotactic equipment without adequate space for the syringe holder requires a special connection tube between needle and syringe (Fig. 7.**5**).

Not only cell material near the needle tip, but also cells detached from the immediate surrounding may be aspirated. As a rule, more than one aspiration biopsy should be obtained from a lesion. After fixation and staining, the cytopathologist can determine immediately whether material is adequately representative while the patient is waiting. If necessary, the aspiration can be repeated. To avoid a hematoma, the puncture site is compressed manually for some time, as is customary for all percutaneous needle procedures.

The Contribution of the Method

FNA cytology is a quick and cost-effective diagnostic method, especially in combination with mammography. The examination is well tolerated by the patient, and complications (such as infection and hematoma) are rare. False negative findings, even in knowledgeable and experienced hands, cannot be avoided. The image-guided FNA cytology of noncystic lesions is read out as follows:

- Inadequate material: repeat FNA.
- Benign: follow-up after 6 months (mammography/sonography).
- Uncertain, atypical: histological examination (core-needle biopsy or surgical biopsy).
- Malignant: core-needle biopsy or excision biopsy.

In normal breast tissue or in benign breast lesions, the multiple passes of the needle may create changes that simulate malignancy on sonography, which remain sonographically visible for several months after the FNA. Therefore, sonography should be performed before rather than after FNA. This also applies to mammography since FNA may also change the mammographic findings. Bleeding, for instance, may preclude mammographic evaluation.

The contribution of FNA cytology may increase in the future when the specimen obtained from FNA can be evaluated by flow cytometry, which may contribute to the differentiation between benignancy and malignancy. This is achieved by determining the DNA content (ploidy) and the percentage of cells in the growth phase of the cell cycle (the S-phase fraction [SPF]).

■ Histological Core-Needle Biopsy

For several decades, percutaneous needle biopsies of the breast have been performed using specially designed needles of the true-cut type. A small cylinder of intact tissue is obtained for histological examination. Different types of needles had been developed in the past, includ-

ing drill and core needles for manual insertion. Drill needles can cause problems by becoming locked in dense tissue structures. If this happens, they have to be untwisted and removed without gaining any material. Functionally better needle systems consist of a sliding mechanism that contains a hollow inner trocar and an outer needle. They have the disadvantage of pushing aside rather than penetrating firm lesions located in normally soft surrounding tissue structures. This can give false negative results. Biopsies with manually inserted 14-gauge needles can be painful. These methods have become obsolete since the introduction of automatic high-speed biopsy guns (Bard, Manan, Biopty, ASAP) (Fig. 7.**7**).

Biopsy guns have a spring mechanism, which first drives an inner trocar with a notch for the specimen (sample chamber) into the lesion and then, following almost instantaneously, an outer needle, cutting out a tissue sample. Its beveled tip causes the inner needle to bend slightly when entering the lesion. The outer needle is less flexible and returns the inner needle to its straight position, pressing its notch into the wall of the puncture channel and filling it with a core of tissue, which is cut by the outer needle. This bending mechanism allows for two or four biopsies through the same puncture site in the skin by turning the gun 180° or 90° degrees between each biopsy (Fig. 7.**8**).

The high speed of the shooting action also penetrates firm lesions instead of pushing them aside. Probably due to the high shooting speed, the biopsy is hardly painful and most patients do not experience this method as burdensome.

Biopsy guns may have different strokes. Some have a long stroke of 22–23 mm, others have a short stroke of about half that length. Long stroke action requires needles with a longer notch. Usually 14-gauge needles are used, but 16-gauge and 18-gauge needles are also suitable.

The biopsy method with a needle inserted by drilling, as used in bone biopsies, is not applicable in all add-on stereotactic devices. Nowadays, drill biopsy is hardly ever used.

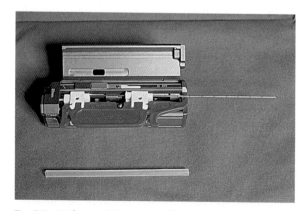

Fig. 7.7   **High-speed biopsy gun** (formerly BIP, now Bard)

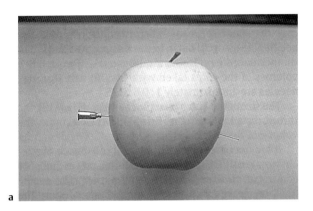

a

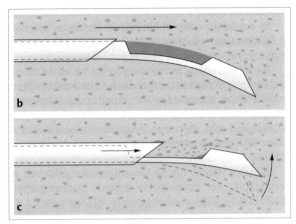

b

c

Fig. 7.**8 a–c** **Bending of the needle caused by the beveled tip**
a Demonstration on an apple
b, c Exaggerated presentation of the action of core-needle biopsy. The beveled tip bends the needle. The needle tip creates a cylindric channel in the tissue so that the notch (sample chamber) remains empty (**b**). The forward thrust of the outer needle neutralizes the bending of the inner needle. The notch is pressed into the wall of the puncture channel (**c**) and filled with tissue, cutting off a tissue cylinder

Technique

The biopsy can be performed freehand for palpable lesions. Nonpalpable lesions require sonographic or stereotactic mammographic guidance.

After disinfection of the skin and infiltration of the skin and subcutaneous tissue with an anesthetic solution, a small nick is made into the skin for needles with a diameter of 16 gauge and less.

The small cutaneous incision is made to facilitate passage of the needle through tough skin, avoiding a subcutaneous hematoma in many cases, and improves the cutting action of the biopsy gun by eliminating the friction between outer needle and skin. The shortest route to the lesion is selected, circumventing the sensitive areola.

With thin needles (e.g., 18-gauge), rotating the needle during insertion is advisable to avoid bending of the needle induced by its beveled tip. Especially in mam-

mographically dense breast tissue, even needles used for core biopsy may deviate by several millimeters. Deviation can also be prevented by using a coaxial needle system.

With the spring of the biopsy gun cocked, the needle is advanced until its tip is positioned close to the lesion. After firing, the middle of the sample chamber must be in the center of the lesion (Fig. 7.**9**).

Firing advances the needle tip by about 2 cm from the position before firing. This throw distance has to be taken into consideration beforehand. Damage or perforation of the chest wall (pneumothorax) and perforation of the fascia pectoralis, which is an important barrier for metastases, must absolutely be avoided. To prevent damage to the thorax, it is advisable to keep the needle parallel to the chest during the procedure. When the freehand approach is used, the operator should protect his or her fingers under the breast with a polystyrene board. In the stereotactic procedure, the polystyrene board is placed under the breast so that the needle tip cannot hit the cassette holder. The software used

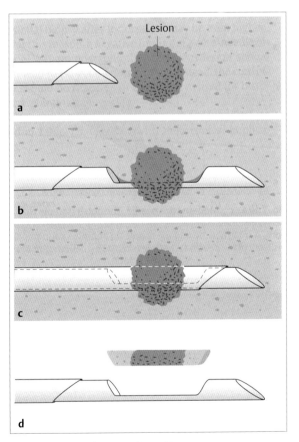

Lesion

a

b

c

d

Fig. 7.**9 a–d** **Mechanism of core biopsy**
a Initial position of the needle tip near the lesion with the biopsy gun in the cocked position
b Forward thrust of the inner needle
c Fired position after forward thrust of the outer needle
d Removed core after pullback of the outer needle

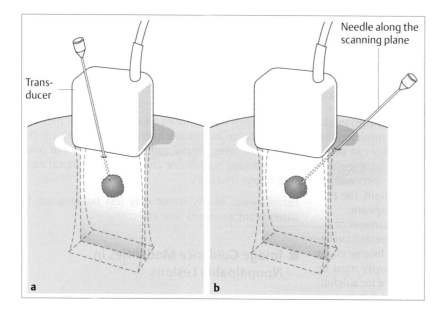

Trans-
ducer

Needle along the
scanning plane

a   b

Fig. 7.**13 a, b** **Two different
methods of sonographic
guidance**
a Needle perpendicular to the
scanning plane
b Needle along the scanning
plane

The first method is more difficult as the needle is pointed at the lesion outside the sonographic image and only becomes visible when its tip reaches the scanning plane (Fig 7.**13 a**).

The second method is easier to perform as the needle tip can be seen as soon as it passes through the skin (Fig. 7.**13 b**). The transducer is placed on the skin with the tumor seen on one side of the image. Since the visibility of the needle improves when it is more horizontally positioned (Fig. 7.**14**), it is advisable to insert the needle as horizontally as possible on the other side of the scanning plane.

Depending on the size of the transducer, one can switch from one method to the other during the procedure.

The supine position is most comfortable for the woman. The ipsilateral arm is raised with the hand placed under the head. The patient may lie flat for puncturing the medial side of the breast and may be turned slightly on the contralateral side for puncturing the lateral side.

Before puncturing, the skin is disinfected. The transducer is packed in a sterile bag filled with sterile gel. Acoustic coupling is achieved with sterile gel or ethanol. The "freehand" method is mostly followed, but guiding systems that determine the site of skin entry and angulation of the needle can be used.

The examination can also be performed by two persons, one for puncturing and one for imaging.

The shortest distance to the lesion is chosen. The entrance of the needle tip into the lesion can be verified by moving the needle back and forth. If the lesion moves with the needle tip, the needle can be assumed to be in the right position. Sonographic guidance generally makes it easy to take specimens from different parts of the lesion. Even for palpable lesions, sonography can be helpful for biopsy of different parts of the lesion.

■ Stereotactic Mammographic Guidance

The first stereotactic breast biopsies were performed with a dedicated unit consisting of a horizontal examination table and the X-ray tube, cassette holder, and stereotactic device beneath the tabletop. Figure 7.**15** shows a modern version. The woman lies prone on the examination table, which has a hole for the breast. The breast can be approached from different directions parallel to the thoracic wall. For lesions situated near the thoracic wall, angulation of the needle is possible, though this adds the risk of injuring the chest wall. These dedicated units, like Mammotest (Fisher Imaging) and Stereoguide (Lorad) (Fig. 7.**15**) can only be used for stereotactic mammographic guidance and not for mammography.

Stereotactic mammography can also be performed by standard mammography units with add-on stereotactic devices (Stereotix, Cytoguide, Fig. 7.**16**).

These units have the same precision with a variance of less than 1 mm and also can approach the breast from all directions parallel to the thorax wall. The biopsies can be performed with the patient seated or lying on the side (Fig. 7.**17**).

Parts of the add-on stereotactic device

- Stereotactic unit with needle guidance system (Fig. 7.**18**)
- Computer system with viewing console

Modern stereotactic equipment works with digital imaging that decreases the duration of the procedure by eliminating film processing. This lowers the risk of any movement of the breast between imaging and biopsy. Even the slightest positional change of the breast can

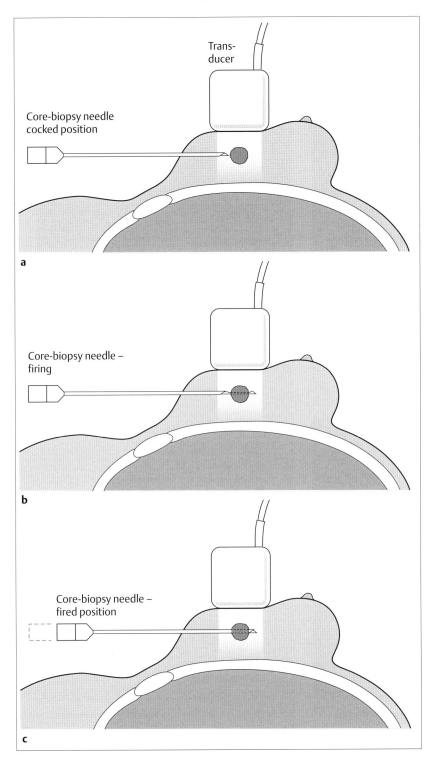

Core-biopsy needle
cocked position

a

Trans-
ducer

Core-biopsy needle –
firing

b

Core-biopsy needle –
fired position

c

Fig. 7.**14 a – c   Procedure of sonography guided core biopsy parallel to the thorax to avoid injury of the thoracic wall**
a The patient is positioned supine with the lesion at the highest point in the breast
b The needle is always inserted parallel to the thoracic wall
c The entire intramammary portion of the needle must be visible

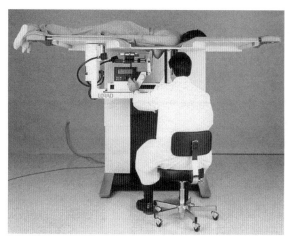

Fig. 7.**15** **Dedicated unit for stereotactic mammographic guidance** (Stereoguide, LORAD)

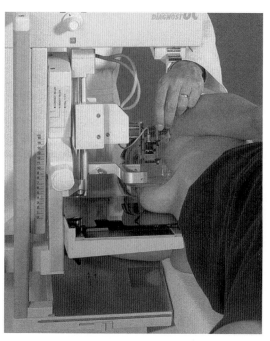

Fig. 7.**17** **Mammographic unit with add-on device, for examination with patient lying on the side**

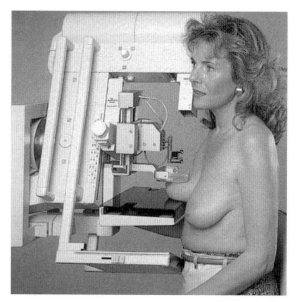

Fig. 7.**16** **Mammographic unit with add-on stereotactic device** (Cytoguide)

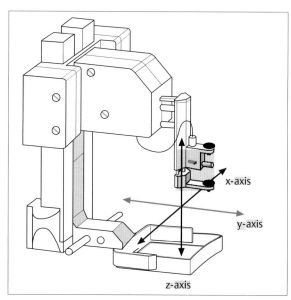

Fig. 7.**18** **Motorized needle holder.** The motorized needle holder is moved in three planes: laterally along the *x*-axis, anteroposteriorly along the *y*-axis, and vertically along the *z*-axis (Cytoguide) (courtesy of Philips Medical Systems, Hamburg, Germany)

Table 7.**4** Advantages and disadvantages of add-on devices and dedicated units for stereotaxy

Type	Advantages	Disadvantages
Add-on device	Lower purchase price	Examination table necessary for examination in prone position
	Space saving	Risk of movement with patients seated
	Nearly all mammographically visible lesions accessible	Risk of vasovagal reactions with patients seated
Dedicated units	Minimal patient movement	Higher purchase price
	Patient does not see the procedure	Impossible to perform standard mammography, therefore not cost effective
		Axillary region difficult to reach
		With angulation, risk of injuring the thoracic wall

lead to a false negative biopsy. Digital images are available within a few seconds and their brightness and contrast can be adjusted for optimal image quality. A disadvantage is a small field of view.

The advantages and disadvantages of the different units are listed in Table 7.**4**.

With a lateral holding device added to dedicated prone tables as well as to add-on units, biopsies can be performed parallel to the compression plate. This can be of advantage in patients with breasts that are too thin under compression for the automated biopsy gun. The lateral holding device also allows the para-areolar approach, i.e., insertion of the needle directed toward but not reaching the thoracic wall. The path is close to the surgical routes to most breast lesions, an especially important consideration in preoperative localizations. This approach also enables the total excision of the needle track.

Technique

When working with dedicated units and add-on equipment, the following points need to be considered.

- The patient has to be placed in a comfortable position to avoid any movement and positional change of the breast.
- The shortest route to the lesion should be selected: craniocaudally for the lesion in the upper half of the breast and lateromedially or mediolaterally for the lesion in the lower half of the breast, depending on the location of the lesion; with add-on devices, the caudocranial approach is also possible.

- Two images are obtained, with the tube assembly swivelled first into the + 15° position from the center position for the first exposure and into the – 15° position for the second stereotactic exposure. It must be ensured that the position of the compressed breast does not change during the movement of the X-ray tube.
- Precise angulation and correct positioning of the cassette are important during radiographic exposure.
- Trigonometric principles are used to determine the depth of the lesion. The center of the lesion and the reference mark of both stereo images are processed by the computer, which determines the three-dimensional position of the lesion in the breast (Fig. 7.**19**).
- A straight line connecting the center of the lesions on both stereo images should run through the translatory movement of the X-ray tube parallel to the longitudinal axis of the film. If this fails, the breast has moved during the acquisition of the stereo images. Anteroposterior displacements are uncovered by most computer systems and lead to an error message.

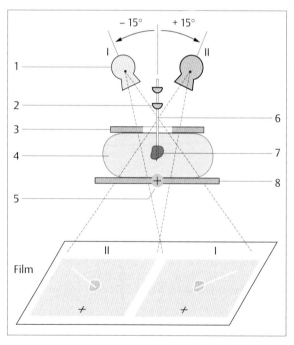

Fig. 7.19 Diagram of the principle of stereotactic imaging (Cytoguide) (courtesy of Philips Medical Systems, Hamburg, Germany)
1 X-ray tube
2 Needle holder, lower guide
3 Compression paddle
4 Breast
5 Reference cross on the support
6 Needle
7 Pathologic lesion
8 Support/film
I Tube position for first exposure
II Tube position for second exposure

This is not the case for any displacement parallel to the thorax wall, which results in an incorrect computer calculation of the lesions's location.

- It is extremely important to enter the exact length of the biopsy needle into the computer. The entire length of the needle from tip to hub is used for localization wire insertion needles and FNA needles. For core biopsies, the needle length entered into the computer is not the length from tip to hub or, respectively, connector of the biopsy gun, but the length from the front of the case of the biopsy gun to the center of the sampling notch of the inner needle in the postfiring position of the gun. After firing of the gun, the tip of the biopsy needle extends into the breast beyond the center of the lesion (Fig. 7.9 c). Consequently, a polystyrene board of at least 2 cm should be placed under very thin breasts to avoid damage to the needle by its hitting the cassette holder.
- The precise inner diameter of the sterile guide cone(s) must tightly fit the outer diameter of the biopsy needle to prevent any unwanted lateral deviation of the needle.
- To avoid any deviation of the needle during insertion for FNA as well as for localizations and core biopsies, the needle should be inserted with slight rotation. Since small firm lesions within soft breast tissue may be pushed back, it is advisable to add about 1 cm to the anticipated depth in localization procedures. This will "harpoon" the lesion and lead to better fixation of the guide wire.
- During the procedure, especially when using add-on devices, the patient must be watched to be sure her breast does not change position.
- Proper function of the stereotactic equipment has to be checked regularly to ensure correct stereotactic alignment of all coordinates. This can even be carried out during the examinations by obtaining stereo images after insertion of the needle. The performance can also be checked by a test phantom provided by the manufacturer.

Coaxial systems allow placement of a guide wire after core biopsy. Corkscrew-shaped guide wires have also been developed. These can be advanced and their depth position adjusted by rotation.

■ Radiology Support for Surgical Excisional Biopsy

- Preoperative localization of nonpalpable or questionable palpable findings.
- Specimen radiograph to confirm that the mammographically suspicious lesion has been excised. This represents an integral part of the localization procedure. Specimen verification can also be achieved with sonography by putting the specimen in a cup containing a physiological saline solution.

■ Preoperative Localization (Marking)

Preoperative localization is obligatory for nonpalpable but mammographically and/or sonographically suspicious breast lesions.

Goals of preoperative localization

- To assure excision of the suspicious area
- To avoid excision of normal surrounding tissue as much as feasible (avoidance of unnecessary mutilation)

Sonographic guidance is obviously preferred for sonographically visible lesions. Other guidance methods use mammography with fenestrated compression plate or stereotaxis.

Methods/Instrumentation

Injection of methylene blue or another vital dye, mixed with an intravenous contrast agent (or carbon particles) is done less and less today. The dye injection method is taxing because it is difficult to estimate the correct amount of dye and to minimize the time between injection and the surgical biopsy to lessen the effect of dye diffusion.

The dye injection techniques have largely been replaced by special needle–wire localizing systems consisting of an insertion needle and a metal localizing wire with an anchoring end. Most localizing wires are solid, but braided wires, which are especially flexible, are available. If wires are cut during surgery, their fragments can become dislodged in the breast and left behind.

Types of localizing wires

- Removable
- Nonremovable

Removable wires have the advantage that they can be withdrawn if the end of the wire is positioned too far from the lesion. However, their fixation in tissue is less stable than the fixation of nonremovable wires. The latter are not well liked by pathologists. If control images obtained after insertion suggest the need for repositioning of the localizing wire, the position of either type of localizing wire can be corrected before anchoring. The insertion needle of some localizations systems remains in situ until surgery.

Several types of needle-wire localization systems are listed below (Fig. 7.**20**).

Frank type (Fig. 7.**20 a**). Standard 25-gauge needle with wire, with a sturdy hook at the end. The needle wire system is inserted with the wire in the needle, and the hook of the wire protrudes from the needle end, which does

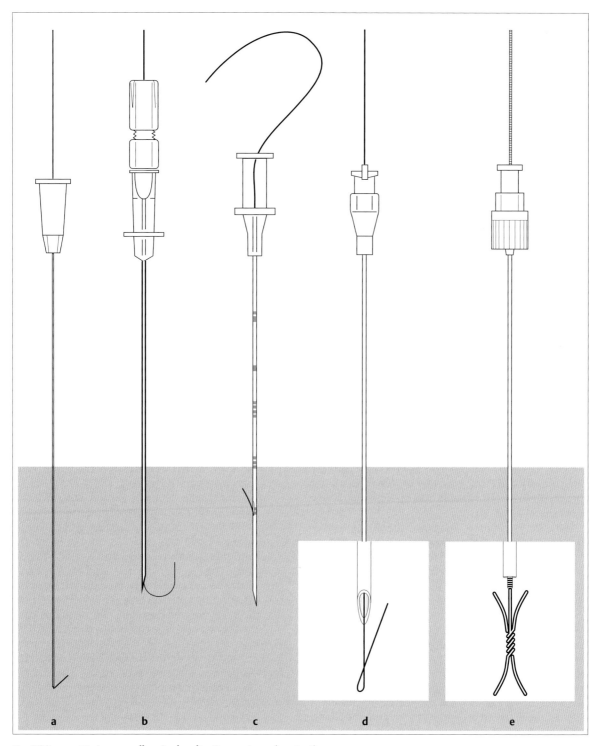

Fig. 7.**20**a – e   **Various needle wire localization systems** (see text)
a Frank type
b Homer type
c Hawkins type
d Kopans type
e X-Reidy type

not affect the insertion. The wire can be withdrawn if the positioning is not correct.

Homer type (Fig. 7.**20 b**). Curved J-wire. Simple repositioning. As wire and needle are fixed, it provides clinically acceptable anchoring strength. Both needle and wire can be felt by the surgeon during the operation.

Hawkins type (Fig. 7.**20 c**). Removable barbed hook. The needle remains in the breast until the operation and is fixed to the skin by a plastic plate.

Kopans type (Fig. 7.**20 d**). Spring hook wire that cannot be removed easily. During insertion the spring hook is located inside the lumen of the needle.

X-Reidy type (Fig. 7.**20 e**). X-shaped hook that cannot be removed easily from the breast tissue.

General Guidelines for Localization

Consultation with the surgeon is recommended before the localization procedure. If possible, the route with the shortest distance to the lesion should be selected for the puncture. Local anesthesia of the skin is often performed but is actually not needed. Premenopausal women in the second half of their menstrual cycle have the most sensitive breasts and local anesthesia might be restricted to this group of patients.

Voluminous breasts and deeply located lesions require a sufficient length of the localizing wire. With release of the breast compression, the distance between puncture site and lesion increases in most breasts, and the end of the wire can disappear in the breast if the wire is too short.

After the procedure is completed, the part of the wire extending from the breast is taped to the skin and the puncture site covered with a sterile bandage.

As most needles for localization are thin and have a beveled tip, the needle might deviate if inserted without being rotated at the same time.

For documentation after the localization procedure, two views perpendicular to each other are obtained and the center of the suspicious area and its mammographic extension is marked on the films for the surgeon. The puncture site may also be marked with a small lead bullet on the skin. Some radiologists mark the position of the tip of the wire on the skin of the breast by means of fluoroscopy of the breast with the patient in the supine position. This makes it easier for the surgeon to take the shortest anteroposterior approach to the lesion.

Localization Methods

- **Sonographic**: Nonpalpable, sonographic visible lesions will be mostly localized with sonographic guidance (Fig. 7.**13**). Sonographic localization can be done preoperatively in the operating room.

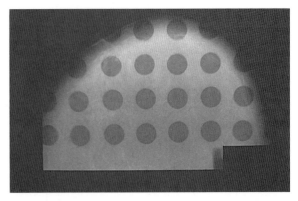

Fig. 7.**21**   **Radiograph of breast and compression plate for localization**

- **Mammographic**: For lesions not visible sonographically or for which sonographic guidance is difficult, such as small lesions in big breasts, mammographic guidance is used.
  - *Method with compression*: Compression paddle with a rectangular window and coordinates or a perforated plate (Fig. 7.**21**). A preliminary radiograph is taken to determine whether the lesion is located under the window or one of the holes. After the exposure, the compression should not be released automatically. If the lesion is not positioned under a hole, the breast must be repositioned until the lesion is accessible through one of the holes. When this is achieved, the X- and the Y-coordinates are determined (Fig. 7.**22 a**). The localizing needle should be aligned with the direction of the X-ray beam. This is ascertained when the shadow of the needle hub cast by the collimator light beam falls onto the entry point on the skin. This establishes the correct X- and Y-coordinates. The Z-coordinate, the depth of the lesion, must now be calculated by measuring the vertical distance on the true lateral view between the overlying skin and the center of the lesion (a), and the diameter of the breast in this projection (b). If c is the thickness of the craniocaudally compressed breast during the localization procedure, the depth of the lesion is $c/b \times a$.

    The needle can also be inserted to penetrate the lesion.

    Using the same compression plate, a second film is now taken perpendicular to the first film. This image shows the position of both the needle tip and the lesion. For the correct localization, the position of the needle tip can be adjusted by being pulled back slightly.
  - *Stereotactic method*: Stereotactic localization is fast and precise (Fig. 7.**23**). Deviation of thin needles with beveled tips can pose a problem. To avoid fainting of the patient, a stereotactic localization with add-on equipment should never be

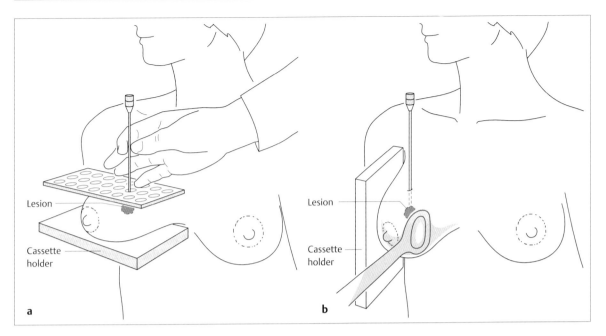

Fig. 7.**22 a, b   Procedure of mammographic localization with fenestrated compression plate** (according to Kopans)
a Insertion of the needle parallel to the thoracic wall up to the   **b** Lateral verification
lesion

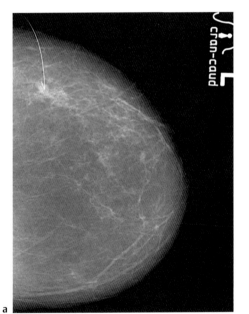

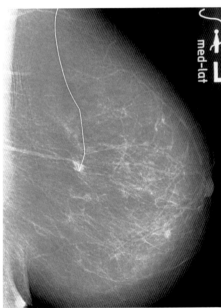

Fig. 7.**23 a, b   Documentation after localization with two films perpendicular to each other**

performed in the sitting position after premedication.

- **Freehand method localization or with coordinates drawn on the skin**: Based on the mammograms, the position of the lesion in the breast is estimated and marked on the skin with ink. This localization method is cumbersome and not always precise.

■ Specimen Radiography

Specimen radiography is an integral part of the localization procedure: it determines whether localization and excision were successful. The radiograph of the entire specimen is made to confirm the presence of the suspicious lesion. Only a second radiograph perpendicular to the first one can establish complete removal or lack of it.

Table 7.**5**   Etiology of sanguineous and serous nipple discharge (in %): galactography, followed by surgery (summary according to Tabar and coworkers)

	Carcinoma	Papilloma Papillomatosis	Cystic hyperplasia	Duct ectasia	Others	Normal	Total
Sanguineous discharge	13[1]	61	12	2	12	0,2	535
Serous discharge	7[1]	35	36	11	6	6	223

[1] Discovered by magnification mammography in $^3/_4$ of the cases

The interpretation is relatively straightforward for fibrocystic mastopathy: many small cysts filled with contrast.

The galactogram should be interpreted within the context of the mammographic and sonographic findings.

The data of Table 7.**5** indicate that a carcinoma is more often found with hemorrhagic discharge than with serous secretion. In the series published by Tabár et al. (1983), only half of the cancers detected by galactography could also be seen on routine mammograms.

Magnification mammography increases the detection rate of retromamillary cancers.

Cancer is found in only in 4–10% of all cases with nipple discharge.

With increasing age of the patient, carcinoma is more often the cause of hemorrhagic discharge.

Remark: The cytological analysis of the secretion is unreliable for the detection of intraductal cancer (Menges et al., 1974; Tabár et al., 1983).

Galactography may be helpful in males with unilateral nipple discharge. Unilateral hemorrhagic nipple discharge in males is caused by malignancy in more than 60% of cases.

Pneumocystography

J. H. C. L. Hendriks and G. Rosenbusch

Pneumocystography (filling the cyst with air after aspiration of the cystic fluid) was often performed in the 1980 s. Because of the higher quality of sonography, especially the development of special transducers for small parts (frequency 7.5 – 12.5 MHz), the method is rarely performed diagnostically, but sometimes therapeutically.

Indications

In symptomatic cysts, after puncturing for drainage, air is injected. This may promote involution of the cyst by desiccating its epithelial lining.

Contraindications

- Inflammatory changes.
- Abscesses.
- Hemorrhage during puncturing.
- Sonographically atypical cysts (irregular margins, internal vegetations) should be excised; puncturing and draining these cysts may make them impalpable and surgically undetectable.

Technique

Cleaning of the skin with alcohol; sterile gloves. Local anesthesia is seldom required.
- Sterile surgical drapes around puncture site; sonographic transducer placed in a sterile cover; sterile coupling gel.

- Puncture of palpable cysts without sonographic or stereotactic mammographic guidance.
- The quantity of injected air should equal the volume of aspirated fluid (Fig. 7.**25**).
- Two views after removal of the needle:
  – CC view
  – MLO or lateromedial (mediolateral)
- The injected air may remain visible for several weeks. Total resorption may take 2 – 3 months.
- If no fluid can be aspirated, FNA should follow immediately.
- Cysts may collapse after pneumocystography: filling with air may have a therapeutic effect.
- Excision if there are
  – atypical cells in the aspirated fluid;
  – irregular margins;
  – intracystic lesions.

Complications

- Hemorrhage: may be falsely interpreted as hemorrhagic cyst fluid.
- Infection.

Interpretation

- The cyst should have smooth margins to exclude a malignancy.

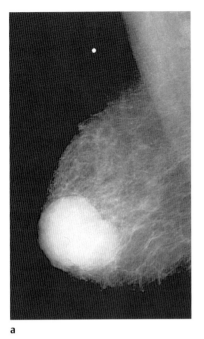
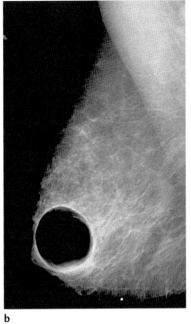
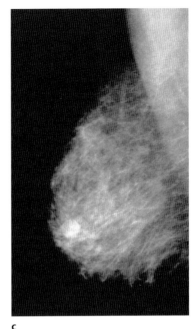

a   b   c

Fig. 7.**25 a - c   Pneumocystography**
a Retromammillary density with mainly smooth margins in a 54-year-old woman
b Pneumocystography shows a smooth inner wall
c After three months there is only a residual density

- Septa in the cysts or superimposed breast structures may compromise the interpretation. Multiple communicating cysts may also exist.
- Adjacent cysts may cause an atypical configuration of the punctured cysts.
- Microcalcifications that were hidden by superimposed cysts become visible after pneumocystography.

Role

- Cytological analysis of aspirated fluid is positive in only a few cases of intracystic cancer: high false negative rate (>50%).
- Color of aspirate: in 5 out of 13 intracystic cancers the aspirate was clear and not hemorrhagic (Tabár et al., 1983).
- Intracystic breast cancer accounts for 0.2 – 1.3% of all breast cancers (Tabár, 1981).

Computed Tomography

J. H. C. L. Hendriks and G. Rosenbusch

Computed tomography (CT) contributes little to breast imaging and has no place at all in breast cancer screening, whether it is performed with or without administration of contrast medium. CT scanners dedicated for breast examinations have not gained acceptance. Because of its relatively high radiation dose, the routine use of CT for breast imaging was abandoned after the introduction of MRI. CT can only be justified when the patient's condition precludes the performance of MRI or when MRI is not available.

Indications (see Introduction)

- Assessment of any infiltration of breast cancer into the thoracic wall.
- Visualization of lesions, mostly those near the thoracic wall, that are seen solely in one mammographic projection.
- Detection of axillary and retrosternal nodal metastases.
- For the detection of recurrence after tumor resection.
- Treatment planning in radiotherapy.
- Breast implants: evaluating surrounding tissue and detecting possible rupture, when mammography and ultrasound are inconclusive.
- Very dense breasts: better definition of lesions.

Remark: Postcontrast CT should be avoided one week before and after menstruation when tumor enhancement is less conspicuous due to a higher iodine concentration in the normal breast tissue.

Technique

- **Patient positioning:**
  - *Supine*: examination of the thoracic wall.
  - *Prone*: examination of breast tissue. Arms above the head; nipples marked with barium paste and symmetrically positioned. Transverse scans of the breast at 0.5 cm intervals before and after the infusion of 300 ml of 30% contrast medium over 10 minutes. During scanning, shallow respiration is advised to reduce respiratory artifacts.
- **Spiral CT**: Spiral acquisition in breath holding for up to 30 seconds, before and immediately after intravenous injection of 100 ml of nonionic contrast medium (300 mg I/g) with an injection rate of 2 ml/ second, with the spiral acquisition repeated after a delay of 60 seconds. Collimator 2–3 mm, pitch 2–3 mm.

Interpretation

- Breast cancers present in fatty breasts as irregular density with spicules (as in conventional mammography).
- Enhancement is observed in carcinomas and also, though less intense, in fibrocystic disease, fibroadenomas, and abscesses.
- The breast cancer appears larger after administration of contrast medium than on precontrast images (extravascular pooling of contrast medium due to neovascularity).
- Local recurrence may manifest itself as follows:
  - Focal skin thickening.
  - Dense subcutaneous tissue.
  - Heterogeneous or irregular remnants of the pectoralis muscle.
  - Nodal metastasis: axillary lymph nodes larger than 1 cm.

- Involvement of brachial plexus: interruption of the fat layer between anterior and medius scalenus muscles, and in the soft tissue around subclavian artery (*caveat*: check for symmetry).
  - Destruction of ribs or sternum is often quite subtle; review of the images using different window settings.
- Retrosternal lymph nodes:
  - Normal lymph nodes along the internal mammary arteries are smaller than 5 mm and are located in fat tissue within 3 cm of the lateral border of the sternum (normally 3–5 lymph nodes on each side in the first three intercostal spaces).
  - Lymph nodes larger than 6 mm are pathological and hard to detect with other imaging techniques; detecting these nodes may affect radiotherapy planning.
- Postoperative findings:
  - Depend on the extent of the resection; many surgical modifications are used with simple as well as radical mastectomy; sometimes remnants of the major pectoral muscle are found at its sternal or costal insertion, even after radical mastectomy (*caveat*: it is important to be informed about the surgical procedure and possible postoperative complications): not to be mistaken for recurrent tumor.
  - The overlying skin measures less than 5 mm and shows no local thickening.
  - Comparison with the unaltered other breast necessary for comparative assessment of muscles after simple mastectomy.
  - Axillary densities measuring less than 5 mm are to be considered normal lymph nodes.
- After radiotherapy:
  - Within three months: generalized skin thickening, streaky densities in the subcutaneous fat; the fat shows increased attenuation; discrete anterolateral pleural thickening and thickening of the subpleural septa (radiation pneumonitis).
  - After six months: platelike atelectases with smooth margins and dilated bronchi; reduced skin thickening.

Sonography of the Breast

Harmine M. Zonderland

In the diagnosis of breast pathology, sonography of the breast plays an important role as supplementary imaging modality. In general, the sonographic examination should be preceded by a complete mammogram. The examiner must be familiar with interpreting both mammography and sonography. Performing the sonographic examination should not be entrusted to technicians.

■ Technical Considerations and Imaging Technique

The automated systems developed in the 1980s for sonography of the breast are currently replaced by high-resolution real-time units. Although modern equipment is preset for imaging small parts, it is nevertheless necessary to understand the technical parameters affecting the image quality.

■ Technical Considerations

Ultrasound Intensity

The ultrasound (US) intensity corresponds to the electric voltage applied to the transducer to produce the US that enters the breast tissue. With the current small parts equipment, it is possible to penetrate 4–6 cm deep into the tissue. If the intensity is too high, the image will be completely saturated and details lost. Furthermore, the concomitant amplification of the side lobes of the US wave will negatively affect the axial resolution. The gain setting is optimal when the pectoral muscle and its fascia can be clearly identified through the breast tissue.

Time-Gain Compensation

The high-frequency sound waves are rapidly absorbed and attenuated by the breast tissue; therefore the reflected returning sound waves must be amplified. To achieve the same amplitude, the echoes of structures far from the transducer must be amplified more than those from nearby structures. The higher the transducer frequency and the more dense the tissue, the steeper the gain compensation must be set. This automatically reduces the depth of field.

Transducers and Focusing

The optimal sound frequency lies between 7.5 and 10 MHz for a penetration depth of 6 to 4 cm, respectively. Transducers with sound frequencies up to 13 MHz are under development.

Several transducer designs are available:

- The electronic linear-array or phased-array transducers contain many small elements that are activated in sequence to produce a real-time image. They have a variable, electronically controlled focusing system, and depth and range of the focal zone can be adjusted to encompass the lesion. A stand-off pad is generally not needed except for very superficial lesions. Electronic transducers have a higher noise level than mechanical sector transducers, making it often more difficult to visualize a cyst as a completely anechoic lesion (Figs. 7.**26a–f**).
- The mechanical sector transducer has only one element, which produces an image by rotation or oscillation. The focusing is set, and a stand-off pad is usually needed for optimal imaging with the lesion located in the focal zone. Modern high-resolution mechanical transducers have a built-in stand-off pad, eliminating noise caused by possible leakage or air bubbles.
- The newly developed annular array transducer applies mechanical sector technology with multiple ring-shaped crystals in a concentric array, enabling emission of a focused beam of, e.g., 6, 8, and 10 MHz. This transducer often has a built in stand-off pad.

■ Imaging Technique

The patient lies supine. The arm on the side to be examined is bent, with the hand lying over her head. This produces flattening of the breast and stabilizes its position. The side to be examined should be raised slightly. For optimal imaging of lesions located in the outer quadrants of large breasts, it may be necessary to turn the patient on her side.

Before beginning a sonographic examination, the mammogram must be available for correlation of both imaging modalities. The examiner should know the clinical history and symptomatology. It is important to follow a standardized protocol to carry out the examination. It is advisable not to examine the entire breast, but to target the examination to the site of the lesion. It can be helpful to examine the lesion from several different directions. The image quality can be improved by slowly compressing the tissue. By shortening the distance between the transducer and the lesion, artifacts like shadowing due to large differences in attenuation can be eliminated. Furthermore, the examination is better endured by patients with a painful lesion, improving the performance of the examination and resulting in a better final assessment of the lesion. Finally, the sonographic findings should be documented in at least two different sonographic planes. The targeted examination requires appropriate labeling of the location of the lesion.

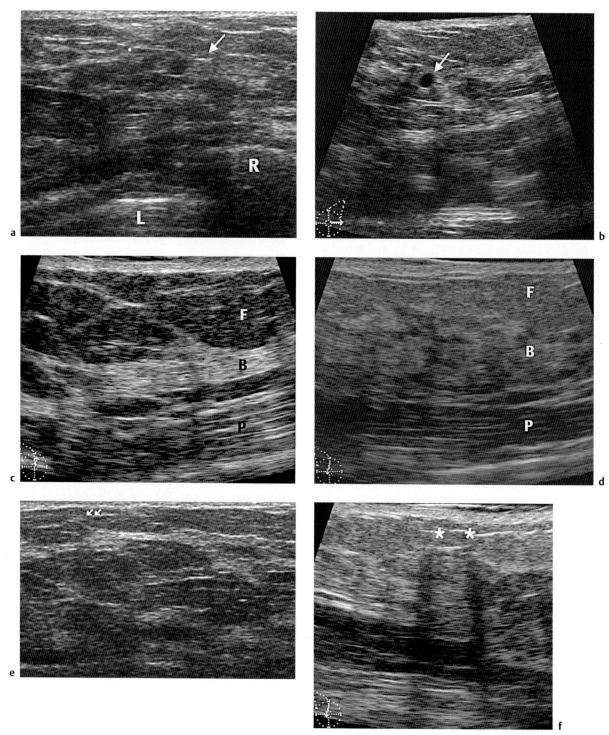

Fig. 7.26 a – f   Normal breast anatomy on sonography

a A 7.5 MHz linear array transducer. Electronic noise makes it difficult to identify a small cyst (arrow). R = rib; L = lung

b A 10 MHz sector transducer with stand-off pad reveals the same cyst (arrow) completely anechoic, but the background is blurred

c A 10 MHz sector transducer with stand-off pad. Normal breast tissue. F = hypoechoic, subcutaneous fatty tissue; B = moderately echogenic breast tissue; P = pectoralis muscle

d A 10 MHz sector transducer with stand-off pad. Breast tissue six weeks postpartum. F = subcutaneous fatty tissue, more echogenic than in (**c**) because of higher depth gain compensation.   B = heterogeneous   breast   tissue;   P = pectoralis muscle

e A 7.5 MHz linear array transducer demonstrates Cooper ligaments (arrow)

f A 10 MHz sector transducer with stand-off pad. Shadowing behind the crossing points of the ligaments (*)

■ Interpretation of Sonographic Images

▇ Normal Anatomy

In contrast to other surface organs examined by high-resolution sonography, breast tissue is not sharply delineated. It is embedded in the fatty tissue of the chest wall and exhibits large variations in its proportion of fatty and glandular tissue. Both components alter with age, nutritional status, and mastopathic changes in the glandular tissue.

The skin is 1–3 mm thick and appears as two echogenic lines. The subcutaneous fatty tissue is composed of ovoid, hypoechoic lobuli, separated from each other by fibrous connective stroma, the Cooper ligaments, which appear as echogenic stripes that arise from the glandular tissue and insert in the skin. These ligaments, especially behind their crossing points, cast acoustic shadows due to abrupt attenuation differences, which disappear when moving the transducer.

The true breast tissue forms a conical disk of ducts and lobuli, interlobular and intralobular connective tissue, and fat. The nipple produces acoustic shadowing. The retromammary lactiferous ducts can often be identified if they are slightly (2–4 mm) distended (Fig. 7.**27**). In general, the branching small ducts and lobuli cannot be identified individually. The breast tissue is discernible from the surrounding fatty tissue by moderately echogenic areas of parenchyma, alternating with hypoechoic fat lobuli and transected by echogenic septa of connective tissue. Only in dense mastopathic breasts are ducts and lobuli recognizable as hypoechoic oval and tubular structures, which are several millimeters in width and interspersed in the echogenic parenchyma. Behind the conical disk of glandular tissue, the retromammary fatty tissue, the pectoralis muscle with its fascia, the ribs, and finally the reflecting surface of pleura and lungs should be evident. If these structures are not visible, compression should be increased, the position of the patient or the transducer changed, or a lower-frequency transducer used.

▇ Lesion Characteristics

Many criteria are available for assessing a lesion. They must be systematically applied to be useful in the differentiation between benign and malignant lesions.

Shape

The shape of a lesion has two different aspects:

- its "intrinsic" border, which can be smooth or irregular;
- its contour, which reflects its demarcation from surrounding tissues and can be well-defined or ill-defined (Figs. 7.**28 a, b**).

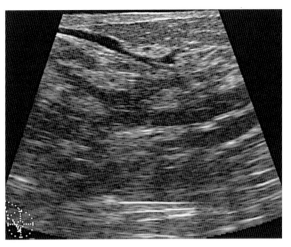

Fig. 7.**27**   **Slightly distended lactiferous duct behind the nipple**

The lateral borders of a lesion can cause bilateral shadowing by refraction of the sound wave, which becomes stronger the sharper and more vertical the lateral borders are. This is an imaging artifact that must be distinguished from shadowing behind the lesion.

Echo Structure

- The echo structure can be anechoic, hypoechoic, or echogenic.
- The structure can also be homogeneous or heterogeneous. If a heterogeneous lesion contains anechoic areas, it generally is called a complex lesion. If a lesion is homogeneously hypoechoic or echogenic, it is usually a solid lesion. An anechoic lesion with smooth borders and a well-defined contour represents an accumulation of fluid, usually a cyst. Not all accumulations of fluid are anechoic: the anterior wall often produces reverberation artifacts, which are projected in the fluid; the fluid may contain debris, which may also produce internal echoes. Since sound waves are less attenuated by the fluid, the posterior wall appears strongly echogenic, referred to as posterior wall enhancement. This decreased attenuation of the sound waves also results in enhanced sound transmission.

Sound Transmission behind the Lesion

The sound transmission depends on the structure of the lesion:

- If the lesion and the surrounding breast tissue have the same structure, the transmission is unchanged.
- Behind a very homogeneous or anechoic lesion the sound transmission can be enhanced in comparison with the sound transmission in the adjacent breast tissue, producing the so-called posterior acoustic enhancement.

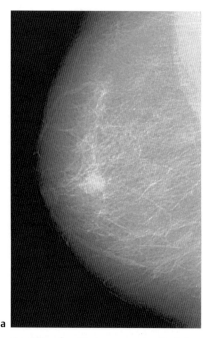

a

Fig. 7.28 a, b   Contour aspects of a lesion
a Nonpalpable lesion in a 63-year-old woman. The contour is not well-defined throughout, but spicules are absent

b

b The border of this homogenous, hypoechoic lesion is somewhat irregular posteriorly, and sound transmission is slightly decreased between the lateral acoustic shadows. The lesion has both benign and malignant characteristics
Histology: duct ectasia

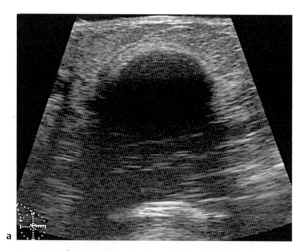

a

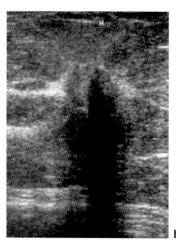

b

Fig. 7.29 a, b   Sound transmission through lesions
a Several months after a trauma, a 68-year-old woman noticed a palpable lesion where a hematoma was present before. Sonography showed strongly decreased through-transmission. A biopsy revealed only fatty material arising from traumatic fat necrosis

b Strong refraction of the sound waves with acoustic shadowing, caused by a scirrhous cancer in a 61-year-old woman

• Absorption and refraction of the sound waves in a lesion with many interfaces reduce the energy of the sound waves behind the lesion, leading to shadowing behind the lesion. If refraction is predominant, as for a lesion with many irregular interfaces, the shadow cast by the lesion may appear more prominent than the lesion itself (Figs. 7.29 a, b).

Changing of the Shape with Compression

Fatty tissue is often pliable. Fluid collections can be occasionally deformed with compression.

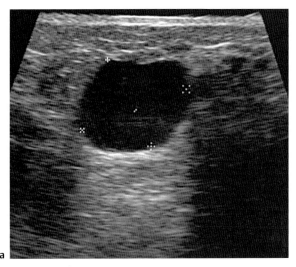

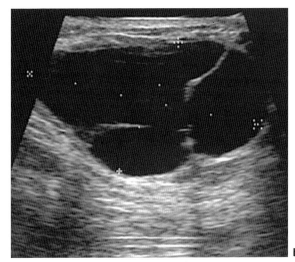

Fig. 7.30 a, b   Uncomplicated cysts
a Uncomplicated cyst with a smooth border and a well-de-fined contour, anechoic contents and posterior wall en-hancement. The bilateral shadowing phenomenon becomes inconspicuous because of the strongly enhanced sound transmission of the cyst

b Uncomplicated cyst with a thin wall and thin septa

Orientation of the Lesion in the Breast Tissue

- The longitudinal axis of the lesion can be either verti-cally or horizontally oriented.
- Determining the extent of a lesion into subcutaneous or retromammary fatty tissue and the fascia of the pectoralis muscle is easy for lesions with normal or enhanced sound transmission, but can be difficult or even impossible for lesions with pronounced acous-tic shadowing.

■ Cystic Lesions

The classic image of an uncomplicated cyst (Figs. 7.**30 a, b**) is a round or oval lesion with a well-defined, smooth contour and a thin wall. It is anechoic with an increased reflection from the posterior wall and enhanced through-transmission. When electronic linear-array transducers are used, cysts can have internal echos due to reverberation artifacts. By change in the direction of the sound beam and increase in the compression, the re-verberation artifacts can be reduced or made more ap-parent. The enhanced through-transmission together with the enhanced posterior wall provides further sup-port for the diagnosis of a cyst. A very small cyst can act like an acoustic lens and focus the sound wave, with re-sultant increased propagation. The fluid in a cyst may contain echogenic material representing fibrin, cells, or blood and occasionally may show layering. Cysts with internal echoes and an ill-defined or thickened wall are classified as *complicated cysts*. Occasionally, cysts leak and the wall may become indistinct, often indicative of an inflammatory reaction. Septa may observed within

cysts (Fig. 7.**31**) or small nodules in the wall, with the lat-ter invariably representing benign *papillomatosis* as manifestation of a mastopathy.

Intracystic papillary cancer is rare (Figs. 7.**32 a, b** and 7.**33 a – d**), but this diagnosis must be considered when a single, complicated cyst is found in a postmenopausal woman. It produces not only solid nodules but also wall thickening.

Other fluid accumulations in the breast that can re-semble an uncomplicated cyst include posttraumatic *oil cysts* (Figs. 7. **34 a, b** and 7.**35**), postoperative *seromas*, and liquefied old *hematomas* (Figs. 7.**36 a, b**). *Galacto-celes* contain debris floating in a more or less liquid con-

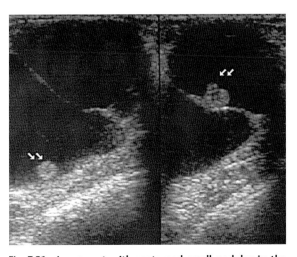

Fig. 7.31   Large cyst with septa and small nodules in the wall (arrow). Histology: benign papillomatosis

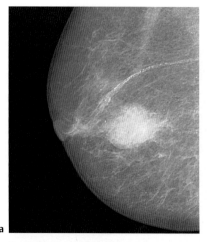
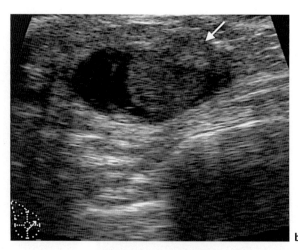

a   b

Fig. 7.**32 a, b**   **Intracystic cancer**
a Oval lesion with partly ill-defined contours in a 77-year-old woman. A calcified artery passes next to the lesion

b Hypoechoic solid lesion arising from the wall of a cyst. The contour is partly ill-defined (arrow). The aspirated fluid was sanguinous
Histology: papillary cribriform cancer

tent. Together with the high proportion of fat, this results in higher echogenicity and less through-transmission of sound.

A *breast abscess* (Figs. 7.**37** and 7.**38 a,b**) and a fresh hematoma contain necrotic debris or coagulated blood, leading to a complex echo structure. Moreover, reactive changes in the adjacent tissue can produce an irregular contour and ill-defined demarcation. If a wall is identifiable, it usually is thickened. Sound transmission can be unchanged or enhanced. The overlying skin is edematous.

■ Solid Lesions, Benign and Malignant Characteristics

Several criteria are applied to differentiate between benign and malignant solid lesions. Although the overlap is considerable and a definitive diagnosis is rarely reached by systematically considering the different characteristics, it is generally possible to classify lesions as suggestive of being benign or malignant.

- A smooth border and a well-defined contour are considered benign characteristics, while an irregular border and an ill-defined contour suggest malignancy.
- Most solid lesions appear hypoechoic relative to the surrounding breast tissue. Solid benign lesions commonly have a homogeneous structure, but a heterogeneous or complex structure can be present in both benign and malignant lesions.
- Benign lesions with a homogeneous structure have normal or enhanced sound transmission. Decreased sound transmission is suspicious for malignancy.
- The orientation of the lesion can also facilitate the differentiation between benign and malignant.

Benign lesions tend to respect the normal tissue layers and tend to have a horizontal orientation, while malignant lesions often invade tissue planes, resulting in a more vertical orientation.
- Malignant infiltration into the surrounding fatty tissue induces an echogenic rim, representing the infiltrated fat surrounding the lesion.

Benign lesions. The most common benign solid lesion is the fibroadenoma (Figs. 7.**39 a – f**). It is a mixed tumor composed of mesenchymal and epithelial components and rarely exceeds 3 cm, except during hormonal stimulation, such as occurring during pregnancy. It changes its histological appearance over time. A new fibroadenoma contains more proliferative epithelial components, while hyalinosis, sclerosis, and calcification appear in older ones. Its border is smooth or gently lobulated, and the contour is well-defined. The structure of a young fibroadenoma is hypoechoic and homogeneous, and the sound transmission through the fibroadenoma is mostly unchanged, occasionally enhanced. The structure of an older fibroadenoma is often heterogeneous. Once sclerosis and hyalinosis appear, the lesion shows weak shadowing without complete obliteration of its posterior border. The acoustic shadowing becomes more prominent once calcifications have developed. The longitudinal axis of the fibroadenoma is usually horizontal, following the anatomic orientation of the tissue structures. The ratio between longitudinal and transverse axes of the lesion is at least 1.4. A fibroadenoma is easily delineated by sonography in dense glandular tissue, but barely in fatty tissue.

A rapidly growing fibroadenoma raises the possibility of a *giant fibroadenoma* (synonym: *juvenile fibroadenoma*) (Figs. 7.**40 a – c**) or a *phyllodes tumor* (Figs. 7.**41 a, b**). The important difference is found in the growth pattern: the phyllodes tumor also consists of

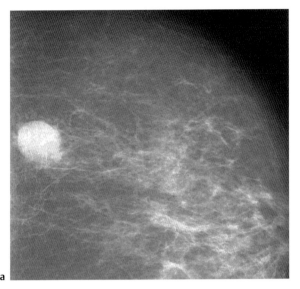

a

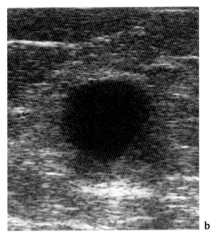

b

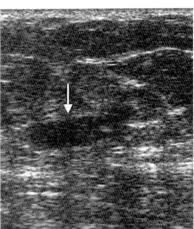

c

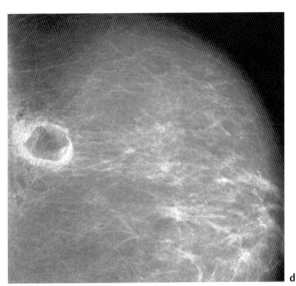

d

Fig. 7.33 a – d   Intracystic cancer
a Round lesion in a postmenopausal woman, partly ill-defined
b Sonography reveals a cystic lesion with a thickened wall

c After aspirating the sanguinous contents, the collapsed wall
is still visible. The fluid contained malignant cells
d Pneumocystography reveals an irregularly thickened wall
Histology: intracystic cancer

mesenchymal and epithelial components, but its histology has a characteristic cauliflower appearance. The phyllodes tumor can grow to a large size, can recur, and has the potential for malignant degeneration. The sonographic appearance of a giant fibroadenoma cannot be differentiated from that of a phyllodes tumor. Regressive changes can render both tumors complex or heterogeneous, with cystlike clefts and echogenic areas. Their large size might make delineating the contour difficult.

The *fibroadenolipoma* (*synonym: hamartoma*) is also a mixed tumor with varying proportions of fatty tissue. Because of the differences in fatty components, the mammographic image is often, but not invariably, characteristic. The fatty components in a fibroadenolipoma produce an echogenic lesion with bright echoes. Its border is smooth or lobulated and the sound transmission is usually decreased by its internal heterogene-

ity. Plasticity due to its fatty components is striking, but never as characteristic as observed radiographically.

If a lesion contains only fatty tissue (lipoma), it is always more hypoechoic than a lesion only partially consisting of fatty tissue.

An *atheroma* (Figs. 7.**42 a,b**) lies immediately under the skin in the subcutaneous fat, has a smooth border and a well-defined contour, is hypoechoic or heterogeneous due to keratin and fat, and is often deformable.

A normal, *intramammary lymph node* is not larger than 1 cm and can be observed mammographically in the upper outer quadrants in 5% of breasts. It is oval in shape and hypoechoic with an echogenic fatty center.

A *papilloma* can completely fill a cyst or a duct, displacing any visible fluid. It has benign but nonspecific features: lobulated border with well-defined contours and a hypoechoic structure. It is rounded and its orienta-

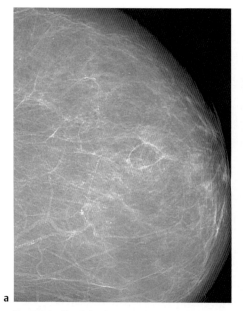

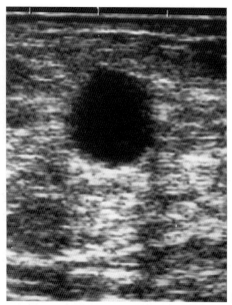

a

b

Fig. 7.**34a, b** **Oil cyst**. Posttraumatic lesion in a 80-year-old woman
a Mammography reveals an oil cyst

b Sonography shows an anechoic cyst, aspiration produced clear oil

Fig. 7.**35** **Oil cyst**. Lesion mammographically identical to the lesion in Fig. 7.**34a**, but sonography shows the lesion to be echogenic. Aspiration produced cloudy oil

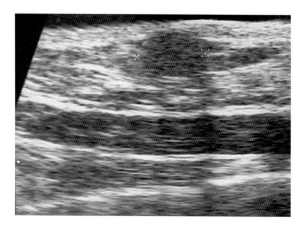

tion is determined by the encasing cyst or duct. It lacks the horizontal orientation of the fibroadenoma.

Mastopathy with local atypical epithelial hyperplasia of the lobuli can present as lesion: a well-defined or ill-defined heterogeneous area, with very small cysts along with hypoechoic ducts and lobuli. The heterogeneity causes decreased sound transmission, almost always inducing acoustic shadowing. Only the presence of cysts suggests the correct diagnosis.

A superficial phlebitis of the breast (*Mondor disease*) induces contraction of the skin overlying the inflamed vein. The vein itself can be identified as a hypoechoic tubular structure.

Malignant lesions. The most common malignant lesion is the *ductal cancer*. The many basic histological types are reflected by different sonographic patterns.

Although a lactiferous duct filled by cancer is sonographically detectable under optimal conditions, most of the malignant lesions detected by sonography are not purely intraductal, but invasive.

Small ductal cancers about 1 cm in size often have a smooth border and a well-defined contour, and show a hypoechoic structure and unchanged sound transmission. They can be differentiated from a fibroadenoma by their indeterminate orientation, although considerable overlap is encountered. With growth of the cancer, the following malignant characteristics become evident:

- Cancers (Figs. 7.**43a–f**) presenting as round or lobulated mass are often the medullary, papillary, or mucinous type. The contours are somewhat ill-defined, the structure is heterogeneous, with hypoechoic or anechoic components due to tumor necro-

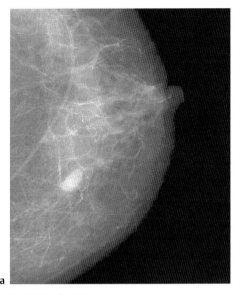

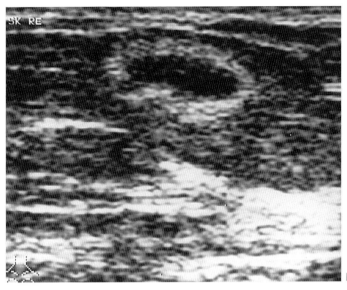

a

b

Fig. 7.36 a, b Hematoma
a Small lesion in a 60-year-old woman on anticoagulation therapy

b Sonography reveals an accumulation of fluid surrounded by an echogenic, thickened wall. Biopsy produced old blood. Spontaneous resolution confirmed by follow-up

Fig. 7.37 Puerperal abscess. Irregular border, ill-defined contour, thickened wall with hypoechoic contents

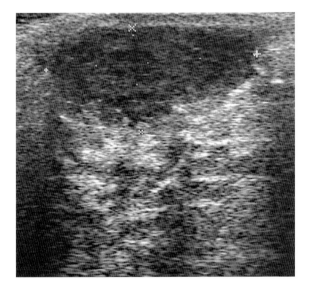

sis or mucinous degeneration. This may increase the sound transmission with acoustic enhancement behind the lesion, but usually it is unchanged. The longitudinal axis is generally undetermined or vertically oriented.

- Cancers presenting as tumor mass with short spiculations are usually solid invasive ductal cancers. The border is irregular, the contour ill-defined, and the structure hypoechoic. Absorption of the sound waves produces weak acoustic shadowing. The mass is vertically oriented, with extension into and fixation by surrounding fatty tissue, which results in a more echogenic aspect.

- Cancers presenting with a predominantly stellate structure are usually scirrhous cancers. Acoustic shadowing is pronounced and can be so severe that the posterior border of the tumor mass can no longer be delineated. Fixation in the surrounding fatty tissue also develops often with this cancer type.

- Cancers with a diffuse growth pattern and rapid spread into the lymphatic system and blood vessels are often poorly differentiated. They distort the architecture. Upon compression, ill-defined, small, bizarre, hypoechoic structures become visible, with decreased sound transmission. Their exact size cannot measured sonographically.

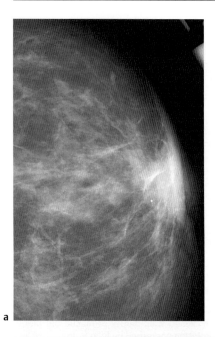

a

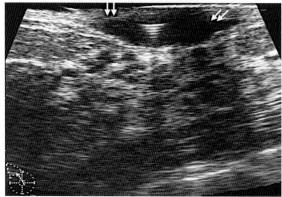

b

Fig. 7.38 a, b   Nonpuerperal mastitis
a Retromammillar density; the skin is thickened locally
b Sonography shows a small retromammillar abscess (arrow)
containing air

Only 10% of breast cancers are of the lobular invasive type (Figs. 7.**44 a,b**). Neither mammography nor sonography permit a definite differentiation from IDC. Sonographically, the subtle, infiltrating growth pattern of most invasive lobular cancers resembles that of diffusely growing ductal cancers. Except for these types, the size of a malignant lesion can be better determined by sonography than by palpation or mammography.

Other breast malignancies are rare, but not unusual. The most common sarcoma is the *angiosarcoma*, a rapidly growing malignant tumor predominantly in young women. It has a smooth or lobulated border, a well-defined contour, and a hypoechoic structure with enhanced sound transmission. Echogenic and complex lesions have been described. At the time of detection, it has already reached a large size and the horizontal orientation of the fibroadenoma is lacking.

All *hematopoietic malignancies* can appear in breast tissue, aside from their well-known involvement of liver, spleen, and lymph nodes (Figs. 7.**45 a,b** and 7.**46 a,b**). Usually, they present as multiple, occasionally even as bilateral lesions with a smooth or lobulated border and a well-defined contour. They can be highly hypoechoic, echogenic, or mixed, but these characteristics do not correspond to specific histological types. Furthermore, benign hematopoietic disorders, such as extramedullary hematopoiesis, can have the same sonographic appearance. The hematopoietic infiltration can also appear more diffuse. Secondary skin edema can arise with distended lymphatic vessels. Because of a rapid growth pattern, highly aggressive non-Hodgkin lymphomas can reach a large size.

Enlarged lymph nodes (larger than 1 cm) in the upper outer quadrants are hypoechoic with loss of their echogenic center. The enlargement is usually caused by metastasis of a ductal cancer, but the primary tumor cannot always be identified. In addition, metastases (Figs. 7.**47 a,b**) of other malignancies, generally adenocarcinomas and malignant melanomas, can produce lymph node enlargement or multiple, occasionally bilateral, round, hypoechoic lesions in the breast tissue itself. Echogenic metastases of a thyroid cancer have been described. Metastases show more benign than malignant characteristics since they do not induce the typical desmoplastic reaction seen with a primary breast cancer.

■ Doppler Sonography

Doppler or color Doppler sonography enables the examination of the vascularity of a lesion. The vessels of interest are small and thin-walled, necessitating a highly flow-sensitive system. Not only is a high-frequency transducer needed but also a high Doppler frequency must be applied to make the small Doppler differences of the slow flow velocities measurable. The pulse repetition frequency and the high-pass filter have to be set very low. The sample volume can be varied and determined by the size of the vessel. The colors allow a quick and exact selection of the sample volume.

Working with Doppler devices is time consuming. The examination must proceed slowly because of the very sensitive settings of the device, as otherwise too many motion artifacts are produced. The number of vessels should be counted, the Doppler spectrum displayed, and the maximum vascularity measured. It is futile to measure the Doppler angle of these winding vessels. Applying color Doppler sonography to lesions in the breasts is based on the assumption that neovascularity is already found in malignant lesions of just a few millimeters in size. Anastomoses and shunts produce a measurable flow even at an early stage. Benign solid lesions, such as fibroadenomas, contain very few vessels. Only fibroadenomas in young women and exceeding 2 cm in size show a moderate flow. Quantitative measurements

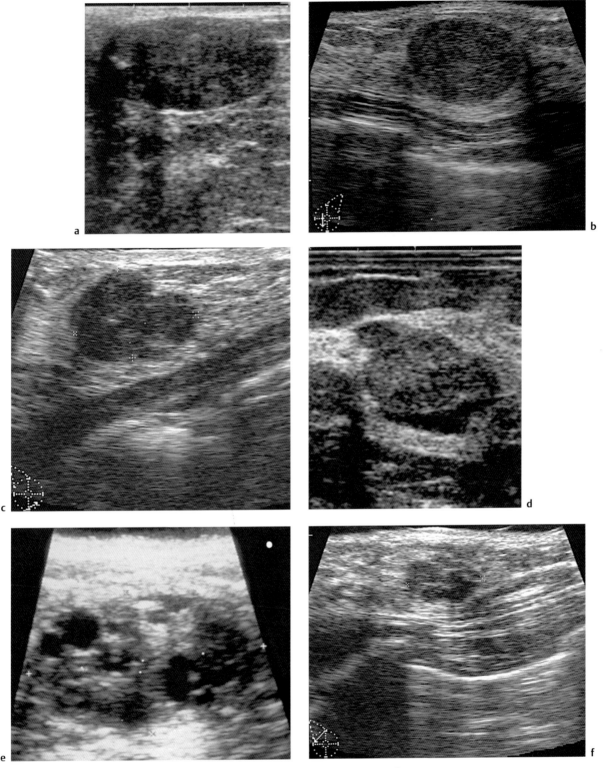

Fig. 7.**39 a – f   Fibroadenoma**

a Horizontally oriented fibroadenoma with macrocalcification in a 35-year-old woman, present for eight years

b Homogeneous fibroadenoma in a 26-year-old woman. The border is smooth and the contours are sharp. Evidence of bilateral shadowing and slightly enhanced sound transmission. The structure is homogeneous

c Lobulated fibroadenoma

d Lobulated fibroadenoma, a small accumulation of fluid surrounding the posterior wall

e Fibroadenoma with cystic components and enhanced sound transmission

f Fibroadenoma with heterogeneous structure due to sclerosis in a 43-year-old woman

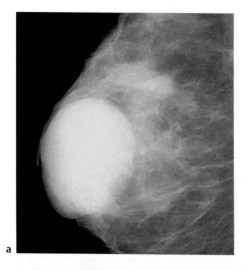

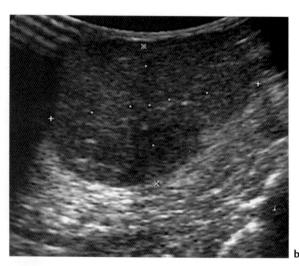

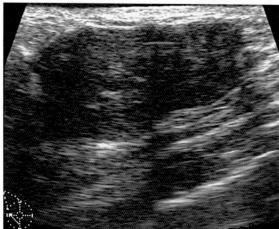

Fig. 7.40 a – c **Giant fibroadenoma**
a Mammography of a giant fibroadenoma with smooth border in a 30-year-old woman
b Sonography with a 5 MHz transducer shows an almost homogeneous, hypoechoic lesion
c Sonography with a 10 MHz transducer of a giant fibroadenoma in a 22-year-old woman. The limited depth penetration of the sound waves leads to shadowing and the appearance of a heterogeneous structure

correspond well with the subjective evaluation of the vascularity, but the Doppler characteristics fail to correlate with real-time images and histological characteristics. In conclusion, Doppler measurements are supplementary, contributing to the separation between benign and malignant lesions, but enabling no definitive differentiation.

■ Indications for Sonography

■ Differentiation between Cystic and Solid Lesions

If the mammogram of a patient with a palpable lesion shows a circumscript density, is often impossible to determine the nature of the lesion. Magnification mammography can be used for better identification, but might not improve delineation of the lesion due to overlying glandular tissue. In these situations, sonography plays a role as supplementary examination:

• Sonography can confirm the diagnosis of an uncomplicated cyst, thereby providing a final diagnosis, without the need for additional diagnostic procedures.
  - Patients with cystic mastopathy are often satisfied with the sonographic diagnosis alone, knowing the spontaneous regression of cysts.
  - Only if the definitive diagnosis of a cyst cannot be achieved, additional fine-needle aspiration (FNA) is mandatory, preferably under sonographic guidance.
  - The advantages are the reduction of false negative aspirations and the prevention of unnecessary recurrences in case of intracystic papillomatosis or intracystic cancer.
• Sonography can confirm the diagnosis of a solid lesion. The suspicion of malignancy will increase when malignant characteristics are found. Because of the overlap between benign and malignant lesions, additional procedures will invariably be required. There are two exceptions:

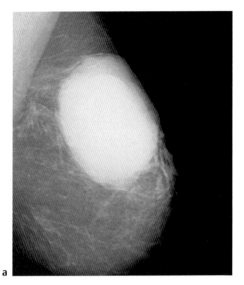

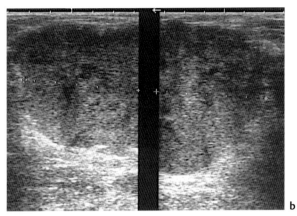

Fig. 7.**41 a, b**   **Phyllodes tumor**
a Mammography of a lobulated phyllodes
tumor in a 49-year-old woman

b Sonography confirms the lobulated border.
Clefts are clearly visible

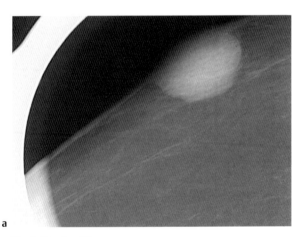

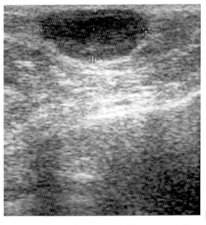

Fig. 7.**42 a, b**   **Atheroma**
a Mammmography shows a well-defined lesion immediately
beneath the skin

b Sonography shows a solid lesion with heterogenous echoes
caused by keratin and fatty components. The mammographic image is more typical than the sonographic image

  – A solid lesion with all the characteristics of a fibroadenoma, smaller than 3 cm in a woman less
than 30 years old.
  – A solid lesion, smaller than 1 cm, with benign
characteristics on mammography and sonography. The possibility of malignancy is 1.4%. Annual
follow-up for three years is considered adequate.

▪ Indeterminate Mammographic Results

If mammography only reveals architectural distortion or
suspicious asymmetry of the glandular tissue at the site
of a palpable lesion, sonography may provide additional
information. Ill-defined, hypoechoic lesions may become visible with graded compression. In general, these

lesions represent cancers with a diffuse growth pattern.
Tangential mammographic views should be obtained,
with a radiopaque marker placed over the suspicious
findings for better identification.

    If sonography fails to identify a lesion, it should be
kept in mind that mammography is superior to sonography for the detection of cancer. Consequently, mammographic findings will supersede sonographic findings.

▪ Palpable Lesion Not Visible with Mammography

A palpable lesion not identified on the mammogram
should be assessed further by sonography (Figs. 7.**48 a,
b**). Even state-of-the-art mammography will miss 5% of

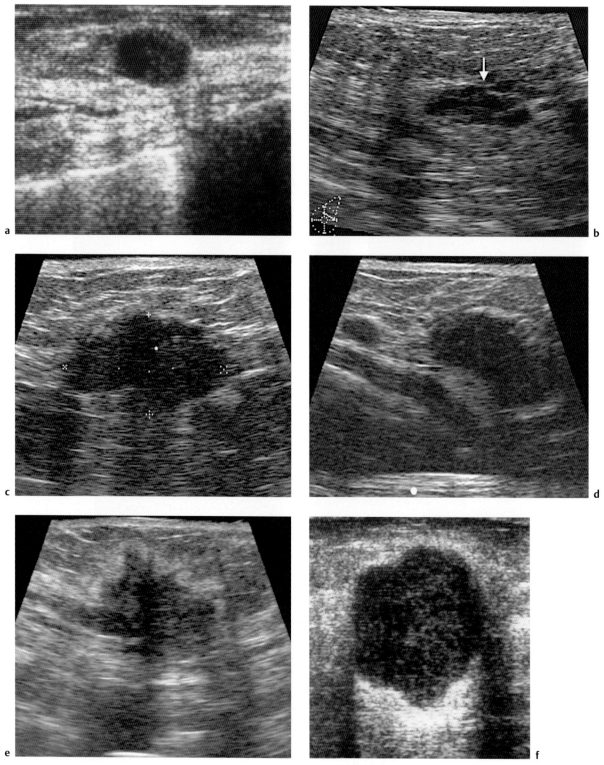

Fig. 7.43 a – f   Malignant lesions

a Ovoid lesion, smooth border and well-defined contour. The structure is somewhat heterogeneous. Histology: tubulo-papillary cancer

b Duct with irregularly thickened wall (short arrow). Histology: well differentiated in situ ductal carcinoma

c Ovoid lesion with irregular border and ill-defined contour. Histology: invasive ductal cancer

d In the vicinity of this malignant lesion, a second, solid lesion is present, not identified by mammography. Histology: satellite focus of cancer

e Scirrhous cancer with infiltration of the surrounding subcutaneous fatty tissue

f Well-defined but irregularly outlined medullary cancer. The sound transmission is strikingly enhanced

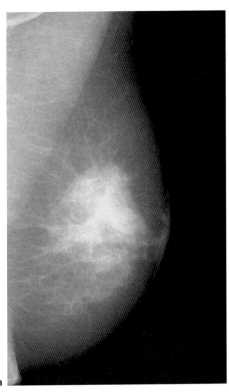

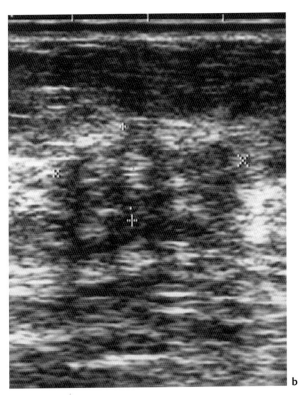

Fig. 7.**44 a, b   Invasive lobular cancer (ILC)**
a Architectural distortion in the upper outer quadrant

b The same architectural distortion appears on the sonogram as a group of tiny shadows, not entirely explained as crossings of fibrous and parenchymal tissue. Histology: invasive lobular cancer

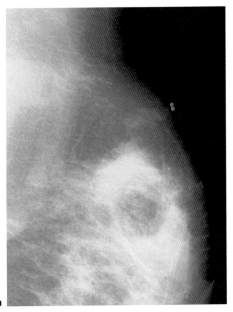

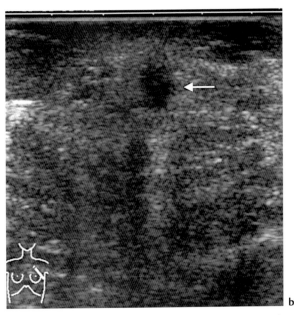

Fig. 7.**45 a, b   Intramammary Hodgkin disease**
a The palpable lesion is identified by the radiopaque marker: a small, ill-defined non-specific density

b Sonography shows an ill-defined, hypoechoic lesion with vertical orientation (arrow)

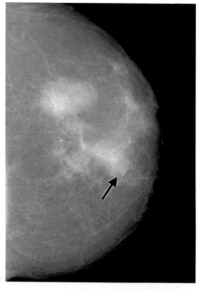
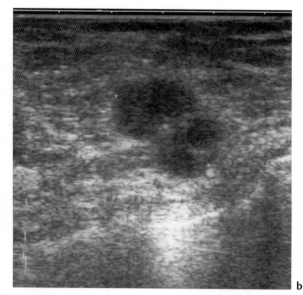

Fig. 7.**46 a, b   Intramammary non-Hodgkin lymphoma**
a Palpable lesion, mammographically lobulated with mostly smooth borders, located somewhat laterally of the nipple. A second small focus is visible medial to the nipple (arrow)

b Sonography also shows a lobulated, solid lesion with heterogeneous structure

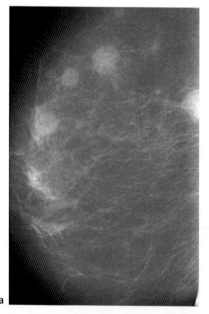
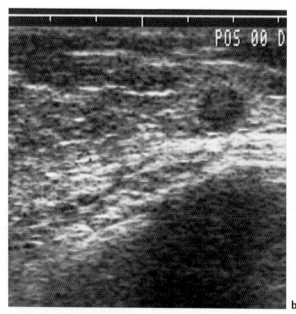

Fig. 7.**47 a, b   Metastases from a malignant melanoma**
a Mammography with multiple, round lesions, partially ill-defined with several small extensions

b Sonographically, the metastases are round, hypoechoic, and homogeneous. The mammogram is more specific than the sonogram

all cancers. These are mainly cancers without desmo-plastic reaction or microcalcifications or located in an area of very dense glandular tissue or in a breast with cystic mastopathy. For this group of patients, sonography is clearly beneficial if it can bring out a discrete solid lesion, but of doubtful value if it only produces a vague solid lesion, because of the false positive rate of the latter.

Sonographic assessment of mastopathy can be difficult since mastopathy lacks specific sonographic features, with the appearance ranging from hypoechoic

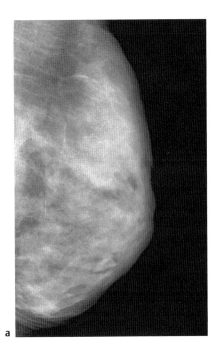

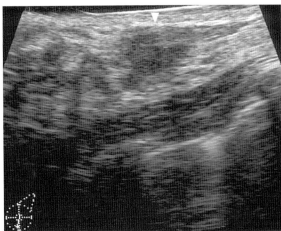

Fig. 7.**48 a, b   Palpable lesion not visible with mammography**
a A 32-year-old woman with palpable lesion behind the nipple, not visible in the dense, retromammillar breast tissue
b Solid lesion (arrow) with irregular border, ill-defined contour and heterogeneous structure. Normal sound transmission. Histology: invasive ductal cancer

solid lesions, including small groups of cysts, to glandular tissue with a normal sonographic pattern. The small solid, hypoechoic lesions in particular often remain suspicious. Even FNA may not exclude malignancy. If the palpation is suspicious, additional histological examination is required. If the palpation is doubtful and sonography is unspecific, the patient should at least be followed clinically. This responsibility lies with the clinician.

■ Nonpalpable Lesion Visible with Mammography (Figs. 7.**49 a, b**)

The responsibility for further analysis lies with the radiologist. After exact localization of the lesion on the mammogram, each quadrant has to be assessed systematically. The sonographic transducer should be slowly moved from the outer border of the breast to the nipple region, gradually rotating between horizontal and vertical sections to obtain a complete set of radial slices of the entire breast. If the lesion can be identified sonographically, its characteristics should be determined. Any solid lesion with indeterminate or suspicious characteristics mandates FNA or histological examination if it is larger than 1 cm and found in a woman older than 30 years.

■ Evaluation of Benign Lesions

■ Young Patients and Pregnancy

Breast cancer hardly ever develops in women younger than 25 years. It is rare in women between 25 and 35 years, and is almost always discovered by palpation. Breast cancer occurring during pregnancy will also be found by palpation. Given the dense breast tissue found in most young women (under the age of 30 years) and the hypertrophy of the breast tissue during pregnancy, problems with the interpretation of a mammogram can be expected and sonography should be selected as initial imaging modality. For complaints other than palpable lesions, such as pain and galactorrhea, imaging is not indicated.

If sonography reveals a solid lesion with all characteristics of a fibroadenoma, follow-up is sufficient. Sonographic differentiation between a large or giant fibroadenoma, phyllodes tumor and lymphoma is not possible and FNA or histological examination is required.

If sonography reveals a solid lesion without typical benign characteristics, mammography is indicated and must be performed with a radiopaque marker placed at the site of the palpable lesion. Even if the lesion itself is not identified, microcalcifications or other features associated with malignancy may be detected. During pregnancy, a galactocele must be included in the differential diagnosis. The fear of radiation-induced damage to the fetus is unjustified with current mammographic technology and is not a valid argument for replacing mammography entirely by sonography.

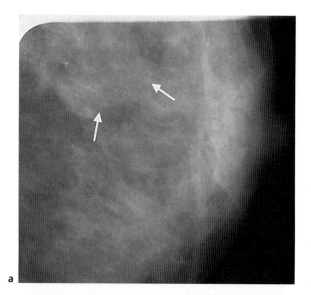

a

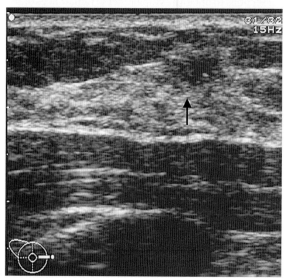

b

Fig. 7.49 a, b   Sonography as supplemental method for nonpalpable lesion with mammography
a Microcalcification suspicious for malignancy, surrounded by slightly increased tissue density (arrows)
b The density can be identified on sonography and suggests infiltrative growth. Histology: small invasive ductal cancer (arrow) in a large DCIS

■ Puerperal and Nonpuerperal Mastitis

Mastitis and *abscess formation* occur in 5 – 11 % of women during lactation as result of a *Staphylococcus aureus* infection of the nipple. The clinical symptomatology is generally unmistakable: skin thickening, warmth, and erythema over a painful, fluctuating swelling. Sonography can differentiate between an inflammatory infiltrate with microabscesses and a unilocular or multilocular abscess.

Retromammillar nonpuerperal mastitis develops from a squamous metaplasia. The larger lactiferous ducts are plugged with keratin, followed by a secondary infection, occasionally with a fistula to the areola. The symptomatology is not always conclusive. The sonographic finding is either typical of an abscess or reveals an atypical, indistinctly outlined, hypoechoic lesion. With cystic mastopathy, a secondary infection of cysts can also develop, leading to the sonographic appearance of complicated cysts.

A mammogram is not indicated for a patient with mastitis: the procedure is not only painful but also unreliable as the skin thickening and ill-defined border of the inflammatory lesion precludes its differentiation from a malignancy. The diagnosis can be established by sonography, to be followed by drainage or aspiration. In any case, mammography should be performed three months later, to exclude the possibility of an underlying malignancy.

■ The Contribution of Sonography

The opinions concerning the role of sonography in the diagnosis of cancer are rather diverse. The initially optimistic attitude regarding the use of sonography soon faded after its introduction in the 1970 s. Sonography performed on the entire breast proved to be inferior to mammography and consequently sonographic screening has long been abandoned. Even for symptomatic patients, the diagnostic performance of sonography is under critical discussion, especially in the Anglo-Saxon literature, as exemplified by the phrase "sonography can see but not find a breast cancer." This cautionary approach is supported by several arguments.

- Benign and malignant sonographic characteristics show considerable overlap. Lesions with clearly malignant characteristics are not controversial. If no lesion can be identified on sonography or lesions show indeterminate or benign characteristics, the indication for additional diagnostic modalities should not depend on sonography alone but on the combination of sonographic findings, patient's age, symptomatology, and mammography results.
- If mammography does not indicate a malignancy, but rather an asymmetric distribution of the glandular tissue, sonography should not replace additional or magnification views. Sonography will often lead to a false positive result.
- Microcalcifications should not be assessed by sonography. Even if a group of microcalcifications (Figs. 7.**50 a – c**) can be identified with sonography, which is often achieved with the current high-frequency transducers, this will not affect the therapeutic procedure. This identification assists only with the localization.
- The imaging of enlarged lymph nodes in the axilla or retrosternally plays a limited role. For definitive stag-

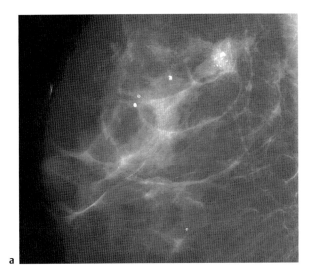

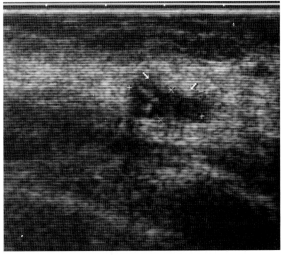

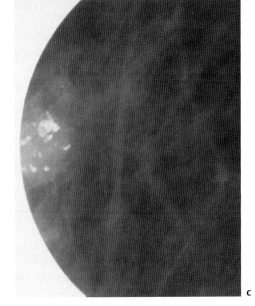

Fig. 7.**50 a – c Sonography of microcalcifications.** Incidental nonpalpable lesion in a 62-year-old woman
a Mammography shows a partially well-demarcated density with relatively coarse calcifications not clearly identifiable as benign or malignant
b Although the microcalcifications are also sonographically evident, sonography does not provide further information
c The suboptimal magnification view shows the ill-defined contour of the lesion and the heterogeneity of the microcalcifications, suggestive for malignancy
Histology: invasive ductal cancer

ing, histopathological examination of the entire axillary lymph node group is essential. Imaging an individual lymph node will not affect the procedure or the prognosis. It is only helpful with the localization for FNA if a primary malignancy cannot be found or if a sentinel node procedure is planned.

■ Summary

Sonography is an integral component of breast imaging and should be used whenever mammography cannot provide a conclusive result:

- Differentiation between cysts and solid lesions.
- Palpable lesion visible at mammography with indeterminate or suspicious characteristics.
- Palpable lesion, not visible at mammography.
- Nonpalpable lesion, visible at mammography.
- Palpable lesion in a patient younger than 30 years of age.
- Benign conditions, such as mastitis and abscesses.
- Finally, sonography is useful as a guidance for interventional procedures.

It is the radiologist who holds the key position in determining the role of sonography in the diagnosis of benign and malignant breast conditions.

Magnetic Resonance Imaging

Sylvia H. Heywang-Köbrunner and Carla Boetes

Principles

Magnetic resonance imaging is a tomographic technique that images the breast in sections without irradiation. The sections are generated using radio waves to excite protons in the water and fat of the tissue in a magnetic field. The excitation energy is released as radio waves that are registered by the imaging unit. Spatial phase and frequency encoding enables the identification of the exact location that emits the radio wave. These are the data points used to reconstruct sectional images. The signal intensity of the individual tissue depends both on the pulse sequence that excites the protons and on the tissue properties, which are determined by the number of protons contributing to the signal and by the relaxation times T1 and T2.

Tissue properties determining the signal intensity of the tissue

- Proton density
- T1 relaxation time
- T2 relaxation time

Depending on the tissue properties elicited by the applied pulse sequence, the images are called proton density, T1-weighted, or T2-weighted images.

By the use of proton density, T1-weighted, or T2-weighted pulse sequences, the same section is displayed with different contrasts. Initially, it was thought that the signal intensities characterize different tissues with a high degree of accuracy, thus enabling a differentiation between benign and malignant changes. This was not substantiated for the so-called *native* or *unenhanced MR mammography*, i.e., MR mammography without administration of contrast medium. Even though the native image has a high intrinsic contrast with the signal intensities corresponding to the amount of fat, water, cellularity, and fibrosis within the different tissues, this information is insufficient for the crucial differentiation between benign and malignant changes.

Consequently, native MR mammography has not found a place in the distinction between benign and malignant lesions or for the detection of malignancy. However, the high contrast of the images has been proved very useful for recognizing ruptured silicone implants, which have become one of the most important indications of plain MR mammography.

Enhanced MR mammography, i.e., MR mammography with administration of contrast medium, has evolved as a new and interesting additional method for addressing selected problems. The entire breast is displayed in sections both before and after intravenous injection of a paramagnetic contrast medium. MRI is very sensitive in demonstrating even slight uptake of contrast medium as enhancement.

Most invasive carcinomas enhance (Figs. 7.**51**–7.**53**). This is attributed to high vascularity, increased permeability of the vascular wall, and, possibly, an enlarged interstitial space, as encountered in malignant tumors due to angiogenesis and factors altering the permeability. Using an optimal technique, 95–99% of invasive malignancies and more than 85% of ductal carcinomas in situ show enhancement (as compared to nonproliferative normal breast tissue). This is especially useful in patients with very dense breasts or with scar tissue in the breast.

Technique

As in mammography, optimal technique is an absolute prerequisite for the detection of small lesions.

The following points are important for enhanced MR mammography.

- A single or double breast coil must be used to achieve good image quality and excellent resolution.
- The examination has to be performed with the patient prone to minimize artifacts introduced by respiratory motion. Furthermore, it is recommended that the breasts be compressed slightly by a tourniquet or by cotton wool to reduce motion artifacts.
- The pulse sequence with the most sensitive display of contrast enhancement must be selected. It is important that the signal intensity correlates linearly with the concentration of the contrast medium in the tissue. Otherwise, enhancement in the nonlinear region of the curve, which may result from signal saturation, may fail to distinguish intermediate from strong enhancement.
- The echo time must be chosen to preclude opposed-phase imaging. As fat and water vectors are opposed, they can cancel each other. Especially in carcinomas in situ (with their possible partial volume effect with surrounding fat), enhancement may not increase the signal intensity but may leave it unchanged or, paradoxically, decrease it. This can lead to considerable misinterpretation of opposed-phase images. Therefore, MR mammography should only be performed with echo times that produce in-phase images (at 1.5 Tesla 5 ms, at 1 Tesla 7 ms, at 0.5 Tesla 14 ms + 25% or less than 3.5 ms). Spoiled 3 D gradient echo sequences (e.g., FLASH 3 D, spoiled 3 D FFE, or GRASS or 3 D-FT) are very suitable for enhanced MR mammography. For instance, excellent contrast is achieved using FLASH-3 D with a repetition time (TR) of 12 ms, an echo time (TE) of 5 ms, and a flip angle (FA) of 25° at 1.5 Tesla, and with a TR of 14 ms, a TE of 7 ms, and a FA of 25° at 1 Tesla.

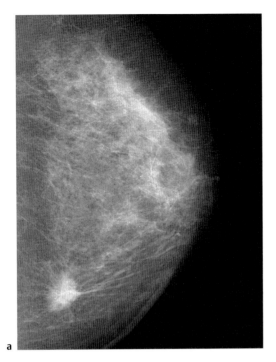

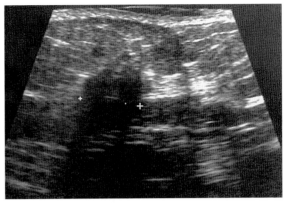

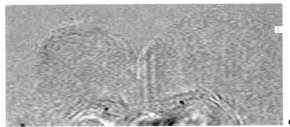

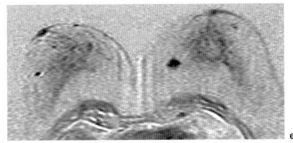

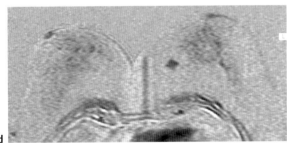

Fig. 7.**51 a–e Invasive tubulo-lobular carcinoma, 2 cm in size, medially in the left breast.** Twenty-two lymph nodes negative
a CC view: In the lower inner quadrant, stellate density with relatively long spicules. No microcalcifications
b Sonography: irregular, hypoechoic lesion, 1.3 cm in size

c–e *MRI (Turbo Flash 2 D, subtraction). Early contrast enhancement of the lesion*
c After 0 sec. Enhancement of the aorta
d After 8 sec.
e After 18 sec.
 (Enhancement was noticed to begin after 4 sec.)

With this pulse sequence, the entire breast (64 or 32 sections of 2 or 4 mm thickness) can be imaged in 87 or 44 seconds.
- The entire breast should routinely be imaged with contiguous slices before and at least twice after intravenous injection of a paramagnetic contrast medium (without changing imaging parameters). In addition to dynamic imaging with acquisitions every 30 to 60 sec., early enhancing lesions can be detected with the first postcontrast measurement (acquired in the first to third minute after the contrast injection) at a good specificity. Late enhancing lesions are detected with measurements acquired about five to seven minutes after the injection. Since many benign lesions enhance late, the specificity of late measurements is low.

Sequences with very high temporal resolution have been designed for a more detailed assessment of the enhancement dynamics. Presently, these sequences can only be applied to a few slices. This approach may help improve the specificity. Since the number of slices are limited, they must be combined with 3 D reconstruction to image the entire breast.

- For reliable interpretation of the images, a standardized window setting is recommended as well as routine subtraction of the corresponding slices of the postcontrast and precontrast sequence. Subtraction series, however, are only reliable with very little to no patient motion between precontrast and postcontrast sequences (Fig. 7.**54**).
- Fat suppression pulse sequences are also possible, but are not required for enhanced MR mammogra-

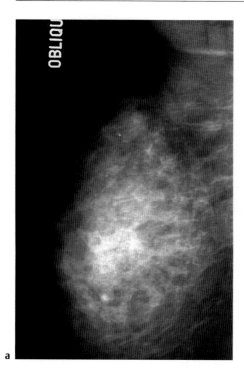

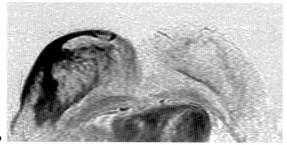

Fig. 7.**52 a, b**   **Mastitis carcinomatosa of right breast**. Stage T4 N1 Mx, 58-year-old woman
a ML view. Skin thickening, no focal lesion
b MRI (Turbo Flash 2 D, subtraction). Strong enhancement of the skin and of the glandular structures

phy. Frequency-selective fat suppression (or water excitation) may lead to interpretation errors due to inevitable heterogeneities of the magnetic field. Since such sequences use narrow bandwidth, water signal (including signal from enhancing areas) may be missed in regions with an insufficiently homogeneous magnetic field. The heterogeneities are caused by both the breast coil and the patient.

- The dosage of contrast medium (Gd-DTPA) must be adapted to the body weight. A dosage of 0.1 – 0.2 mmol/kg body weight has been recommended. We prefer a higher dosage because of a more conspicuous enhancement. The dosage must be mentioned in the report or posted on the images.

For the detection or exclusion of ruptures of silicon implants, the following should be observed.

- A combination of at least three pulse sequences is recommended: e.g., a T1-weighted high-resolution pulse sequence with or without fat suppression, and a T2-weighted high-resolution pulse sequence. If a fluid collection is visible, a silicone-only sequence or a silicone-suppression or water-suppression sequence should be used for further differentiation.
- The section thickness should be less than 5 mm. At least one pulse sequence should allow sections smaller than or equal to 2 mm.
- The examination should be performed in different planes (transverse, sagittal, and, if deemed necessary, coronal).

Criteria for Interpretation

The criteria for the interpretation of MR mammography vary, depending on the quantitative assessment recommended by different authors.

A low threshold and only restrained consideration of the dynamic information can achieve a high sensitivity (95 – 99%), but yields only a moderate specificity (30 – 70%).

A high threshold and inclusion of the dynamic information increases the specificity (70 – 90%) but decreases the sensitivity (about 90%). The lower sensitivity using this approach is caused by classifying about 10% of the slower enhancing malignancies as "benign."

Awareness of the accuracy achieved by the chosen criteria has consequences for the correct interpretation of the MRI findings.

The final diagnosis should not be based solely on the findings of enhanced MR mammography but should be reached by taking into account the mammographic findings and clinical presentation.

The following interpretation criteria for enhanced MR mammography are recommended.

- *No enhancement* rules out an invasive malignancy larger than the section thickness with a very high degree of certainty (sensitivity for invasive malignancy 95 – 99%). About 80 – 90% of ductal carcinoma in situ (DCIS) show some type of contrast enhancement. Early contrast enhancement is encountered in about 40 – 50% of DCIS, late contrast enhancement in about 40%. Because of the high percentage of ductal carcinoma in situ with either late or no enhancement, it is always necessary to evaluate MR mammography together with conventional mammography (mammographically, ductal carcinoma in situ can be recognized by microcalcifications).
- *Irregularly outlined focal enhancement* can be caused by malignancy (or mastopathy, fibroadenoma, papilloma, or necrosis) and usually should be followed by a biopsy, even in the absence of a mammographic finding. Early enhancement speaks more for a malignancy, but late enhancement does not exclude it. A biopsy for histological analysis should always be taken whenever malignancy is suspected, either clinically or mammographically.

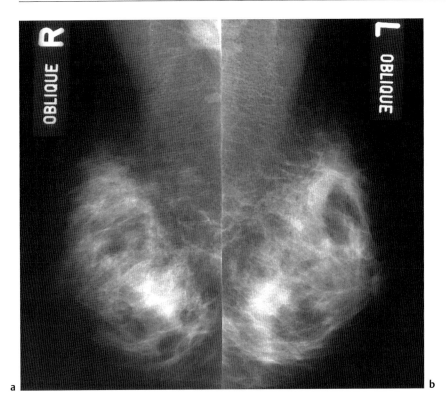

a, b

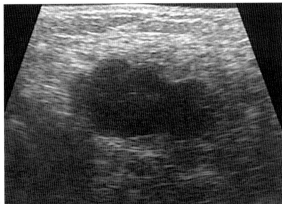

c

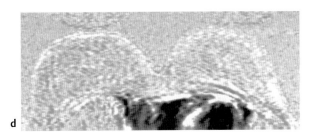

d

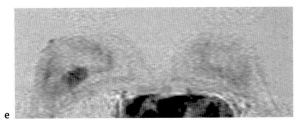

e

Fig. 7.**53 a – e** **IDC, 4 cm in size, concomitant with a poorly differentiated DCIS**. Mitosis activity index 32. Fifteen axillary lymph nodes without metastases. This 36-year-old woman discovered a lump in the right breast one month ago
a, b ML views. No lesion visible in the relatively dense breast
c Sonography: irregularly shaped hypoechoic lesion measuring 2.8 cm in diameter
d, e MRI (Turbo Flash 2 D, subtraction). Early enhancing tumor
d Enhancement of the aorta (time 0 sec.)
e Strong enhancement of the lesion after 8 sec.

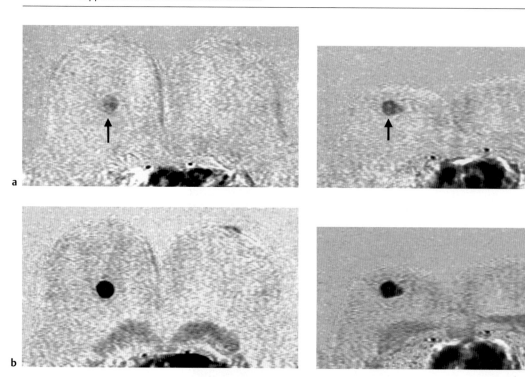

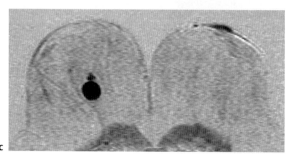

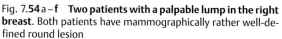

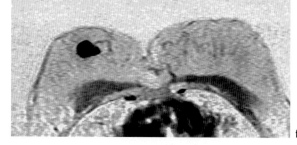

Fig. 7.54 a–f   **Two patients with a palpable lump in the right breast**. Both patients have mammographically rather well-defined round lesion

a–c A 39-year-old woman. (Turbo Flash 2D subtraction). Centrifugal enhancement. Histology: fibroadenoma

d–f A 62-year-old woman. (Turbo Flash 2 D, subtraction). Centripetal enhancement.
Histology: IDC

- *Well-circumscribed focal enhancement* can be caused by a fibroadenoma, a papilloma or, though rarely, a malignancy. If the lesion is visible mammographically or sonographically or is palpable and lacks clearly benign findings, further evaluation by core biopsy or open biopsy with histological analysis is mandatory. If the lesion is clinically asymptomatic, does not appear suspicious, or is not seen by conventional imaging and has no early wash-out or centripetal enhancement, we recommend a follow-up MR mammography within six months (to avoid false positive results).
- *Diffuse enhancement* is mostly seen in benign disorders but does not rule out malignancy. In these cases, MR mammography does not help and should not influence other diagnostic decisions.
- If an early dynamic enhanced examination is performed and shows an enhancement in the lesion

within 11.5 sec. after enhancement of the aorta, the lesion is highly suspicious for malignancy.
- Silicone implants are seen as smoothly outlined cushions of homogeneous signal intensity as long as they consist of one lumen. Double-lumen implants have a smaller central lumen embedded in a second larger lumen. The signal intensity of the outer and inner lumina depends on their contents (saline solution in the outer and silicone gel in the inner lumen or vice versa). A very small line with a low signal intensity between inner and outer lumina represents the envelope of the inner lumen. The outer lumen of the implant is also surrounded by a thin line of low signal intensity, consisting of the silicone envelope and a fibrous encapsulation, which are visually inseparable as long as the implant is intact. If silicone gel or other fluid (transudate around the implant) leaks outside

the outer silicone envelope, it separates the fibrous tissue from the outer envelope of the implant, visualizing the fibrous capsule and the silicone envelope as separate structures. Tissue fluid (transudate) and silicone gel can be distinguished by their different signal intensities, especially on T2-weighted images with silicone-suppression or water-suppression. The following signs are important for recognizing a ruptured silicone implant:

- *Linguine sign.* The outer envelope of the silicon implant is ruptured and completely collapsed, with the silicon gel usually contained within the fibrous capsule. The collapsed outer envelope of the implant is visualized on tomographic images as bands of dark signal intensity within the silicon gel.
- *C-sign.* This describes a localized separation of the fibrous capsule from the outer envelope of the implant.
- *Keyhole sign.*
- *Teardrop sign.* This sign occurs with a rupture of the envelope that separates the two lumina of a double-lumen implant. Since the contents of the inner and outer lumina (silicone gel and saline solution) do not mix, droplets of silicone gel are visualized within the saline solution or vice versa.

Two types of ruptures can occur: intracapsular and extracapsular rupture. The latter describes a rupture with extruded silicon gel seen outside the reactive fibrous capsule, while the former describes a rupture of the outer envelope of the implant only (see signs 1 – 3), with the silicone gel contained within the reactive fibrous capsule. Intracapsular ruptures must be distinguished from "sweating." Some (mostly older) implants release small amounts of silicone gel, which may become visible as a small rim of silicone gel between the fibrous capsule and the outer envelope of the implant, even without a rupture. This release of silicone gel is called "sweating." In general, the amount of silicone gel visible between the outer envelope and the fibrous capsule is smaller with sweating than with frank ruptures, but exact distinction may not be possible by imaging. A transudate between fibrous capsule and outer silicone envelope can be distinguished by the sufficiently different resonance frequencies with the use of sequences with selective silicone-suppression or water-suppression.

Patient Preparation

No special preparation is necessary for enhanced MR mammography. Patients are allowed to eat or drink. Only for patients with a known history of the rare allergic reaction to MR contrast agent, premedication need be considered.

The patient should be informed about the nature of the examination and be aware of the importance of not moving for the approximately 15 minutes it takes to perform the examination.

Manifestations of Different Breast Changes

Normal breast tissue, nonproliferative and *nonhyperplastic changes,* and, in part, even *proliferate changes* usually do not enhance after injection of contrast medium.

Since normal breast tissue may show nonspecific focal or diffuse enhancement in the first and third weeks of the menstrual cycle, it is recommended that the examination be performed in the second or third weeks of the cycle. Hormone replacement can induce enhancement in normal breast tissue, especially if high amounts of gestagens are included. Since this can lead to diagnostic problems, hormone administration should, if at all possible, be discontinued for 6 to 12 weeks before the MRI examination

Cysts do not enhance.

Scars do not enhance after they are completely fibrosed, which means three months after surgery or 12 to 18 months after radiation, and at that stage can easily be differentiated from malignant lesions.

Granulomas may enhance strongly, especially if active as in fresh *fat necroses.* It can be difficult to differentiate granulomas with early and focal enhancement from malignant lesions. Granulomas are mostly round and relatively smooth in outline, whereas fat necroses are irregularly outlined. However, granulomas that are fibrosed and inactive do not enhance.

Benign tumors, such as *fibroadenomas* or *papillomas,* fail to show any appreciable enhancement if they are completely sclerosed (especially in older women). Nonsclerosing benign tumors, however, can enhance both moderately to strongly and early or late, making it difficult to differentiate them from rare circumscribed malignancies (Fig. 7.**55**).

Inflammatory changes mostly enhance diffusely (an abscess focally) and late (seldom early).

Invasive carcinomas enhance with rare exceptions (caution is in order when dealing with lobular sclerotic malignancies or mucinous malignancies). In 85 – 90% of the cases, enhancement is fast and focal but, depending on the histology, can be diffuse (diffusely growing malignancies or malignancies surrounded by diffusely distributed benign proliferative or hyperplastic changes) and even late (for instance, medullary, tubular, or papillary carcinomas).

Ductal carcinoma in situ (DCIS) may show moderate to strong enhancement in 80 – 90% of the lesions. In about half of the them, the enhancement is diffuse or late, making it difficult to differentiate this enhancement from the enhancement seen in proliferative benign changes.

Therefore, enhanced MRI is not recommended for further evaluation of microcalcifications. Moreover, a biopsy remains necessary whenever mammography or clinical findings are suspicious for malignancy, particularly if MR mammography shows late or diffuse enhancement (Fig. 7.**55**).

Ruptures of silicon implants can be recognized by looking for the signs described above. MR mammogra-

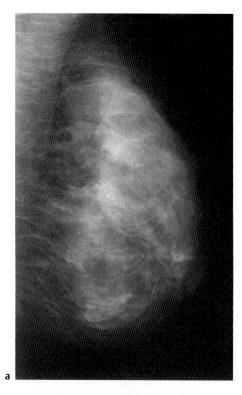

Fig. 7.55 a – d **Small palpable lump in the left breast in a 45-year-old woman**
a ML view of the left breast: no intramammary lesion visible. It is also not seen on the CC view. A few axillary lymph nodes are visible
b Sonography: a 6 mm hypoechoic lesion with acoustic shadowing
c, d MRI (Flash 3 D subtraction). Strong enhancement of area extending from thoracic wall to the mamilla: (**c**) transverse; (**d**) sagittal
Histology: IL covering an area of 9 cm

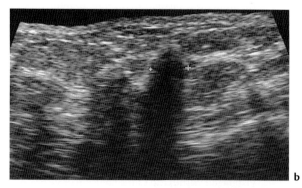

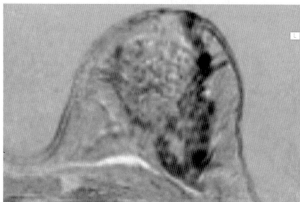

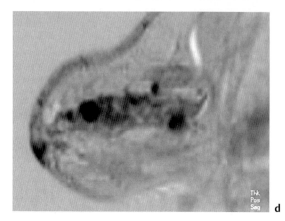

phy is very sensitive for detecting even small ruptures of the implant envelope with only minimal leakage of silicone gel. However, false positive and false negative findings are occasionally observed.

The clinical relevance of asymptomatic small ruptures is not clear at this moment. The formerly described adverse effects, such as headache, generalized autoimmune reaction, and connective disorder, could not be conclusively attributed to silicone since the same symptoms have been observed in a similar percentage of patients without silicone implants.

Indications

Enhanced MR mammography provides supplementary information when other methods are inconclusive in patients with increased risk of breast cancer and the following diagnostic problems:

- Extensive surgical scarring.
- Status following breast-conserving surgery and irradiation.
- Silicone implant in place.
- Search for a primary tumor in mammographically dense breasts (Fig. 7.**57**).
- Assessing multimodality and multicentricity and assessing the exact extent of the malignancy in dense breast tissue if breast-conserving surgery is planned.

The following indications are currently under investigation:

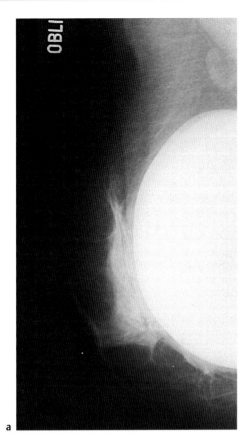

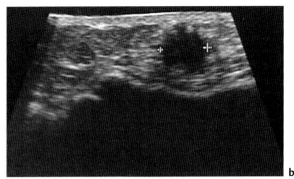

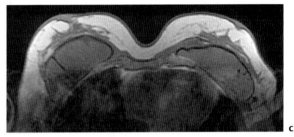

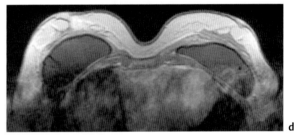

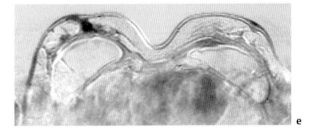

Fig. 7.56 a–e   A 44-year old woman with bilateral breast implants. A lump in the right breast was felt several days before the mammogram was performed
a ML view: subpectoral implant, no other changes
b Sonography: solid lesion, 1 cm in size. Granuloma? Malignancy?
c–e *MRI (MPR-3 D)*
c Before administration of contrast medium, retromammary tumor with low signal intensity
d After intravenous administration of Gd-DTPA, strong enhancement
e Subtraction image shows the lesion to better advantage
Histology: 1.8 cm ILC, 25 lymph nodes negative

- Detection or exclusion of malignancy in women with dense breast and increased risk of breast cancer (family history, genetic risk)
- Exclusion of a malignancy in the contralateral breast

Enhanced MR mammography is not indicated for the evaluation of microcalcifications (limited sensitivity for ductal carcinoma in situ, problems concerning differentiation of moderate enhancement). Furthermore, MR mammography is not recommended for the evaluation of benign changes with known enhancement, as found in fibroadenoma in young patients, inflammation, or proliferative changes, since a differentiation from malignancy is not possible.

Enhanced MR should not be used when a diagnosis can be made with a more cost-effective method. Dense breast tissue alone is not an indication for enhanced MRI. For inconclusive mammographic findings, ultrasound is the method of choice. Finally, enhanced MRI is not recommended during pregnancy or lactation since hormone-induced increased metabolism must be expected to cause diagnostically confusing enhancement.

Contraindications and Adverse Effects

Contraindications. MR mammography cannot be performed in patients with a pacemaker, intracerebral clips, magnetic foreign bodies, certain types of artificial cardiac valves, and electronic pumps.

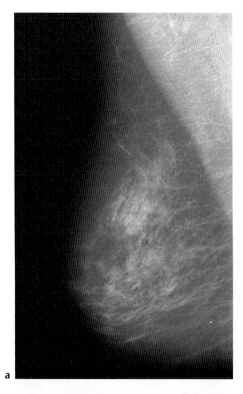

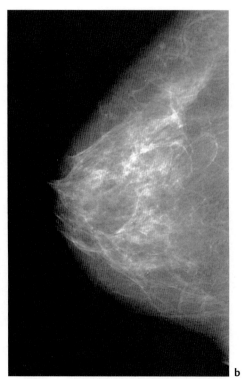

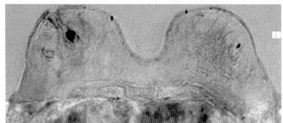

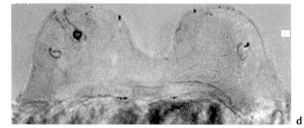

Fig. 7.**57 a – d**   **A 55-year-old woman with palpable axillary lymph nodes on the right**. Histology of axillary lymph node: metastases of adenocarcinoma
a, b *Mammography, right:*
a ML view of the right breast. Enlarged axillary lymph nodes, no intramammary lesion

b CC view of the right breast. No abnormality
c, d MRI (Flash-3 D, subtraction). Centrifugal enhancement of the lesion in the right breast
Histology: IDC

As long as patients with these contraindications are excluded, MR mammography can be expected to be free of any adverse effects.

Adverse effects. Adverse effects induced by the paramagnetic contrast medium are extremely rare, as supported by extensive data addressing the tolerance of Gd-DTPA. In spite of these data, Gd-DTPA should not be given to patients with severe hepatic or renal insufficiency.

In the very few patients known to have an allergy to Gd-DTPA, the indication must be critically reviewed and, if it has been decided to proceed, adequate prophylactic measures must be taken.

Conclusion

Contrast MR mammography offers new pathophysiological information not available with other methods and conceivably valuable in certain clinical problems. The technique for performing MRI and the guidelines for interpreting the findings are both still evolving. Understanding the method of MRI and knowing how to integrate MRI with conventional methods are necessary to optimize the diagnostic process, especially by avoiding false positive results and unnecessary biopsies. Contrast MR mammography should be used only if the complementary information can be expected to contribute to the diagnosis. If evaluation with conventional methods is limited, MRI can be expected to increase the accuracy.

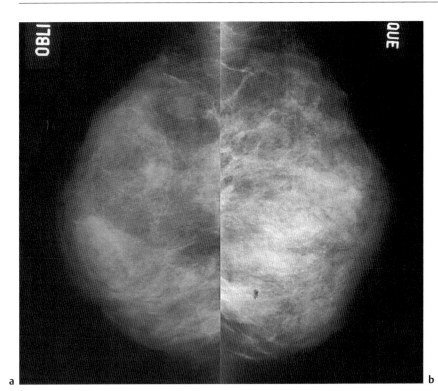

a

b

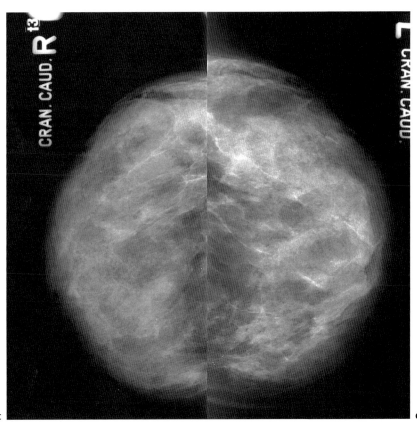

c

d

Fig. 7.**58 a – e**   **A 37-year-old woman without palpable breast lesion**. Family history of multiple premenopausal breast cancers

a – d ML and CC views show dense breasts. No lesion detectable. Because of the limited interpretation of the mammograms, MRI was performed

Fig. 7.**58 e** See next page

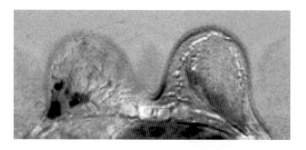

Fig. **7.58 e** MRI (Flash-3 D, subtraction). The right lower lateral quadrant shows multiple enhancing lesions (apparent skin thickening due to motion blurring)
Histology: IDC. Lymph nodes negative

Obsolete Methods

J. H. C. L. Hendriks

■ Transillumination

Passing (red) light through the breast is called diaphanoscopy or transillumination. On the basis of their neovascularity, cancers should absorb more light than normal breast tissue and appear as black shadows. In addition, very intense bright light has been used. This method has the following deficiencies:

- The breast cancer detection rate was not higher than 30–60%.
- The differentiation between cyst and solid lesion is far inferior to sonography.

In summary, this method should be rejected as a screening method for breast cancer and as a diagnostic method for further assessment of unclear findings. Neither electronic amplification nor computerization has brought any new justification for this method.

■ Thermography

Thermography visualizes the temperature of the body surface by measuring infrared radiation.

The infrared method uses *tele-thermography with a heat-sensitive camera* and *contact thermography* using a special plate placed on the breast.

The plate contains liquid crystals that emit light of different colors, with the difference in colors corresponding to the subtle difference in temperature.

The early reports on detecting and differentiating breast cancer by thermography were quite encouraging. Microcalcifications, however, were not imaged. Not all breast cancers emit heat, whereas some benign lesions do. Even when it was combined with physical breast examination, only half of all breast cancers were detected.

Thermography has not been proved to add information to radiographic mammography. With the advances of mammography, thermography has became obsolete as diagnostic procedure for the breast. Both its sensitivity and specificity are too low.

References

Magnification Mammography:

McSweeney, M. B., P. Sprawls, R. L. Egan: Magnification Mammography. Recent Results in Cancer Research, Vol. 90. Springer, Berlin 1984
Reuther, G., R. Hoffmann, B. Bier: Digitale Vergrößerungsmammographie. Radiologe 33 (1993) 260–266
Sickles, E. A.: Further experience with microfocal spot magnification mammography in the assessment of clustered breast microcalcifications. Radiology 137 (1980) 9–14
Teubner, J., J. Z. Lenk, K. U. Wentz, M. Georgi: Vergrößerungsmammographie mit 0,1 mm Mikrofokus. Radiologe 27 (1987) 155–164

Percutaneous Diagnostic Procedures, Preoperative Localization, and Specimen Radiography:

Azavedo, E., G. Auer, G. Svane: Stereotactic fine needle biopsy in 2594 mammographically detected non-palpable lesions. Lancet 13 (1989) 1033–1036
Ciatto, S., S. Catarzi, D. Morrone, M. Rosseli del Turco: Fine-needle aspiration cytology of non-palpable breast lesions: US versus stereotaxic guidance. Radiology 188 (1993) 195–198
Dronkers, D. J.: Stereotaxic core biopsy of breast lesions. Radiology 183 (1992) 631–634
Evans, W. P.: Stereotaxic fine needle aspiration and core biopsy. RSNA categorical course in breast imaging. RSNA, Oak Brook 1995 (pp. 151–160)
Fornage, B. D., J. D. Coan, C. L. David: Ultrasound guided needle biopsy of the breast and other interventional procedures. Radiol. Clin. N. Amer. 30 (1992) 167–185
Gordon, P. B., S. L. Goldenberg, N. H. L. Chan: Solid breast lesions: diagnosis with US-guided fine-needle aspiration biopsy. Radiology 189 (1993) 573–580
Harter, P. P., J. S. Curtis, G. Ponto, P. H. Craig: Malignant seeding of the needle track during stereotaxic core needle breast biopsy. Radiology 185 (1992) 713–714
Helvie, M. A., D. E. Baker, D. D. Adler, I. Andersson, B. Naylor, K. A. Buckwalter: Radiographically guided fine-needle aspiration of non-palpable breast lesions. Radiology 174 (1990) 657–661
Hendrick, R. E., S. H. Parker: Stereotaxic imaging. RSNA categorical course in physics. RSNA, Oak Brook 1994 (pp. 263–274)
Jackson, V. P., H. E. Reynolds: Stereotaxic needle-core biopsy and fine-needle aspiration cytologic evaluation of non-palpable breast lesions. Radiology 181 (1991) 633–634
Jackson, V. P.: Needle localization to guide excisional biopsy. RSNA categorical course in breast imaging. RSNA, Oak Brook 1995 (pp. 161–166)

Liberman, L., D. D. Dershaw, P. P. Rosen, A. F. Abramson, B. M. Deutsch, L. E. Hann: Stereotaxic 14-gauge breast biopsy: How many core biopsy specimens are needed? Radiology 192 (1994) 793–795

Liberman, L., W. Ph. Evans, D. D. Dershaw, L. E. Hann et al.: Radiography of microcalcifications in stereotaxic mammary core biopsy specimens. Radiology 190 (1994) 223–225

Liberman, L., D. D. Dershaw, P. P. Rosen, C. S. Giess et al.: Stereotaxic core biopsy of breast carcinoma: accuracy at predicting invasion. Radiology 194 (1995) 379–381

Löfgren, M., I. Andersson, L. Bondeson, K. Lindholm: X-ray guided fine-needle aspiration for the cytologic diagnosis of non-palpable breast lesions. Cancer 61 (1988) 1032–1037

Moritz, J. D., S. Luftner-Nagel, J. P. Westerhof, J. W. Oestmann, E. Grabbe: Microcalcifications in breast core biopsy specimens: disappearance at radiography after storage in formaldehyde. Radiology 200 (1996) 361–363

Parker, S. H., J. D. Lovin, W. E. Jobe, J. M. Luethke et al.: Stereotactic breast biopsy with a biopsy gun. Radiology 176 (1990) 741–747

Parker, S. H., J. D. Lovin, W. E. Jobe, B. J. Burke et al.: Non-palpable breast lesions: stereotactic automated large-core biopsies. Radiology 180 (1991) 403–407

Parker, S. H., W. E. Jobe, M. A. Dennis, A. T. Stavros et al.: US-guided automated large-core breast biopsy. Radiology 187 (1993) 507–511

Parker, S. H., F. Burbak, R. J. Jackman et al.: Percutaneous large-core breast biopsy; a multi-institutional study. Radiology 193 (1994) 359–364

Parker, S. H., M. A. Dennis, A. T. Stavros, K. K. Johnson: Ultrasound-guided mammotomy, a new breast biopsy technique. J. diagn. Med. Sonogr. 12 (1996) 113–118

Sickles, E. A.: Management of probably benign lesions. RSNA categorical course in breast imaging. RSNA, Oak Brook 1995 (pp. 133–138)

Galactography:

Cardenosa, G., C. Doudna, G. W. Eklund: Ductography of the breast: technique and findings. Amer. J. Roentgenol. 162 (1994) 1081–1087

Menges, V., A. Troxler, R. Stadelmann, W. Wirth: Galaktographie: Indikation und diagnostische Aussage. Fortschr. Röntgenstr. 120 (1974) 381–388

Tabár, L., P. B. Dean, Z. Pentek: Galactography: the diagnostic procedure of nipple discharge. Radiology 149 (1983) 31–38

Pneumocystography:

Cardenosa, G., G. W. Eklund: Interventional procedures in breast imaging (part II), ductography, cyst aspiration and pneumocystography and fine needle aspiration. In Taveras, J. M., J. T. Ferrucci: Radiology, Diagnosis, Imaging and Intervention. Lippincott, Philadelphia 1993

Hoeffken, W., C. Hintzen: Die Diagnostik der Mammazysten durch Mammographie und Pneumozystographie. Fortschr. Röntgenstr. 112 (1970) 9–18

Pentek, Z., I. Balogh, B. Bako: Maligne Papillomatose in einer riesigen Brustzyste. Fortschr. Röntgenstr. 120 (1974) 756–759

Tabár, L., Z. Pentek, P. B. Dean: The diagnostic and therapeutic value of breast cyst puncture and pneumocystography. Radiology 141 (1981) 659–663

Computed Tomography:

Chang, C. H. J., D. E. Nesbit, D. R. Fisher, S. L. Fritz et al.: Computed tomographic mammography using a conventional body scanner. Amer. J. Roentgenol. 138 (1982) 553–558

Kopans, D. B.: Computed breast tomography. In Kopans, B.: Breast Imaging. Lippincott, Philadelphia 1989 (pp. 312–319)

Sonography of the Breast:

Bassett, L. W., C. Kimme-Smith, L. K. Sutherland, R. H. Gold, D. Sarti, W. King: Automated and hand-held breast ultrasound: effect on patient management. Radiology 165 (1987) 103–108

Bassett, L. W., C. Kimme-Smith: Breast sonography: technique, equipment and normal anatomy. Semin. Ultrasound 10 (1989) 82–89

Cooperberg, P. L.: Artefacts in US. In Rifkin, M. D.: Special Course: Ultrasound 1991. Radiological Society of North America, Oak Brook 1991 (p. 57)

Cosgrove, D. O., R. P. Kedar, J. C. Bamber, B. Al-Murrani et al.: Breast diseases: color Doppler US in differential diagnosis. Radiology 189 (1993) 99–104

Feig, S. A.: Breast masses: mammographic and sonographic evaluation. Radiol. Clin. N. Amer. 30 (1992) 67–92

Jackson, V. P.: The current role of ultrasonography in breast imaging. Radiol. Clin. North Am. 33 (1995) 1161–1170

Kolb, T. M., L. Lichy, J. H. Newhouse: Occult cancer in women with dense breasts: detection with screening US—diagnostic yield and tumor characteristics. Radiology 207 (1998) 191–199

Liberman, L., C. S. Giess, D. D. Dershaw, D. C. Louie, B. M. Deutsch: Non-Hodgkin lymphoma of the breast: imaging characteristics and correlation with histopathologic findings. Radiology 192 (1994) 157–160

Shaw de Paredes, E., L. P. Marsteller, B. V. Eden: Breast cancers in women 35 years of age and younger: mammographic findings. Radiology 177 (1990) 117–119

Skaane, P., K. Engedal: Analysis of sonographic features in the differentiation of fibroadenoma and invasive ductal carcinoma. Am. J. Roentgenol. 170 (1998) 109–114

Stavros, A. T., D. Thickman, C. L. Rapp, M. A. Dennis, S. A. Parker, G. A. Sisney: Solid breast nodules: use of sonography to distinguish between benign and malignant lesions. Radiology 96 (1995) 123–134

Venta, L. A., C. M. Dudiak, C. G. Salomon, M. E. Flisak: Sonographic evaluation of the breast. Radiographics 14 (1994) 29–40

Zonderland, H. M., G. Coerkamp, J. Hermans, M. J. van de Vijver, A. E. van Voorthuisen: Diagnosis of breast cancer: contribution of US as an adjunct to mammography. Radiology 213 (1999) 412–422

Magnetic Resonance Imaging:

Beatty, S. M., S. G. Orel, M. D. Schnall et al.: MR imaging detection of occult breast carcinoma manifesting as axillary metastases. Radiology 201 (1996) (P) 129

Boetes, C., R. D. M. Mus, R. Holland, J. O. Barentsz et al.: Breast tumors: comparative accuracy of MR imaging relative to mammography and US for demonstrating extent. Radiology 197 (1995) 743–747

Boné, B., P. Aspelin, B. Isberg et al.: Contrast-enhanced MR imaging of the breast in patients with silicon implants after cancer surgery. Acta radiol. 36 (1995) 111–116

Die, van L. E., C. Boetes, J. O. Barentsz et al.: Additional value of MR imaging of the breast in women with pathologic axillary lymph nodes and normal mammograms. Radiology 201 (1996) (P) 241

Everson, L. I., H. Parantainen, T. Detlie et al.: Diagnosis of breast implant rupture: imaging findings and relative efficacies of imaging techniques. Amer. J. Roentgenol. 163 (1994) 57–60

Fischer, U., R. Vosshenrich, A. Probst et al.: Preoperative MR mammography in patients with breast cancer – useful information or useless extravagance? Fortschr. Röntgenstr. 161 (1994) 300–306

Gilles, R., J. M. Guinebretière, O. Lucidarme, P. Cluzel et al.: Non palpable breast tumors: diagnosis with contrast-enhanced subtraction dynamic MR imaging. Radiology 191 (1994) 625–631

Gilles, R., J. M. Guinbretière, L. G. Shapeero et al.: Assessment of breast cancer recurrence with contrast-enhanced subtraction MR imaging: preliminary results in 26 patients. Radiology 188 (1993) 473–478

Gorczyca, D. P., E. Scheider, N. D. DeBruhl, T. K. Foo et al.: Silicone breast implant rupture: comparison between three point Dixon and fast spin-echo MR imaging. Amer. J. Roentgenol. 162 (1994) 305–310

Harms, S. E.: MRI in breast cancer diagnosis and treatment. Curr. Probl. diagn. Radiol. 25 (1996) 193–215

Heinig, A., S. H. Heywang-Köbrunner, P. Viehweg: Wertigkeit der Kontrastmittelmagnetresonanztomographie der Mamma bei Wiederaufbau mittels Implantat. Radiologe 37 (1997) 710–717

Heywang-Köbrunner, S. H., R. Beck: Contrast-Enhanced MRI of the Breast. Springer, Berlin 1996

Heywang-Köbrunner, S. H., P. Viehweg, A. Heinig, Ch. Küchler: Contrast-enhanced MRI of the breast: accuracy, value, controversies, solutions. Europ. J. Radiol. 24 (1997) 94–108

Heywang-Köbrunner, S. H., H. D. Wolf, M. Deimling et al.: Misleading changes of the signal intensity on opposed phase MRI after injection of contrast medium. J. Comput. assist. Tomogr. 20 (1996) 173–178

Kuhl, C. K., H. B. Bieling, J. Gieseke et al.: Healthy premenopausal breast parenchyma in dynamic contrast-enhanced MR imaging of the breast: normal contrast-medium enhancement and cyclical-phase dependency. Radiology 203 (1997) 137–144

Monticciolo, D. L., R. C. Nelson, W. T. Dixon et al.: MR detection of leakage from silicone breast implants: value of silicone selective pulse sequence. Amer. J. Roentgenol. 163 (1994) 51–56

Morris, E. A., L. H. Schwartz, D. D. Dershaw et al.: Breast MR in patients with occult primary cancer. Radiology 201 (1996) (P) 129

Müller-Schimpfle, M., K. Ohmenhäuser, P. Stoll et al.: Menstrual cycle and age: influence on parenchymal contrast medium enhancement in MR imaging of the breast. Radiology 203 (1997) 145–149

Mumatz, H., M. A. Hall-Craggs, T. Davidson et al.: Staging of symptomatic primary breast cancer with MR imaging. Amer. J. Roentgenol. 169 (1997) 417–424

Oellinger, H., S. Heins, B. Sander et al.: Gd-DTPA enhanced MR of breast: the most sensitive method for detecting multicentric carcinomas in female breast? Europ. Radiol. 3 (1993) 223–226

Orel, S. G., M. D. Schnall, C. M. Powell et al.: Staging of suspected breast cancer. Effect of MR imaging and MR-guided biopsy. Radiology 156 (1995) 115–122

Orel, S. G., M. H. Mendonca, C. Reynolds et al.: MR imaging of ductal carcinoma in situ. Radiology 202 (1997) 413–420

Schulz-Wendtland, R., S. Krämer, K. Döinghaus et al.: MR mammography in the diagnosis of local recurrences in breast cancer. Europ. J. Radiol. 7, Suppl. (1997) Poster 243

Soderstrom, C. E., S. E. Harms, D. S. Copit et al.: Three-dimensional RODEO breast MR imaging of lesions containing ductal carcinoma in situ. Radiology 201 (1996) 427–432

Obsolete Methods:

American College of Radiology: College policy reviews use of thermography. Amer. Coll. Radiol. Bull. 40 (1984) 13

Bartum, R. J. Jr., H. C. Crow: Transillumination light-scanning to diagnose breast cancer: a feasibility study. Amer. J. Roentgenol. 142 (1984) 409–414

Gautherie, M., C. M. Gros: Breast thermography and cancer risk prediction. Cancer 45 (1980) 51–56

Gros, Ch. M.: Les maladies du sein. La transillumination. Masson, Paris 1963 (pp. 260–262)

Gros, C., M. Gautherie, P. Bourjat: Prognosis and posttherapeutic follow-up of breast cancers by thermography. Bibl. radiol. 6 (1975) 77–90

Moskowitz, M., S. H. Fox, R. Brun del Re, J. R. Miller et al.: The potential value of liquid-crystal thermography in detecting significant mastopathy. Radiology 140 (1981) 659–662

Sickles, E. A.: Breast cancer detection with transillumination and mammography. Amer. J. Roentgenol. 142 (1984) 841–844

Threatt, B., J. M. Norbeck, N. S. Ullman, R. Kummer, P. F. Roselle: Thermography and breast cancer: an analysis of a blind reading. Ann. N.Y. Acad. Sci. 335 (1980) 501–509

8 Mammographic Findings and Their Interpretation

Strategy for Viewing the Mammogram

Petra A. M. Bun

Recognizing any major change on a mammogram presents no difficulty to the experienced radiologist. Detecting subtle changes to keep the number of false negative diagnoses low requires a systematic approach to viewing the mammogram. Furthermore, more than one abnormality might be present and, after finding one, the additional abnormalities elsewhere in the same or in the other breast are easily overlooked (the so-called "happy eye phenomenon").

A systematic approach with a consistent viewing order is recommended when reading mammograms.

Hanging the Films on the Viewbox

The mammograms should be hung conforming to a consistent format. The room lights should be dimmed to prevent interfering reflections of ambient light.

Normally, both breasts show a symmetric distribution of the glandular tissue. This should be taken advantage of by hanging the matched oblique and CC views of the breasts back to back as mirror images. The image of the left breast is placed on the right and that of the right breast on the left side, as if the observer were facing the patients, which is the customary arrangement for viewing radiographic images.

The images should be properly masked to eliminate any glare from extraneous light. This helps the assessment of the periphery of the breast and also improves perception of low-contrast abnormalities.

The following patient data should be verified:

- Correct name
- Date of birth
- Date of examination

It is important to know the patient's age when analyzing any mammographic changes.

The films should be marked right or left; cranial should be clearly identified on the oblique views, and lateral or medial on the CC views.

Previous Mammograms for Comparison

The patient's preceding mammogram is crucial in tracing subtle changes and should be hung the same way as the current mammogram. If even earlier mammograms are available, they also should be included in the analysis. Minor changes might only become evident after longer intervals.

In general, comparison is confined to the most recent previous mammogram. The old oblique and CC views are best placed above and not adjacent to the corresponding images of the current mammogram. This quadratic arrangement of the images offers the advantage of comparing the mammograms at a glance.

Viewing the Mammogram

Assessing the technical quality. Before analyzing the mammogram, it should be verified whether positioning and exposure are adequate. Suboptimal positioning due to the patient's condition (e.g., thorax deformity, frozen shoulder, breast implants, pacemaker) should be noted by the radiographer.

Many modern units record the exposure parameters while the mammographic films are taken. This is essential for good reproducibility of subsequent mammograms.

Classifying the analyzability of the mammogram. The analyzability of an optimal mammogram depends on the ratio of glandular to adipose tissue. Changes are easier to detect in a breast almost entirely consisting of fat than in a breast filled with glandular tissue. The glandular tissue generally undergoes involution with advancing age. Classifying the analyzability of the mammograms as good, moderate or bad implies the confidence level of the reading.

Symmetry. Comparing both breasts for symmetry makes it easier to detect changes. The following should be kept in mind when assessing the parenchyma:

- Asymmetry of the amount of glandular tissue as a normal variant. Well-known normal variants, which may appear on both sides, are:
  - axillary ectopic glandular tissue, corresponding to the so-called first breast anlage,
  - mediocaudal ectopic glandular tissue, corresponding to the so-called third breast anlage, sometimes with its own nipple visible upon inspection of the breast (see embryology, milk line).

Procedure. First, the images are observed from a distance, to look for any major asymmetries. Major changes should not be missed. The masking method is helpful in disclosing more subtle asymmetries: corresponding parts of both breasts are covered or their block-out imagined. Successive strips are made visible in horizontal or oblique direction, enabling the comparison of small symmetric zones with each other.

To a certain degree, a magnifying glass can have the same effect since only part of the breasts is seen when looking through it.

As a normal variant, one breast can have more glandular tissue than the other breast, with a difference in compressibility of the breasts and ensuing difference in mammographic density of the glandular tissue. It must be ascertained, however, that such a difference is only caused by an unequal amount of glandular tissue and not by any other components. This means that the architecture of the parenchyma and distribution of the adipose tissue must be comparable and the trabecular pattern unaltered.

Asymmetry associated with clinical symptoms, such as a palpable abnormality or pain, requires further analysis.

Asymmetric densities may indicate a benign or malignant change:

- *Focally asymmetric density in glandular tissue*: This can be seen in both projections and is more or less demarcated from surrounding structures. The density is not diffuse, but shows a dense center and gradually decreases toward the periphery.
  Common tumor-bearing sites, e.g., upper outer quadrant or retromamillary area require special attention.
- *Focally asymmetric density outside glandular tissue*: Care must be taken to analyze not only the glandular tissue, but also areas of glandular tissue replaced by fat. Above all, this applies to the axillary area, which can bear normal or pathologically enlarged lymph nodes as well as primary malignancies.
  Usually a rim of fatty tissue of variable width is interposed between the glandular cone and thorax wall, to be carefully scrutinized for densities. This applies to the zone along the anterior border of the pectoralis muscle on the oblique and CC views.
- *Asymmetric distortion or retraction of the parenchyma itself or its contours:* The breast tissue is evenly distributed along the lactiferous ducts that converge toward the nipple. They are crossed by the curvilinear Cooper bands, causing a wavy parenchymal contour where they extend into the overlying subcutaneous tissues. Distortion of this normal pattern, e.g., retraction, interruption or straightening of these lines, requires further analysis and must be explained. Sometimes, these changes are apparent on one view only. If they cannot be confirmed on images in a different projection and on additional images obtained at slight angulation, they can be presumed to be caused by superimposition or summation. Unless this is the site of previous surgery, any changes found to be three-dimensional requires a biopsy.
  Along the parenchymal contour, an architectural distortion may also represent a local contraction of structures arising eccentrically from the mamillary region or an inward contraction of the contour induced by a deeply seated malignancy. This causes the so-called "tent sign" along the dorsal surface of the parenchyma. It usually is visible in one view only and often obscured by normal glandular tissue.
- *Asymmetrically prominent lactiferous ducts:* This usually is a normal variant, unless associated with palpable changes or signs of malignancy, such as microcalcifications.
- *Asymmetric vessels*: The intramammary vessels normally are symmetric as to size and distribution. Sometimes, arteries can be distinguished from veins

by mural calcifications and a narrower diameter. Diffusely dilated veins on one or both sides may indicate cardiac decompensation. A single dilated vein is uncommon and usually a normal variant or possibly caused by difference in compression. Only rarely does this indicate malignancy or inflammation.
- *Asymmetry of the skin and subcutaneous tissues:* Bilateral or unilateral skin thickening of the entire breast may indicate systemic disease, e.g., edema due to cardiac decompensation. However, unilateral skin thickening, especially with a local component, may be a secondary sign of malignancy in the breast (see p. 215)
  Before calling such changes or even subcutaneous changes (e.g., an indistinct interface between skin and subcutaneous fat) pathological, it must be established whether they are actually unilateral or local.

Calcifications. After review of the images for analyzing densities, the entire breast must be scrutinized for calcifications with a magnifying glass, with special attention to groups of calcifications. Adequate magnification is essential to avoid missing very small calcifications.

All phases of this part of the examination must be completed, even after an abnormality has been found. The abnormality may be different in either breast. The additional value of the mammogram may be the detection of a simultaneous, clinically occult and curable lesion.

After passing through each of the above-mentioned phases step by step, the areas found to contain changes shall be analyzed a second time before entering the interpretation phase. By doing this, less striking changes may be found and the various already detected changes (e.g., a density with microcalcifications, parenchymal distortions, pathological lymph nodes or local skin thickening) can be linked together.

With experience, this can be done more or less simultaneously.

Interpretation Phase

Further Analysis of the Changes

After a change has been detected, the following questions should be addressed:

- *Is the change really in the breast or in or on the skin?* This can be answered by inspecting the skin and, if necessary, by an additional, usually tangential image with or without lead marker placed on the skin. A wart causing a density in projection of the breast can be recognized by its typical cauliflower-like appearance, accentuated by the surrounding air. Groups of skin calcifications, zinc ointment, talcum powder or tattoos are sometimes difficult to be recognized as such without additional images.
- *Is the change real or coincidental due to superimposition?*

Occasionally, the outline of a change may be more apparent in one than in another view, e.g., a radial scar or a surgical scar. A "tent sign" in one view is always suspicious. A malignancy appears as asymmetric density in the other projection. An additional image obtained at a slightly different projection than the original projection that detected the abnormality may provide the answer. If this additional view fails to show the abnormality, superimposition appears to be the likely cause. Frequently, it becomes necessary to obtain a spot-compression magnification view to confirm or exclude an abnormality. If a palpable finding is absent and the mammographic finding corresponds to normal glandular tissue, the examination is completed.

If palpation of the glandular tissue raises any doubt, a breast ultrasound may provide help.

Mammographic changes found to be real and located in the breast are classified into one of the following groups:

- Circumscribed densities
- Stellate densities
- Calcifications (micro- and macrocalcifications)
- Distortion of the architecture and asymmetry
- Changes of the skin (thickened skin syndrome)
- Lymph nodes
- A combination of two or more of the above changes

The diagnostic investigation of these changes continues in context with the clinical findings, including additional spot-compression magnification views, sonography, aspiration etc.

Clinical Context

For the interpretation of the changes it is necessary to learn about the patient. Many questions have come up already when a change is discovered in the interpretation phase:

- *What is the patient's age?*
  A relatively benign appearing lesion detected on the mammogram of a postmenopausal patient is much more suspicious for malignancy than in a young woman, especially if it is new or has grown.
- *Is the patient on hormone replacement or on other medication?*
  This may explain a diffuse growth of glandular tissue, together with an increasing size of benign densities (cysts). A unilateral growth in post-menopausal women not taking any hormones is suspicious for malignancy.
- *Did the patient undergo surgery or radiotherapy?*
  Changes showing the feature of a scar can be attributed to a scar if they correspond to a scar clinically. The same applies to any diffuse architectural distortion. Radiotherapy can induce a diffuse increase in glandular density or local/diffuse skin thickening. Naturally, these changes should only shrink with time. Any progression is suspicious for malignancy.

- *Are there any skin changes which may explain the mammographic changes?*
  It must be determined whether the changes on the mammogram coincide with the changes of the skin (see p. 215).
- *Are there any risk factors?*
  Risk factors, such as positive family history and former malignancy in the same or other breast, make certain changes more suspicious and should increase the alertness when scrutinizing both breasts.
- *Is there a palpable finding?*
  A palpable finding may explain the abnormality found on the mammogram. It is mandatory to correlate the palpable finding with the mammographic finding. A lesion located in the upper half of the breast may project in the center or even the lower half of the breast on the oblique mammographic view. Repeat imaging after the palpable change has been marked with a lead marker may provide the answer, though most cases must undergo sonography for clarification.

Analyzing the mammogram based on the indication for the examination leads to the following questions:

From a clinical point of view:

- Does the patient have any complaints or symptoms or is it a screening examination, possibly because of risk factors?
- Are there any complaints or symptoms such as a palpable findings? Is this area sufficiently visualized or are additional mammographic views required, such as a "Cleopatra view," a lateromedial or mediolateral view, or a spot-compression magnification view?
- Does the mammogram explain the complaints or are additional diagnostic steps required? A conventional mammogram may be sufficient to evaluate pain. A palpable finding, however, requires further evaluation until a conclusive explanation has been found. Sonography is the first additional examination to be performed for a palpable finding.

From a mammographic point of view after an abnormality was detected on the mammogram:

- Does the detected change explain the symptoms?
- Is this an accidental finding unrelated to the patient's complaints and symptoms? In this case, the finding has the same significance as if it were detected by screening mammography.
- Is there more than one abnormality? What is the mammographic group? Is it a multifocal process or part of a diffuse process?

When analyzing the changes, the effect of the diagnosis on the treatment should be considered. The decision whether the patient may have breast-conservation therapy or total mastectomy should be made jointly by radiologists, surgeons and radiotherapists.

Circumscribed Lesions

J.W.Th. Muller

Eccentrically located lesions might be visible in one projection only.

> **Classification of circumscribed densities**
>
> - Nodular lesions,
> - Stellate lesions

Optimal evaluation requires two mammographic views in different projections, sometimes supplemented by spot-magnification views. Plain mammography cannot differentiate between solid and cystic lesions. This is only possible by adding other methods such as sonography or aspiration. A cyst aspiration immediately before mammography may change the mammographic finding, interfering with the interpretation. This also applies to sonography performed after puncture of the breast.

■ Nodular Lesions

The following factors are substantial for the diagnostic evaluation of nodular lesions (Fig. 8.**1**):

Margin

The margin provides the most important criterion for the differentiation between malignant and benign. A nodular density with an entirely or partially ill-defined margin is suspicious for malignancy, especially when spicules are present. The margin of benign lesions is generally smooth and well-defined.

There are exceptions, however. Small ductal carcinomas may present as small, well-defined round lesions. Furthermore, the infrequent mucinous carcinoma may exhibit a sharp margin. In contrast, superimposed structures, such as trabeculae, ducts or vessels, might make a well-defined margin appear locally ill-defined.

Density

Most nodular lesions are radiopaque. Compared with the surrounding breast tissue, the lesion may be hypodense, isodense or hyperdense. Many malignant lesions are hyperdense, but some can be isodense. Evaluating the nature of the tumor on the basis of its density alone is limited.

Circumscribed radiolucent lesions consist of fat and are generally benign. This also applies to mixed lesions that are partly radiolucent and partly radiopaque.

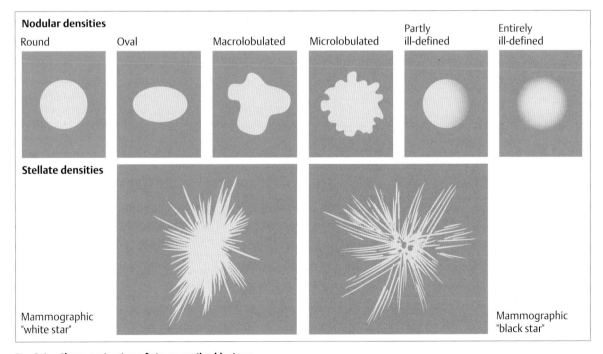

Fig. 8.**1**   **Characterization of circumscribed lesions**

Shape

The shape of nodular lesions varies from round to oval. Fibroadenomas may be coarse-lobulated. Coarse lobulation generally indicates a benign lesion, while fine lobulation is suspicious for malignancy. Cysts with low fluid tension are usually oval. Occasionally, band-like densities may be caused by prominent ducts and intraductal cancer.

Size

The size of a lesion generally does not imply the nature of the lesion, with a few exceptions. A large, well-defined lesion suggests a giant fibroadenoma, phyllodes tumor, sarcoma or cyst. Furthermore, a medullary carcinoma may have reached a large size when first detected.

The radiolucent lipoma can be very large, also the typical mixed radiolucent/radiodense fibroadenolipoma. Whether a lesion is palpable or not depends not only on size and consistency of the tumor but also on the size and the consistency of the breast. Most palpable breast tumors are larger than 1.5 cm.

Location

Malignant and benign tumors can appear anywhere in the breast. Most breast cancers, however, are located in the upper outer quadrant and, less frequently, in the retromamillary area, where they are difficult to see. A carcinoma may also be located along the periphery of the glandular cone or in an area with fatty involution (Fig. 6.17).

Spatial Orientation

According to Tabár and Dean, alignment of oval tumors along the normal trabecular structure of the breast favors a benign process while orientation at random suggests malignancy.

Multiplicity

Both benign and malignant lesions may occur multiple, even bilaterally.

About 1–2% of breast cancers are bilateral when detected. In essence, breast cancer is a unilateral, segmental disease. Within an affected segment, the carcinoma may be unifocal or multifocal. In foci smaller than 5 mm, multifocality may be undetectable by mammography. Other foci may escape detection despite their size.

Age

Breast tumors in women may appear at any age. Breast cancer is very rare under the age of 25. Breast cancer incidence increases with age.

Fibroadenomas occur mainly in the second and third decade of life and become less frequent at a higher age.

Cysts are predominantly seen between the age of 30 and 50 years.

If a nodular lesion or its vicinity contains microcalcifications with a malignant aspect, the lesion itself must be considered malignant, independent of its contour. Fibroadenomas typically contain characteristic coarse calcifications (p. 204).

A number of nodular lesions are difficult to classify, despite good assessment according to the above mentioned criteria. The radiologist must always keep in mind that nodular lesions, especially when they are new or growing, may represent a carcinoma.

■ Nodular Lesions with Well-defined Margins

Diagnostics and Incidence

A sharp margin generally suggests a benign lesion. The sharp edge of the tumor can be accentuated by a small radiolucent halo representing compressed fat. It has been shown that in particular growing benign and malignant tumors exhibit a more distinct halo. In the past, the halo was attributed to the Mach effect. The halo itself is generally considered a sign of benignity. Small, well-defined lesions occur frequently. Stomper et al. (1991) noticed small, well-defined lesions in 7% of the cases undergoing mammography screening. To avoid unnecessary biopsies, it is necessary to recognize benign densities. Most small, well-defined lesions represent cysts or fibroadenomas.

Cysts. A cyst is usually a distended TDLU, explaining its smooth inner wall. When the fluid tension within the cyst is high the cyst generally is round, while a cyst with a lower fluid tension may be oval. Cysts are often multilocular and appear macrolobulated on mammograms. They are mostly multifocal and bilateral, can be asymptomatic and remain unchanged over many years. Cysts may spontaneously regress or recur. Curvilinear calcification can develop in the wall of larger cysts. Before the introduction of sonography, it was common to aspirate cysts and fill them with air to exclude possible intracystic proliferations (so-called pneumocystography) (p. 148). The sonographic criteria (smooth margin, anechoic with an increased reflection from the posterior wall and enhanced sound transmission) are sufficient to determine whether it is a simple cyst without any intracystic proliferation. Multiple, small cysts (microcysts) produce a fine nodular pattern on the mammogram (p. 17).

Fibroadenomas. A fibroadenoma is a local fibroepithelial proliferation. As fibroadenomas mainly arise in the second and third decades of life when sonography is performed more often than mammography, they are often diagnosed by sonography. The shape of the fibroadenoma is variable. It frequently is round, but can be oval or macrolobulated. Degeneration produces typical coarse calcifications (Fig. 8.**22**), but can lead to completely calcified fibroadenomas. Some fibroadenomas may undergo hyalinization, which can induce indistinctness and even spiculation of their margins, making it impossible to distinguish them from a carcinoma. Fibroadenomas vary in size. The giant fibroadenoma (Fig. 3.**6**) and the benign phyllodes tumor are fast growing tumors, often accompanied by internal hemorrhage and cystic degeneration. Mammographically, both tumors present as smoothly marginated, often deeply lobulated density. Sonography shows a well-defined solid lesion (p. 156 and Fig. 7.**39**) that can contain cysts or cystlike lesions. The phyllodes tumor has a malignant variant (see p. 20).

Carcinomas. Only a few sharply marginated lesions are malignant, for instance the intracystic carcinoma. Moreover, a small carcinoma may still have an nearly well-defined margin (Fig. 8.**2**). Some types of breast cancer, like medullary and mucous cancer, may also exhibit a more or less well-defined margin and appear mammographically benign. The *medullary cancer* largely constitutes a homogeneous mass with lymphocytic infiltrates and a more expansile than infiltrative growth pattern. The *mucinous* or *colloid carcinoma* mostly consists of mucin collections around clusters of mucin-producing tumor cells and frequently is less dense. The mucinous carcinoma also shows a predominantly expansile rather than infiltrative growth pattern. Their resemblance of this category of carcinoma to benign tumors give rise to differential diagnostic problems.

DCIS can mammographically present as nodular lesion without microcalcifications. A relatively well-defined margin is found in 5% of these lesions. Malignancy can only be excluded histologically. Moreover, *metastases* and *lymphoma* may emerge in the breast as tumors with mammographically benign features. In the axillary region, round lesions with a smooth margin raise the possibility of nodal metastases or lymphoma. It is extremely rare for the breast to harbor metastases from tumors arising in other organs. If they occur, they appear as rather dense lesions with a sharp margin and are indistinguishable from fibroadenomas or cysts. A *malignant lymphoma* in the breast is also rare and appears as nodular or lobulated lesion with sharp margins. Even though a lesion with sharp margins only occasionally turns out be malignant, such a nodular lesion,

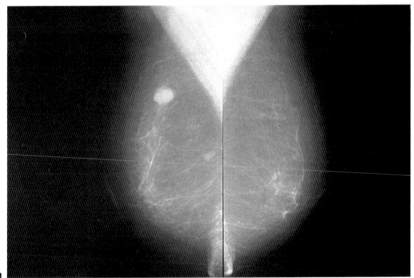

a

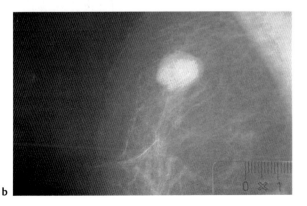

b

Fig. 8.**2 a, b** **Relatively smoothly marginated round density on the right**
a MLO view
b Detail of (**a**)
Histology: IDC with a diameter of 12 mm; negative lymph nodes

especially when found in screening mammography and growing, must always be viewed with suspicion.

Papillomas. An intraductal papilloma is a benign proliferation within the lumen of a lactiferous duct. It generally is nonpalpable and presents clinically as serous or sanguine discharge. If the papilloma does not cast a density on the mammograms, it is only detectable by galactography as intraductal filling defect. Larger papillomas become visible as density that lacks specific features and cannot be distinguished from other benign lesions. The location may help since most papillomas occur in the retromamillary area, where they are seen as oval or lobulated lesions aligned with the structures converging toward the nipple. A papilloma can also develop in a cyst and is as intracystic lesion mammographically indistinguishable from the cyst itself. Sonography can delineate intracystic papillomas. Hemorrhagic discharge indicates that the cyst containing the papilloma communicates with one of the ducts. Papillomas can be solitary or multiple as papillomatosis. The mammographic feature of papillomatosis is a beadlike density and its differentiation from a longitudinal intraductal carcinoma can be difficult. Papilloma may show typical calcifications (Fig. 8.**24**).

Lesions composed entirely or partly of fat:
- *Lipoma*: A lipoma is a usually slowly growing solitary tumor of fat tissue (Fig. 8.**3**) and may be difficult to detect amidst the fat tissue of involuted breasts. It is round or oval and frequently encapsulated by a thin layer of connective tissue, which is seen as a delicate rim around the fat-containing lesion. The lipoma must be differentiated from normal fat tissue that is partly traversed by trabecular structures.
- *Fibroadenolipoma* (*FAL, adenolipoma*): The fibroadenolipoma (Fig. 8.**4**) is also known as hamartoma. It feels like a large soft lump, often defying exact delineation. Its well-defined capsule of connective tissue surrounds fat tissue encompassing areas of fibroglandular tissue. It may be traversed by internal septa and sometimes contains coarse calcifications. Its mammographic appearance is characteristic and surgical incision is not indicated. It seems to arise more frequently in areas where ectopic glandular tissue is prevalent, i.e., upper outer and inner lower aspect of the breast.
- *Oil cyst:* The oil cyst is a type of fat necrosis, mainly resulting from trauma (surgery). The development of oil cysts is characterized by the local destruction of fat cells and release of viscous lipids, explaining the oil-like material found in the central cavity. The radiolucent center is surrounded by a thin capsule, which frequently calcifies resulting in the typical image of a calcified fat necrosis (liponecrosis calcificans macrocystica or microcystica).
- *Lymph nodes* (p. 217): Lymph nodes are seen on most mammograms in the axillary region, but can also be intramammary in location. A lymph node is a nodular

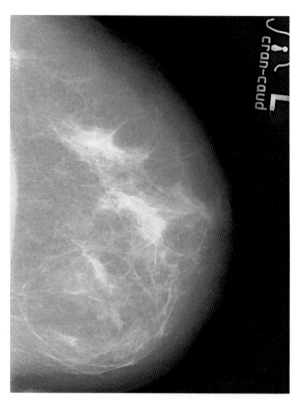

Fig. 8.**3**   **Large round lesion with a thin capsule, typical of a lipoma**

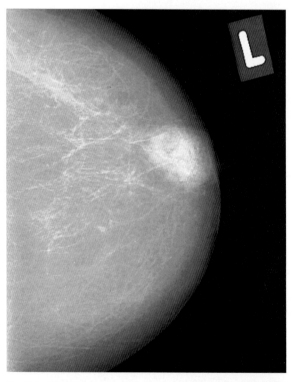

Fig. 8.**4**   **Nodular lesion with central radiolucency due to fat tissue** (42-year-old woman). Histology: Fibroadenolipoma

density characterized by a fatty hilus seen as typical central radiolucency in the tangential projection. Lymph nodes without fat cannot be differentiated from cysts, fibroadenomas, or even carcinomas.

- *Galactocele:* A galactocele develops during lactation and is actually a cyst filled with milky fluid. Depending on the composition of its content, the galactocele is radiopaque or radiolucent, sometimes even containing calcium particles. It is best diagnosed by sonography. It may be hyperechoic because of its high fat content.

Pseudo-lesions. Lesions seen on mammograms may also be pseudo-lesions, representing superimposed extramammary lesions on the skin, such as warts, nevi, fibromas, papillomas, and sebaceous cysts.

▣ Nodular Lesions with Ill-defined Margin

Lesions with ill-defined margins are often malignant. Early breast cancer, however, may present as small nodular density with well-defined margins (Fig. 8.**5**) without spicules. Unrestrained proliferation of cells in an irregular directional pattern make the margin of the lesion ill-defined, though differentiation from benign

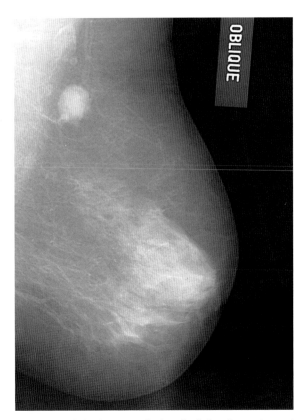

Fig. 8.5 Nodular lesion with sharply-defined margins and small satellite focus. In addition, fatty involuted lymph nodes of varying sizes. Histology: IDC with a diameter of 17 mm; all axillary lymph nodes negative

tumors may be difficult in the early stage. With continuing growth, the blurring of the margin may increase and the center of the lesion may become quite dense. The lesion may assume a bizarre contour. Short spicules with a broad basis represent infiltration of the tumor into adjacent normal tissue (Fig. 8.**6**).

Benign-appearing macrocalcifications in a lesion with ill-defined margins raise a differential diagnostic problem. They may indicate a hyalinized fibroadenoma, but can also develop in a carcinoma. Therefore, histological analysis is always necessary.

In fatty involuted breasts, nodular lesions with a diameter of about 0.5 cm are generally clearly visible on a mammogram. Before menopause, the superimposing normal glandular structures interfere with the detection of such lesions. Mild or advanced fibrocystic disease (mastopathy) worsens the situation. Fibrocystic disease can be likened to dense fog obscuring the contours of objects. Spot-magnification views are essential to gain additional information. A solitary lesion can exhibit secondary malignant features, such as local retraction of the glandular tissue and thickening and retraction of the skin, revealing the true character of the lesion.

In addition to presenting as solitary nodular or stellate lesion, breast cancer can also manifest itself as architectural distortion of glandular structures or as asymmetry. When the tumor has the same density as the surrounding breast tissue, it may remain mammographically invisible (radiologically occult tumor). Invasive lobular cancer (ILC) is notorious for this phenomenon. Asymmetry of the glandular structures might be the only sign of the presence of an ILC. The development of asymmetry in a previously normal mammogram is especially suspicious, even more so when associated with a local increase in density.

Some small carcinomas cannot be differentiated from vague ill-defined densities of less than 1 cm (so-called minimal signs, pp. 245 – 247). This explains why small carcinomas may escape mammographic detection. Another cause for missing small carcinomas is their localization: retromamillar in dense structures, posterior to the visible glandular tissue or in the axillary region.

Differential Diagnosis

Not all lesions with an ill-defined margin are cancers. Some lesions can be classified as probably benign with the differential diagnosis based on clinical history or findings.

Hematoma. A hematoma may develop after trauma or surgery, but may also arise spontaneously in women on anticoagulation therapy. Mammographically, a hematoma generally appears as an ill-defined density, initially without calcifications. Most hematomas resolve within several weeks. Some resolving hematomas develop a central radiolucency, indicating the formation of an oil cyst, or a fat necrosis with calcifications. They may be-

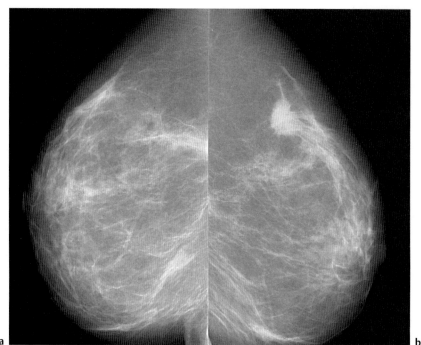

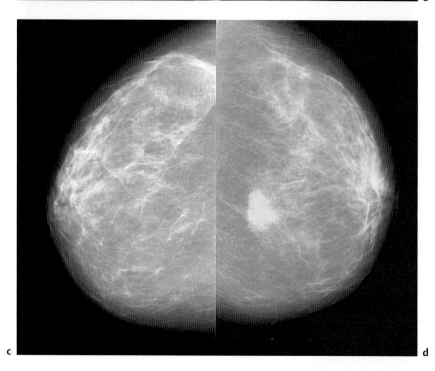

Fig. 8.**6a–d   Nodular density in the left breast with small spicules** (49-year-old woman with palpable tumor
a, b MLO views
c, d CC views
Histology: IDC with a diameter of 19 mm; axillary lymph nodes negative

come fibrotic, producing a stellate lesion (p. 222). A hematoma after lumpectomy for cancer requires careful mammographic follow-up, not only to document resolution, but also to detect early any possible tumor recurrence. Fibrosed hematoma and recurrent carcinoma may have identical mammographic features.

Abscess. The ill-defined density of an abscess is often mammographically indistinguishable from a cancer. In most cases, the clinical diagnosis is obvious. A painful swelling with erythema develops within short period of time. Sonography and aspiration confirm the diagnosis.

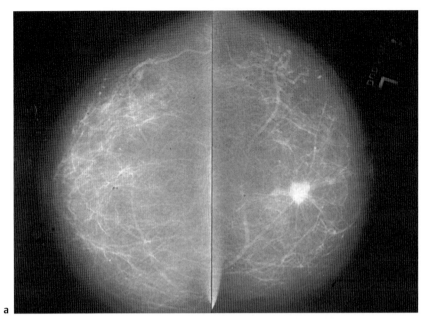

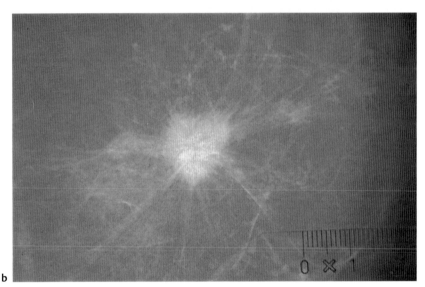

Fig. 8.**7 a, b   Nodular lesion with spicules in the left breast**
a CC views
b Detail from (**a**)
Histology: IDC with a diameter of 10 mm; axillary lymph nodes positive

■ Stellate Lesions

No principal difference exists between ill-defined nodular lesions with spiculated margins and stellate lesions (Fig. 8.**7**).

A lesion with spicules longer than the diameter of its central density is referred to as stellate lesion (Fig. 8.**8**). Breast cancer frequently presents as stellate structure, the so-called scirrhus.

The central density plays a critical role in the analysis of stellate lesions. In the early phase, the tumor might be so small that the spicules are barely discernible. Targeted spot-magnification views in two projections are essential. In the later phase, central density and spicules enlarge and become better discernible (Figs. 8.**9** and 8.**10**).

The length of the spicules varies strongly, and a direct relationship between the diameter of the tumor and the length of the spicules might not exist. The spicules represent a fibrotic reaction of the adjacent breast tissue to the carcinoma. This so-called *desmoplastic reaction* consists of connective tissue proliferation as a defense against the tumor cells. A strong desmoplastic reaction, therefore, might be considered a favorable prognostic sign. In a more advanced stage, however, tumor cells can be found in the spicules.

Roebuck (1990) makes a distinction between spicules and tentacles. Spicules are short and broadbased at the tumor margin, possibly representing tumor infiltration into adjacent breast tissue. Tentacles are longer and evenly thin along their entire length. They more likely manifest a desmoplastic reaction.

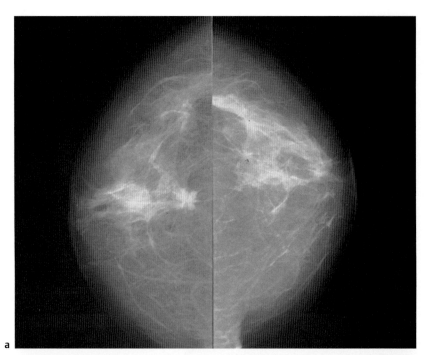

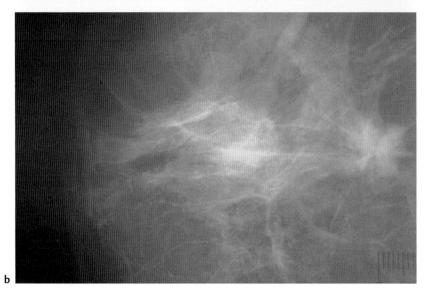

Fig. 8.**8 a, b**   **Stellate lesion in the right breast**
a CC views
b Detail from (**a**)
   Histology: IDC with a diameter of 10 mm, axillary lymph nodes negative

The spicules of stellate cancers may reach the skin or mamilla (skin thickening caused by local edema, mamillary retraction).

Stellate lesions may lack a distinct central mass. Such lesions often contain small central radiolucencies, which can assume a linear appearance. The spicules usually begin as bundles and then diverge into different directions, casting the picture of the so-called *radial scar*. This is also known as benign sclerosing ductal proliferation (Figs. 8.**38** and 8.**39**) and is encountered on screening mammograms as an incidental nonpalpable finding. Biopsy is indicated since its differentiation from breast cancer is difficult or even impossible (p. 19).

Other benign stellate lesions include surgical scar, hyalinized fibroadenoma and fibrosed fat necrosis (for instance, after surgical excision). Mammographically, skin retraction is often seen near the lesion.

■ Mammographically Occult Cancers

Some palpable and nonpalpable cancers have the same density as breast tissue. Unless they induce any secondary findings, these cancers are barely or not at all visible by mammography (Fig. 8.**12**), especially if located within breast parenchyma (Fig. 8.**13**), but even if they are sur-

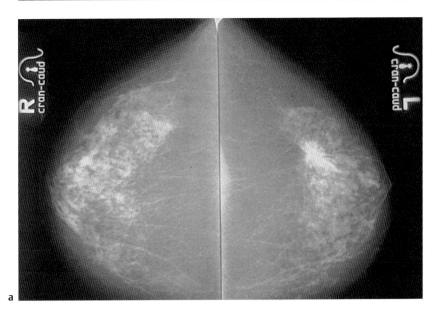

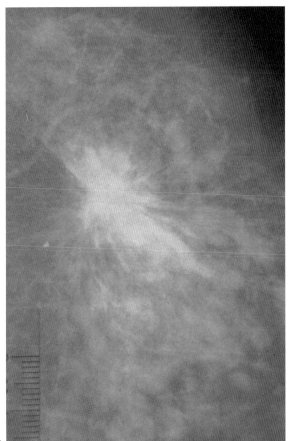

b

Fig. 8.**9 a, b   Stellate lesion in the left breast, easily characterized by the long spicules**
a CC views
b Detail from (**a**)
Histology: IDC with a diameter of 13 mm; axillary lymph nodes negative

rounded by fatty involution (Fig. 8.**40**). They are called mammographically occult cancers. ILC and intraductal carcinomas without microcalcifications are notorious for being mammographically occult. Of all palpable breast cancers, 5–7% are mammographically occult. Therefore, a palpable lesion without corresponding mammographic findings mandates further diagnostic evaluation by sonography.

Palpable lesions. Palpable nodular lesions with an ill-defined margin on supplemental spot-magnification views are suspicious for malignancy and require further

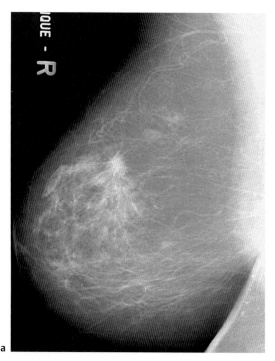

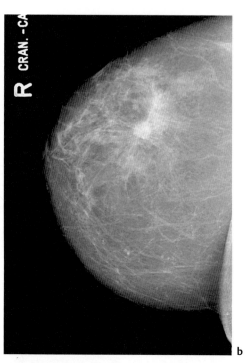

Fig. 8.**10 a, b   Stellate lesion in the right breast**. Screening detected in 69-year-old woman. Not palpable
a MLO view

b CC view. Histology: IDC with a diameter of 11 mm; axillary lymph nodes negativ

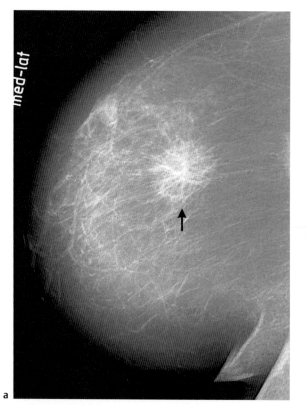

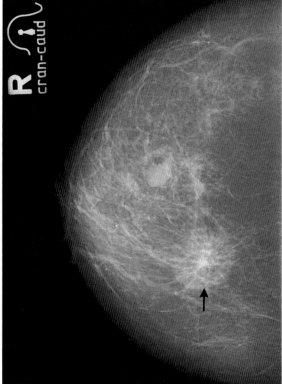

Fig. 8.**11 a, b   Structural change, resembling a radial scar**. Detected at screening, nonpalpable. Histology: ILC with a diameter of 15 mm; one axillary lymph node positive

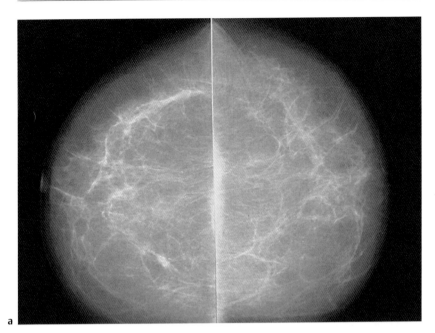

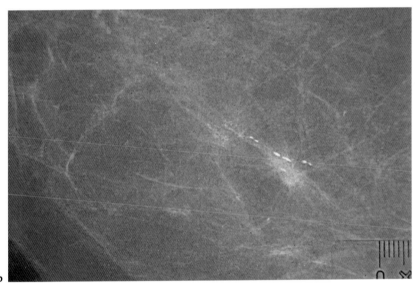

Fig. 8.**12 a, b   Small ILC in the right breast, barely distinguishable from breast tissue**
a CC view
b Detail from (**a**)

assessment by sonography and/or needle biopsy. Lesions with a well-defined margin are principally benign, but may also need further investigation with sonography and/or needle biopsy. Depending on the outcome of the diagnostic work-up, either surgical excision or expectant follow-up is indicated. Proven fibroadenomas still require surgical excision if they are clinically symptomatic, such as causing pain or anxiety. Furthermore, growth of the palpable lesion observed under follow-up is an indication for excision. Nodular lesions that have coarse calcifications characteristic for a fibroadenoma and lesions that are partly or entirely composed of fat do not require further diagnostic assessment or surgical excision since the mammographic features alone sufficiently attest to the benign character of the lesion.

Nonpalpable lesions. In general, the criteria valid for palpable lesions are applicable to nonpalpable lesions. Lesions with an ill-defined margin mandate a histological diagnosis. Small densities without microcalcifications and with a well-defined margin should be considered probably benign. Following sonographic evaluation (detection of cysts), they can be followed by mammography. The likelihood of malignancy is very low (positive predictive value 1.4%; Sickles, 1994; Maes et al.,1997) and the prognosis of a carcinoma detected in such a way favorable. Screen-detected cancers that had minimal signs two years earlier appeared to have a relatively favorable prognosis, probably related to their slow growth rate.

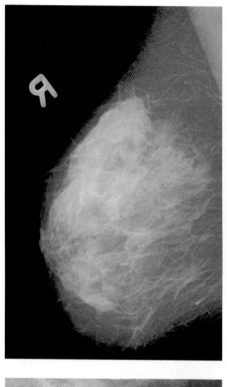

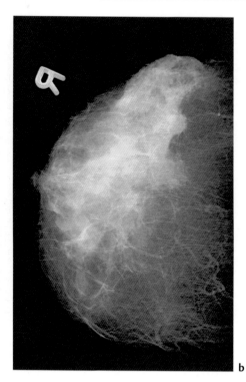

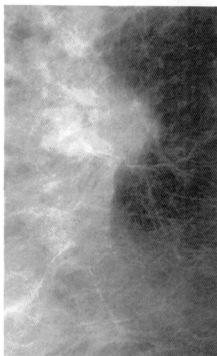

Fig. 8.**13a–c** **ILC**
a On the MLO view barely distinguishable from breast tissue
b CC view. Contour of the cancer visible at the posterior border of glandular tissue
c Detail from (**b**)

Calcifications

Petra A. M. Bun

A special magnifying glass is indispensable (refractive power + 3 diopter, diameter at least 12 cm) for analyzing calcifications discovered on the mammogram. Cases of possible malignancy also require magnification views in two projections, for assessing the calcifications further and for detecting additional calcifications.

Malignant as well as benign breast lesions may show calcifications. Furthermore, calcifications can be physiological. As many calcifications can have malignant or benign features, precise analysis of the calcifications is essential in the differential diagnoses.

Calcifications must be identified as to their location, i.e., identification of the pathoanatomic origin, and to their process of formation. Calcifications mirror the outcome of a benign or malignant process.

Location

Calcifications may develop anywhere in the breast. The calcifications relevant for the differential diagnosis mainly occur in the characteristic element of the fibroglandular tissue, the TDLU.

Pathogenesis

- Calcifications of necrotic cell material (dystrophic calcifications)
- Crystallization of inspissated cellular secretion
- Calcifications caused by degenerative processes or inflammations
- Calcifications caused by scarring
- Calcifications caused by parasites or foreign bodies

■ Analysis of Calcifications

By analysis of size (including density), number, form, distribution (e.g., clustering), and any associated soft tissue density, the pathoanatomic site and genesis can be determined and the underlying benign or malignant process inferred.

Size

Calcifications exceeding 2 mm are referred to as *macrocalcifications*. They are almost always benign (see p. 200). Calcifications smaller than 1 mm are referred to as *microcalcifications*. Microcalcifications may indicate malignancy, but are not invariably caused by a malignant process.

Numerous microcalcifications confined to a small area may deceptively appear as (benign) macrocalcifications effected by superimposition of individual microcalcifications.

In general, the size also determines the density of microcalcifications. Variation in density and size is a sign of malignancy. A distinct radiolucency within a calcification denotes inclusion and indicates a benign process.

Number

The differential diagnosis is not much aided by the absolute number of calcifications, but by the relative number of it is in relation to size, shape, etc. Finding an increased number of calcifications or a newly developed group of microcalcifications on a follow-up examination often indicates malignancy.

Shape

In many cases, site and mode of the development of the calcifications determine shape as well as margin (Fig. 8.**14**).

Depending on the pathogenesis, macrocalcifications can assume quite different shapes.

The smallest microcalcifications are *involutional calcifications*. They are often difficult to detect. Involutional calcifications are round, multiple, and dispersed over large areas, and are referred to as powdery. They develop in atrophied lobes. *Secretory calcification* in normal or enlarged lobes leads to small round, homogenous, sharply demarcated pearl-like microcalcifications. They are multiple and situated closely together as a group, only separated by two abutting normal thin lobular (acinar) walls (Fig. 8.**30**).

These typically lobular calcifications are benign. They characteristically occur in sclerosing adenosis. Then they are often somewhat smaller and spread apart by the fibrosis.

The calcium content of the secretion in the dilated lobes may become so high that it forms so-called "milk of calcium" (Figs. 8.**14 d** and 8.**15**). The corresponding mammographic findings are typical:

- With vertical projection, round calcifications are seen.
- With horizontal projection, semicircular or crescentic calcifications, caudally convex, are seen, resulting in the so-called "teacup phenomenon" (Lanyi, 1986).

Microcalcifications of irregular shape and different size and density are referred to as *granular*. They appear crumbled and often indicate malignancy.

A distinction is made between *coarse granular microcalcifications*, which are easily visible without a magnifying glass, and *fine granular microcalcifications*, which are smaller and only clearly identifiable with a magnifying glass. Coarse granular microcalcifications mostly develop in the necrotic center of a malignant process within the ductal system. Together with a cloud of fine

Longitudinal sections **Transverse section**

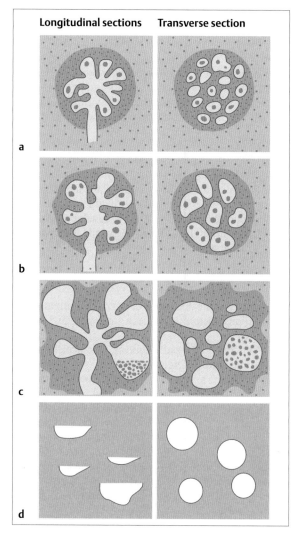

Fig. 8.14 a – d   Lobular calcifications in adenosis
a Blunt duct adenosis
b Microcystic adenosis
c Advanced microcystic adenosis
d Schematic presentation of the radiographic image
   Horizontal and vertical projection

calcium particles around the calcified center of the necrosis, this accounts for the irregular shape and indistinct margin of these microcalcifications on the mammogram.

The accumulation of coarse granular microcalcifications in the center of the tumor necrosis within the duct forms a branching calcific cast that follows the ductal system. It is generally directed toward the mamilla, accounting for the so-called ductal configuration. This pathogenesis also explains the irregular margin of these calcifications. These branching linear calcifications used to be referred to as casting-type or comedo-type calcifications (Fig. 8.**16**).

The fine granular microcalcifications develop through crystallization in the inspissated secretion be-

tween the tumor cells within the lobules (Fig. 3.**11**). They occur in small groups. Contrary to benign lobular calcifications, these calcific particles characteristically are not situated close to each other since they are spread apart by tumor tissue. Sometimes, they may be pearl-like round or oval and are then difficult to distinguish from (benign) lobular calcifications.

Distribution

Calcifications may be regularly dispersed over the major portions of the breast parenchyma of both breasts. This is a sign of benignity. Sometimes, calcifications are restricted to a certain region of the breast, resulting in a segmental or lobar arrangement that raises the possibility of malignancy. Finally, the calcifications may be clustered in a small group. Depending on the shape, size, and orientation as well as on the distance between them, they may point to malignancy, especially if multiple small groups are present in the same breast segment.

■ Benign Macrocalcifications

- Secretory: plasma cell mastitis (Fig. 8.**17**).
- Fat necrosis: liponecrosis (liponecrosis microcystica or macrocystica calcificans) (Fig. 8.**18**).
- Calcifications in the skin and sebaceous glands (Fig. 8.**19**).
- Vascular calcifications (Figs. 8.**20** and 8.**21**).
- Calcifications in fibroadenomas (Figs. 8.**22** and 8.**23**), papillomas (Fig. 8.**24**), hemangiomas. The calcifications in fibroadenomas are:
  - Coarse lumps, located centrally in round or oval soft-tissue densities. These are calcifications in fibrosed or hyalinized stroma.
  - Calcified secretion in cysts and ductlike structures within the fibroadenoma, but not arranged as regularly as in normal fibroglandular tissue. Sometimes they are equidistant from each other since they are separated by a septum constituting two or more layers of cells. During their evolution, these calcifications are most difficult to distinguish from malignant microcalcifications. The differentiation becomes easier with time because of growth and resultant increase in size.
  - A combination of the above (Lanyi, 1986; Sickles, 1986).
- Calcification in scars.
- Calcifications in lymph nodes (e.g., tuberculosis), pseudocalcifications in lymph nodes after gold therapy.
- Finding mimicking calcifications: tattoos (Fig. 8.**25**), ointments (Fig. 8.**26**) and traces of powder (Fig. 8.**27**), film artifacts, foreign bodies (Figs. 8.**28** and 8.**29**).

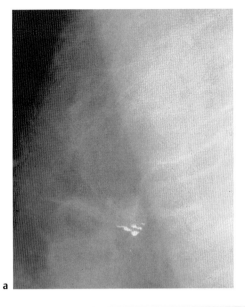

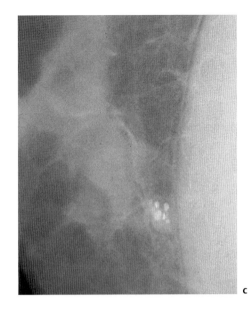

a

c

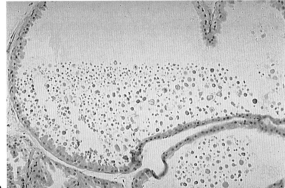

b

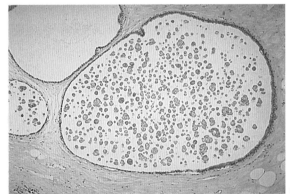

d

Fig. 8.15 a – d   Milk of calcium in microcysts
a Oblique view: crescentic calcium densities due to sedimentation (teacup phenomenon)

b Histological section, corresponding to (**a**)
c CC view shows round densities
d Histological section showing sedimented calcium particles

■ Benign Microcalcifications

- Lobular calcifications (Fig. 8.**30**) including milk of calcium and sclerosing adenosis
- Involutional calcifications

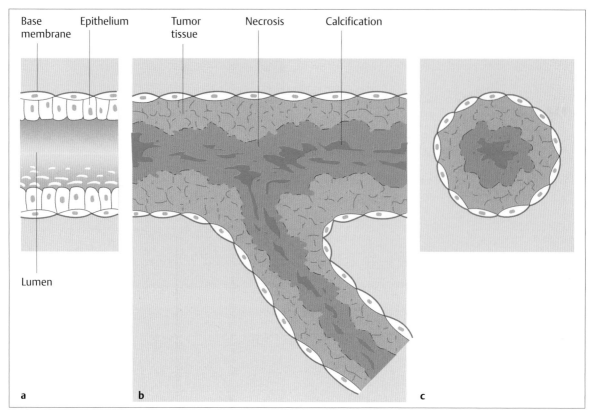

Fig. 8.**16 a – c   Malignant intraductal calcifications**
a Normal duct

b, c Granular to castlike calcifications in poorly differentiated DCIS. The calcifications are irregular, fragmented, and directional. (**b**) Longitudinal section. (**c**) Transverse section

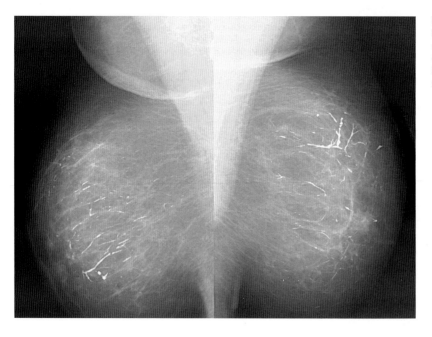

Fig. 8.**17   Plasma cell mastitis.** Bilaterally linear, homogeneously dense calcifications with smooth contours and mostly not branching, representing calcified inspissated secretion

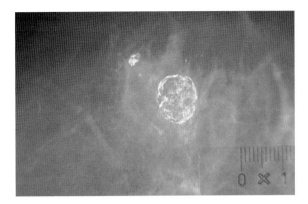

Fig. 8.**18 Fat necrosis with calcification**. Coarse calcifications in the wall of an oil cyst

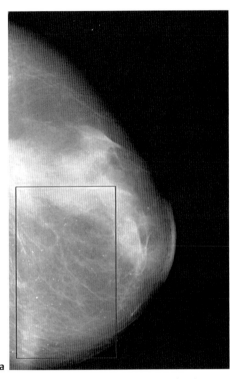

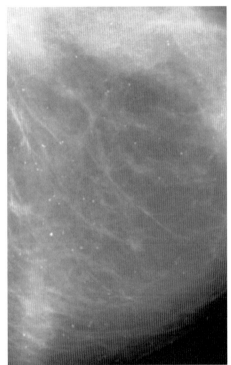

a

b

Fig. 8.**19 a, b   Calcified sebaceous glands**
a CC view
b Magnification view for detail

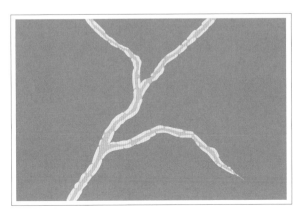

Fig. 8.**20   Diagram of calcifications in arterial walls**

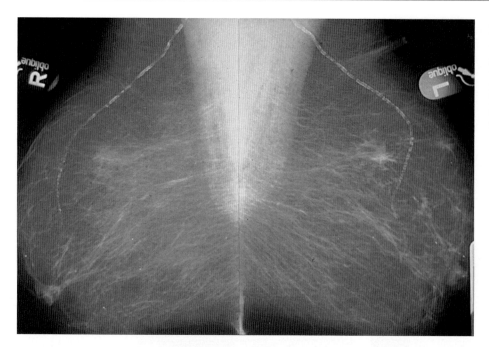

Fig. 8.**21 Calcifications in arterial walls, bilateral**. In addition, a screen-detected stellate lesion on the left. Histology: IDC with a diameter of 15 mm; lymph nodes negative

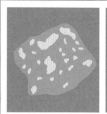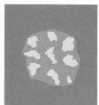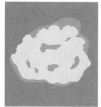

Cluster of polymorphic calcifications

Relatively polymorphic calcifications, mostly peripheral

Coarse calcifications

Almost completely calcified

Fig. 8.**22 Various types of calcifications found in fibroadenomas**

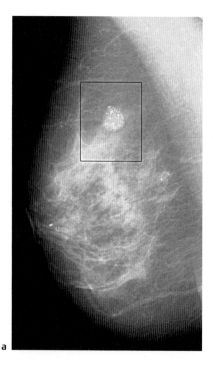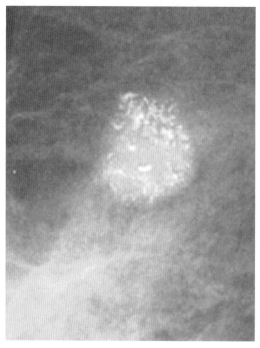

Fig. 8.**23 a, b Atypical polymorphic calcifications in a fibroadenoma**. The calcifications in fibroadenomas generally are bigger than shown here

a

b

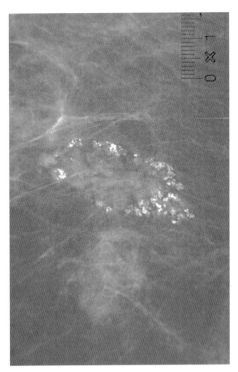

Fig. 8.**24   Papilloma with calcifications.** Mostly peripherally
arranged, coarse calcifications in the soft-tissue density

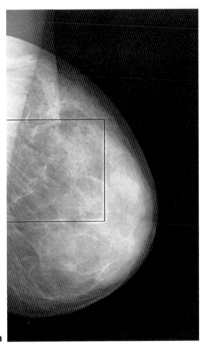

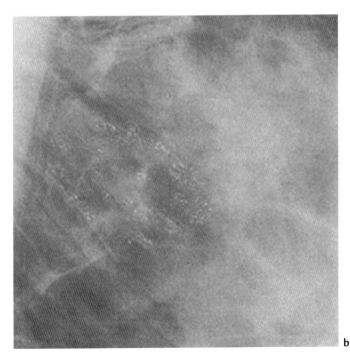

a   b

Fig. 8.**25 a, b   Tattoo.** Radiopaque particles in the skin
a CC view   **b** Magnification view for detail

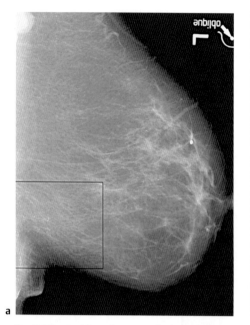
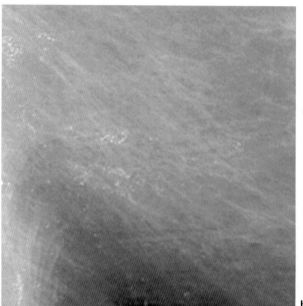

Fig. 8.26 a, b   Zinc ointment along the inframammary skinfold of the left breast
a Oblique view   b Magnification view for detail

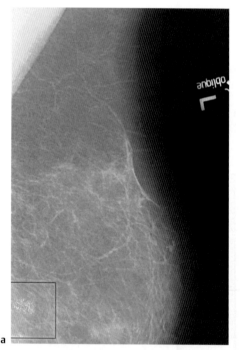
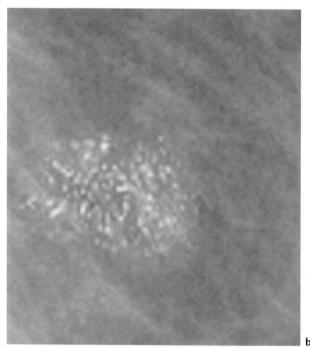

Fig. 8.27 a, b   Nevus with talcum powder
a Oblique view left   b Magnification view for detail

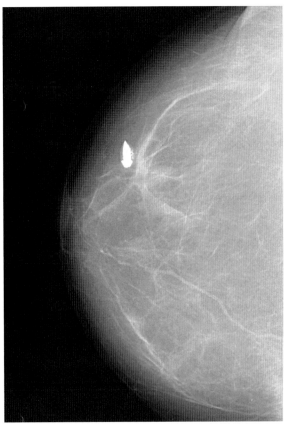

Fig. 8.**28**   Shrapnel splinter

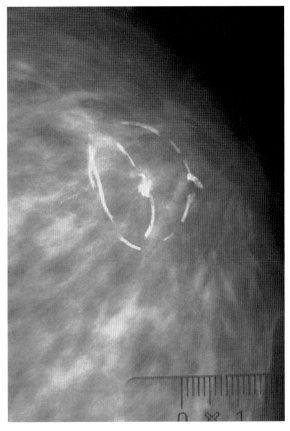

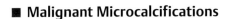

Fig. 8.**29**   Calcified catgut suture

■ Malignant Microcalcifications

The presence of microcalcifications alone indicates a high probability of DCIS. An added soft-tissue density may point to invasive growth. Sometimes, a carcinoma in situ induces a desmoplastic reaction that can also increase the density at the site of the microcalcifications. Consequently, a density next to the microcalcifications does not invariably imply infiltrative growth. Malignant microcalcifications in or around the soft-tissue density of an invasive carcinoma often represent additional foci of a carcinoma in situ:

- Coarse granular (ductal) microcalcifications in a linear arrangement (Fig. 8.**31**) as manifestation of a poorly or moderately differentiated DCIS.
- Fine granular (lobular) microcalcifications, also referred to as cribriform microcalcifications (Fig. 8.**32**) as manifestation of a well-differentiated DCIS (Table 8.**1**).

All suspicious microcalcifications demand a histological diagnosis. Branching linear microcalcifications point to a poorly differentiated ductal carcinoma. Coarse granular calcifications imply a higher probability of a poorly differentiated carcinoma than fine granular calcifications, especially when they form a single cluster. Multi-

ple clusters of fine granular microcalcifications are indicative of a well-differentiated ductal carcinoma.

Table 8.**1**   Malignant microcalcifications (DCIS): classification[1]

Former classification (based on necrosis)	
• Comedo type	• Noncomedo type
Current classification (cytonuclear and architectural differentiation)	
• Poorly differentiated	• Well differentiated
Microcalcifications	
• Amorphous calcifications	• Pearl-like calcifications
• In necrosis	• In secretion
• Branching linear	• Multiple clusters
• Coarse granular	• Fine granular
• In ducts	• In lobuli
Size of the process	
• Mammographic size equals the size in the histopathological section	• Mammographically smaller than in the histopathological section
	• The size on the mammographic magnification view equals the size in the histopathological section
Invasion risk	
• Considerable	• Small

[1] Intermediate forms are possible as well (intermediately differentiated).

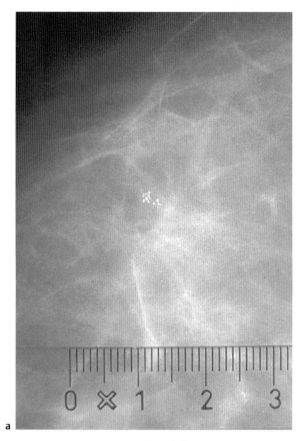

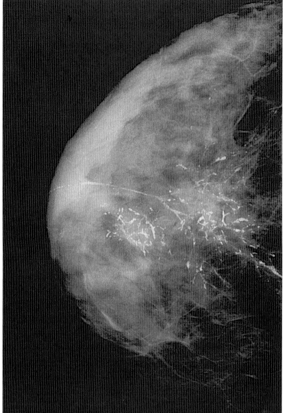

a

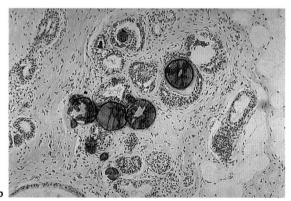

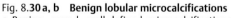

b

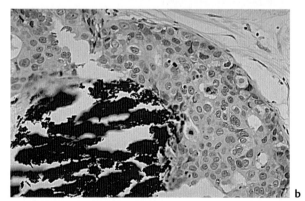

b

Fig. 8.**30 a, b   Benign lobular microcalcifications**
a Benign, round, well-defined microcalcifications on detail mammogram
b Histology: well-defined, lamellated calcifications (HE)

Fig. 8.**31 a, b   Poorly differentiated DCIS with microcalcifications**
a Coarse granular and linear, partly branching microcalcifications, typical of a continuously growing poorly differentiated DCIS
b Transverse section of a duct containing a poorly differentiated DCIS with centrally located dystrophic calcifications (von Kossa and HE stain)

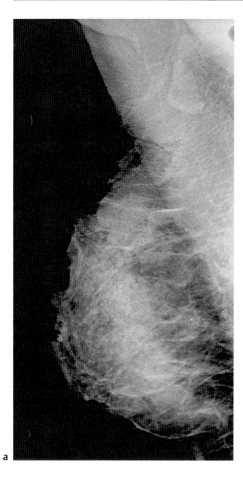

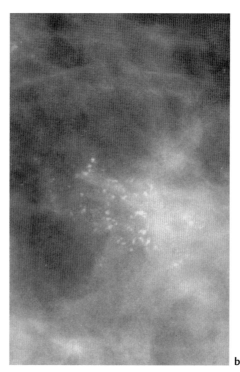

Fig. 8.**32 a, b** **Fine granular microcalcifications as manifestation of a well-differentiated DCIS**
a Oblique view
b Magnification view in oblique projection

Architectural Distortion and Asymmetry

D. J. Dronkers

Aside from its typical manifestations, such as suspicious microcalcifications and/or indistinctly outlined or stellate densities, a malignancy can also have a more subtle mammographic appearance.

The stellate density characteristically found with a breast cancer consists of a central tumor mass surrounded by a radiating structure, the spicules (Fig. 8.**33**).

When the central tumor mass is small relative to the encompassing radiating structure, the lesion is mammographically less obvious. The lesion is even less obvious when a distinct central tumor mass is absent and only the radiating structure is present. Even if the radiating structure is no longer visible as such, a slight architectural distortion or asymmetry of the fibroglandular tissue may be the only mammographic sign of malignancy. The mammographic detection of such subtle changes is extremely difficult.

The fatty involution of normal fibroglandular breast tissue causes the stroma of the glandular tissue to appear mammographically as network of distinct and indistinct trabecular densities. This reticular pattern represents the superimposition of different connective tissue structures:

- Interlobar and interlobular septa.
- Saccular fasciae enveloping the glandular body, with anterior tentlike extensions (superficial fascia) to the skin (Cooper ligaments).
- Trabecular cords arising from the inner surface of the deep fascia and converging toward the mamillary region.
- Retromammilar lactiferous ducts rendered mammographically visible through periductal collagenous connective tissue.

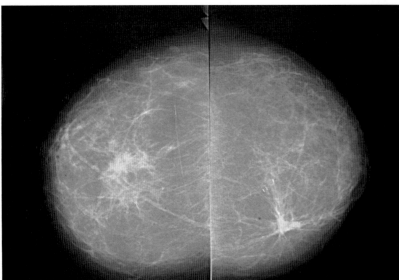

a

Fig. 8.**33 a, b**   **Typical stellate density of breast cancer with relative long spicules in the left breast medially** (59-year-old patient)
a CC views
b Detail enlargement of (**a**)

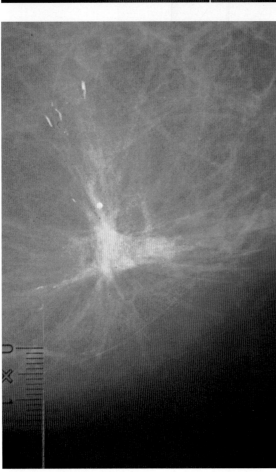

b

Pathology

The normal reticular pattern can be disturbed in different ways:

- The trabecular cords can be *displaced or compressed* by expansively growing processes such as
  - lipomatosis: local proliferation of fat tissue;
  - cysts;
  - phyllodes tumor;
  - fibroadenoma, lipoma, and fibroadenolipoma;
  - expansively growing malignant tumors.

These processes displace and compress surrounding breast structures. Around areas of lipomatosis this might produce abnormal densities and asymmetry. It is therefore advisable to look for nearby causal lipomatosis whenever asymmetry is found (Fig. 8.**34**). Asymmetry can also occur without underlying expansile processes (Fig. 8.**36**). The rudimentary accessory breast is a special case of asymmetry. A distinction is made between the so-called "first breast" located in the upper outer quadrant and sometimes clearly separated from the central glandular body, and the so-called "third breast" located in the lower inner quadrant within the glandular body. The fatty involution of the glandular tissue affects the accessory breasts later than the main part of the breast, causing the accessory breast tissue to become visible as ill-defined density, which might be misinterpreted as tumor (Fig. 8.**35**).

This "congenital" asymmetry (ectopic breast tissue) should be kept in mind as a possible cause of unilateral densities.

- Nearly all breast cancers, whether invasive or in-situ, induce fibrosis and elastosis as desmoplastic reaction of the immune system, causing the tissue to *shrink* regionally. This regional volume loss alters the nor-

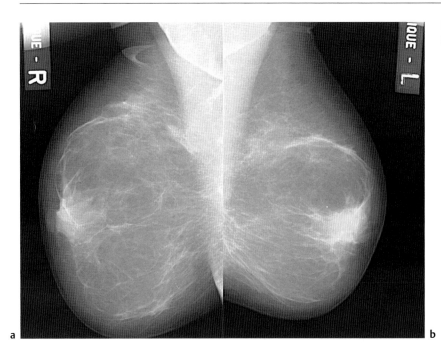

Fig. 8.**34 a, b** **Bilateral local fat proliferation**. MLO views

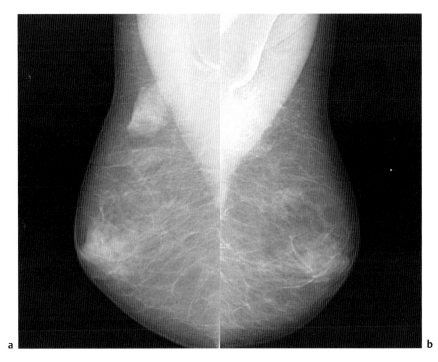

Fig. 8.**35 a, b** **Ectopic fibroglandular tissue with delayed fatty involution in the axillary aspect of the right breast**

mal breast architecture of the tumor-bearing area (Fig. 8.**37**). The trabecular cords may become stretched and lengthened (straight structures are rarely found on mammograms) or may contract, leading to a stellate configuration with a paucity of surrounding structures. This indicates retraction due to local shrinkage of structures and always suggests a malignancy. This often occurs in ILC, which is a relatively rare tumor characterized by diffuse infiltration without destruction of the local structures. Almost one-third of the cases of ILC are only detected by locally altered architecture or by asymmetry. The tumor manifests itself on the mammogram only indirectly by the induced desmoplastic reaction. ILC relatively often induces thickening of the skin as well as retraction of skin and mamilla. When interpreting mammograms, attention should not only be given to the dense glandular and connective tissue structures

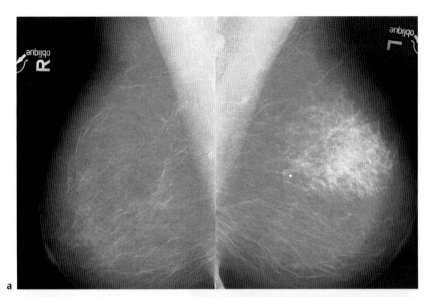

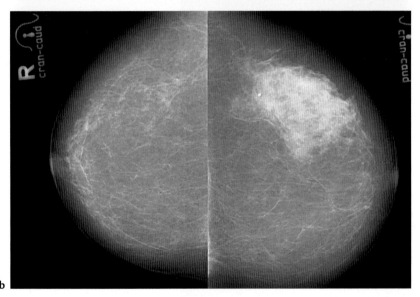

Fig. 8.**36 a, b**   **Benign asymmetry of fibroglandular tissue**
a MLO views
b CC views

but also to the symmetric distribution of the fatty structures.

Shrinkage with retraction can also occur in a benign lesion, such as a radial scar (Fig. 8.**38**).

Radial scar (p. 19): This benign lesion is usually non-palpable. Mammographically, it can appear as radial structure in one projection and, due to its flat orientation along one plane, assume a different configuration in another projection. The discrepancy between definite mammographic abnormality and absent palpable mass is often striking, even when the radial scar is located subcutaneously. In most cases, a central mass is not seen mammographically, but the center may contain one or more radiolucent areas representing fatty tissue. Radiolucent lines indicating fat may parallel the spicules. Thickening or retraction of the skin is not observed, but atypical microcalcifica-

tions can occasionally be encountered. This increases the suspicion for malignancy (Fig. 8.**39**).

Basically, the lesion consists of a benign stellate fibrotic change with central fibroelastosis. The many different names reflect the various opinions about the nature of this lesion. The most frequent synonyms are listed on p. 19.

A small percentage of these lesions have been found to contain malignancy. Furthermore, invasive tubular carcinoma may have the same mammographic appearance. Conversely, a radial scar sometimes exhibits a central mass. Consequently, suspecting a radial scar is an indication for excisional biopsy. An expectant follow-up cannot be justified. It is advisable to inform the pathologist of the mammographic findings that prompted the biopsy, especially in view of a possible false positive reading of frozen sections, which may result in over-treatment. Benign adenosis

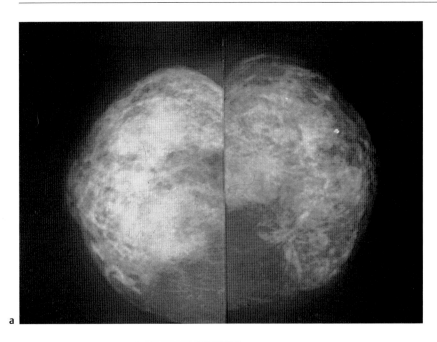

a

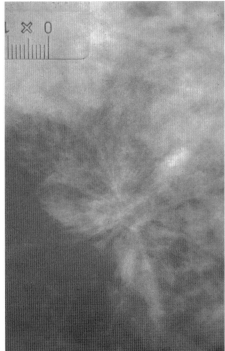

b

Fig. 8.**37 a, b** **Asymmetry due to shrinking medially in the left breast**
a CC views
b Detail magnification of (**a**) (left breast) Histology: DCIS with a diameter of 8 mm; axillary lymph nodes negative

found in a radial scar may mimic a tubular cancer on frozen section.

Surgical scar: Fibrosis or desmoplastic reaction after breast surgery is more an exception. It can lead to a contracted contour of the glandular body ("tent sign"), with locally corresponding loss of volume and increase in density. Frequently, this is associated with a suggested radiating reticular pattern. These post-surgical changes normally disappear within one or two years.

Fibrosed fat necrosis: Fibrotic reactions induced by fat necrosis also lead to architectural distortion or stellate configuration of the breast tissue. Fat necrosis may be caused by surgery, trauma (seatbelt injury of the breast in motor vehicle accidents) or repeated microtraumas as occurring in the so-called "bra syndrome" (repetitive damage of the lateral breast tissue caused by the indenting metal frame of an undersized brassiere).

Local fibrosis after inflammation, bacterial infection, tuberculosis, etc.: Mondor disease is easily diagnosed clinically by the longitudinal retraction of the skin overlying the superficial thrombophlebitis of the thoracoepigastric veins (Fig. 8.**43**). It can be the cause of mammographically visible retraction.

- *Interrupted* trabecular cords as a result of local destruction by tumor may be a sign of malignancy that, according to Roebuck (1990), is often rather difficult to discern. The mammographic findings can be rather subtle.

Amidst dense fibroglandular tissue, these mammographic changes will only be visualized with adequate compression of the breast, optimal exposure and good contrast. In cases with indeterminate findings, targeted magnification views may offer useful additional information.

Tumor-induced fibrosis and elastosis may cause local loss of elasticity at the tumor site. At a stage before these processes cause a local density, they probably can only be detected with optimal compression. With compression, the lost elasticity of the lesion renders it visible as architectural distortion within stretched surrounding tissue.

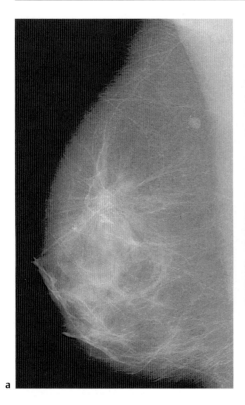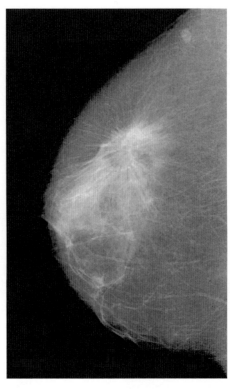

Fig. 8.**38 a, b   Radial scar in the right breast**. The lesion is visible in both projections
a MLO view
b CC view

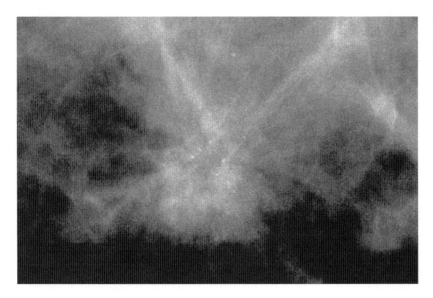

Fig. 8.**39   Radial scar with microcalcifications**. Histology: highly differentiated DCIS (49-year-old patient). Detail magnification of CC view

Differential diagnosis of radiating densities:

- Invasive ductal carcinoma
- Tubular carcinoma
- ILC
- Radial scar
- Fibrotic healing of fat necrosis

- Hyalinized fibroadenoma (mostly nodular center)
- Postsurgical scar
- Radiating type of fibrosing sclerosing adenosis
- Sclerosing type of tuberculosis
- Superimposition of normal breast structures

Changes of the Skin

D. J. Dronkers

The bright light is essential to evaluate the mammogram for skin changes. Local edema, inflammation, trauma (previous surgery), or superficial malignant processes may cause subcutaneous changes and thickening of the skin. The subcutaneous changes appear as a blurring of the normally sharp interface between skin and subcutaneous fat. Furthermore, fine radiopaque lines may appear. The thickened skin can become retracted through infiltration of a subcutaneous carcinoma, but mammographic thickening of the skin is no absolute sign of cutaneous tumor infiltration. Skin thickening may be the only evidence of an otherwise mammographically occult breast cancer (Fig. 8.**40**).

Not infrequently, it represents an invasive and often palpable lobular carcinoma (ILC). This local skin thickening may be caused by tumor obstructing the superficial lymph drainage. Moreover, the areolar thickening (Fig. 8.**41**) seen on the mammogram may be secondary to lymphatic obstruction by an otherwise mammographically occult cancer.

Generalized thickening of the skin, a reticular pattern in the connective tissues and/or a diffuse increase in the density of the parenchyma indicate mastitis and, in older women, an inflammatory carcinoma (mastitis carcinomatosa). Frequently, a soft-tissue density caused by the underlying tumor can be detected. The partial or generalized skin thickening after radiation therapy of the breast is well known. It represents lymphedema with resultant diffusely increased density of the breast tissue, thickening of the reticular pattern, and diffuse subcutaneous changes. If these signs do not disappear within one to one and a half years, tumor recurrence has to be considered.

This mammographic appearance is also known as *thickened skin syndrome of the breast* (Tabár, 1983). The skin thickening begins in the lower part of the breast, and the overall density of the breast increases due to fluid accumulation. It indicates lymphedema caused by axillary lymphatic or venous obstruction. The breast enlarges and the skin resembles a peau d'orange. Mammography alone cannot differentiate between benign inflammatory mastitis and inflammatory carcinoma.

Causes of thickened skin syndrome

- Mastitis carcinomatosa
- Acute mastitis, abscesses, psoriasis
- Axillary lymph obstruction by metastases, malignant lymphadenopathy, mediastinal lymphatic obstruction, etc.
- Local inflammation around the breast
- Edema due to backward failure of the right ventricle, venous obstruction, etc.

Other causes of local skin thickening

- Sebaceous retention cyst, mostly solitary (Fig. 8.**42**); neurofibroma (von Recklinghausen disease), often multiple
- Mondor disease (p. 22) (Fig. 8.**43**)
- Skin folds mimicking local skin thickening
- Thickening of the mamilla as occurring in Paget disease (p. 32) (Fig. 8.**41**).

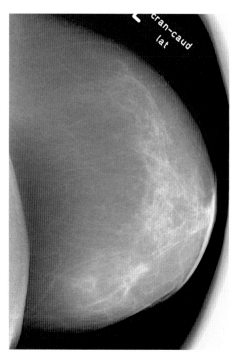

Fig. 8.**40 Local skin thickening associated with otherwise mammographically occult invasive lobular carcinoma, which was palpable**. Histology: ILC, 30 mm in diameter, with skin fixation

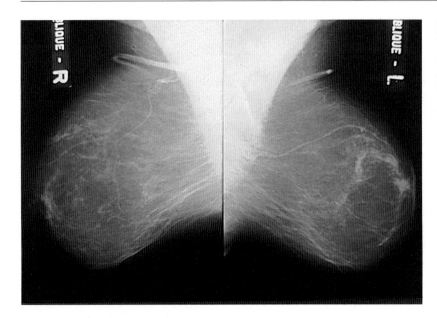

Fig. 8.**41   Skin thickening of the left areola at screening of a 69-year-old woman**. Eight months later, ulceration of the mamilla and a palpable retroareolar tumor. Histology: IDC, 30 mm in diameter, with Paget disease. Lymph nodes negative

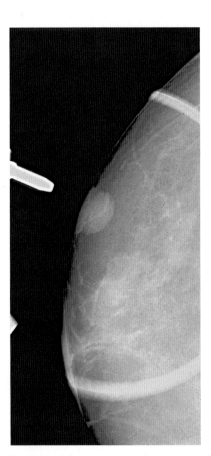

Fig. 8.**42   Sebaceous retention cyst at the level of the marker**

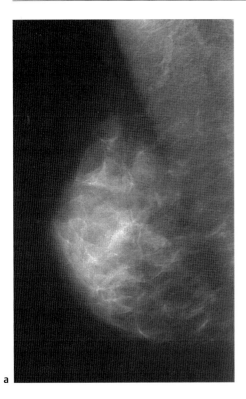

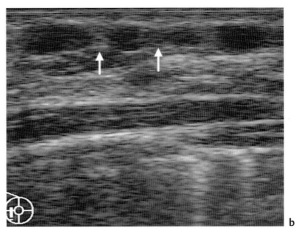

Fig. 8.**43 a, b   Mondor disease of the right breast**
a Mammography: prominent vein
b Sonography: thrombotic vein (arrows)

Lymph Nodes

D. J. Dronkers

■ Axillary Lymph Nodes

The MLO views frequently show the low axillary lymph nodes, which differ in number and size (Fig. 8.**44**). The variable positions of the lymph nodes account for the multifarious appearance in different projections, varying from typical bean-shaped to spherical. The diameter ranges from 5 to 20 mm. The number and size of mammographically visible lymph nodes are subject to individual variations.

The normal involution of lymph nodes begins with fat deposited in the hilar region and continues with intranodal deposition of fat. Eventually, the entire node is replaced by fat, sparing only a thin rim along the nodal periphery. Lymph nodes that are almost completely replaced by fat generally appear quite large and rounded.

The deposited fat in normal lymph nodes contributes to their mammographic and sonographic identification (Fig. 8.**45**).

Metastases replace intranodal fat with dense tumor tissue. The lymph node not only changes to a homogeneously dense structure but also enlarges and frequently assumes a round configuration. Extranodular tumor extension causes local loss of the normally sharp margin of the lymph node. Spiculated lymph nodes indicate perinodal tumor infiltration. Microcalcifications are rarely encountered in metastatic lymph nodes. Deposits of gold have been observed in axillary lymph nodes following gold therapy for rheumatoid arthritis. Tuberculosis may be the best-known cause of nodal calcifications (Fig. 8.**46**).

Bilaterally enlarged and abnormally homogeneous axillary lymph nodes are seen in generalized lymphadenopathy, as occurring in non-Hodgkin lymphoma, lymphatic leukemia, etc., but are also found in rheumatoid arthritis and dermatological disorders, such as psoriasis. No mammographic differentiation can be made between benign lymphadenopathy and nodal metastases from cancer of the breast, pancreas, esophagus, and ovary.

Observation of one or more enlarged, homogeneous, dense axillary lymph nodes together with a suspicious breast lesion suggests a breast cancer with nodal metastases. Mammographically normal-appearing axillary lymph nodes, however, do not exclude metastases. On one hand, involved lymph nodes may harbor micrometastases and, on the other hand, most of the axillary lymph nodes are not included on standard views of routine mammography. Because of the low specificity of nodal mammographic findings, axillary views to target axillary lymph nodes are no longer included in modern routine mammography.

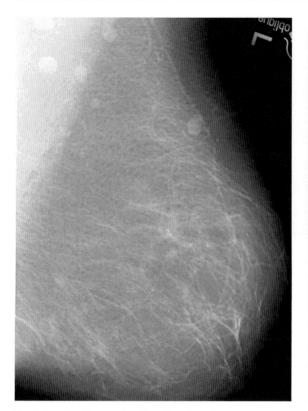

Fig. 8.**44**   **Small normal axillary lymph nodes**

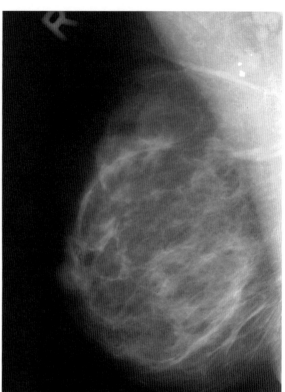

Fig. 8.**46**   **Calcific deposits in axillary lymph nodes after tuberculosis**

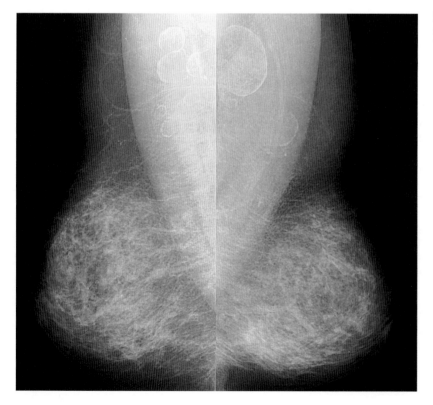

Fig. 8.**45**   **Bilateral enlarged axillary lymph nodes due to fatty involution**

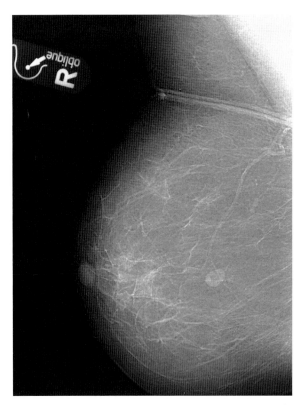

Fig. 8.**47** **Typical image of an intramammary lymph node with fatty involution**

Retrosternal lymph nodes are only visible with CT or scintigraphy.

■ Intramammary Lymph Nodes

It is not rare for intramammary lymph nodes to appear on mammograms as solitary, bean-shaped or round, well-defined densities. They can be found anywhere in the breast (Fig. 8.**47**), most frequently in the upper outer quadrant near the posterior margin of the fibroglandular cone, and are often bilateral and symmetric.

In middle-aged and older women, a centrally located, well-defined radiolucent area caused by deposited fat in the hilar region makes it easy to identify intramammary lymph nodes. Intramammary lymph nodes are usually smaller than axillary lymph nodes and seldom larger than 10 mm.

Suspicion for malignancy must be raised if a known intramammary lymph node becomes more homogeneous and, at the same time, increases in density and size, unless mastitis or dermatitis is clinically present.

Mammographic Findings after Surgery and Radiation Therapy

Harmine M. Zonderland

Surgery for diagnostic, therapeutic or plastic/corrective purposes leaves changes that are evident upon inspection and mammography. An operation limited to the removal of a palpable or mammographically suspicious lesion is called an *excisional biopsy* or *lumpectomy*. Generally, skin is not taken, except for possibly a small oval flap. If the operation removes the associated quadrant of fibroglandular tissue along with the lesion, it is called a *quadrantectomy*. Breast conservation techniques have been used for 20 years to resect malignancies whenever possible. Lumpectomy or a quadrantectomy can replace a mastectomy if

- the result is cosmetically acceptable;
- the malignancy can be removed in toto;
- the operation can be combined with *dissection of the axillary lymph nodes* and *postoperative radiation therapy*.

The cosmetic result is the most important criterion. Large tumors in large breasts and positive axillary lymph nodes do not present an absolute contraindication to breast-conservation surgery. Usually, a few clips are left in the tumor bed to guide the radiotherapy planning. To achieve good cosmetic results, the excisional defect has to fill in by itself. For this reason, purely subcutaneous and cutaneous sutures should be used and no drains inserted. Plastic surgery or corrective operations are performed after mastectomy (*breast reconstruction*) or for aesthetic reasons (*breast reduction* or *augmentation*). Knowledge of technique, time, and site of the surgery is important when interpreting the mammograms. In addition, it must be ascertained whether the patient's complaints are related to the surgery performed. Comparison with all previous mammograms is mandatory.

■ Excisional Biopsy and Breast-conservation Therapy

Every incision produces reversible skin thickening and local distortion of the mammographic architecture (Fig. 8.**48**). Hematoma (Fig. 8.**49**), seroma, fat necrosis, calcification, and fibrosis are secondary findings that can arise in the vicinity of the scar. After core-needle biopsy, all mammographic traces of the procedure should resolve within a short time (weeks to months).

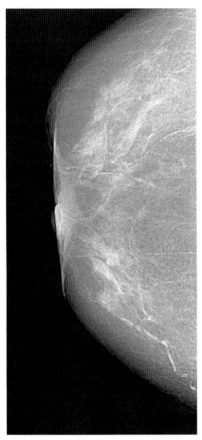

Fig. 8.**48**   **Mammographic appearance ten years after retroareolar excisional biopsy because of intraductal papillomatosis**

■ Skin Thickening and Edema

Normal skin varies in thickness from 0.8 to 3 mm and is thicker on the medial and lower sides of the breasts than on the lateral and upper sides. Skin thickening lasts for four to six weeks after a small excisional biopsy, and persists longer after more extensive surgery (Fig. 8.**50**). The edema is especially extensive if axillary lymph node dissection, which interrupts the normal lymph drainage, is followed by radiation therapy. In this situation, the edema is not limited to the scar, but extends to the region of nipple and areola. Surgical technique and individual variations in wound healing play an important role.

The bright light should be used to evaluate the skin thickness on the mammogram, since the skin is often overexposed. The subcutaneous tissue consists of thickened reticular fibrous structures. Initially, the fibroglandular tissue is indistinctly outlined, but later returns to a sharp outline. After resolution of the skin reaction, shortening of Cooper ligaments and thinning of the subcutaneous fatty tissue layer may still be evident.

Negroid women have a particular tendency to skin thickening secondary to keloid formation. This is caused

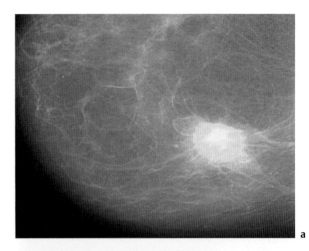

a

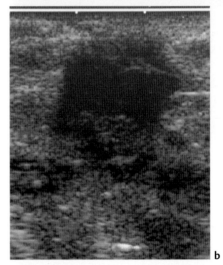

b

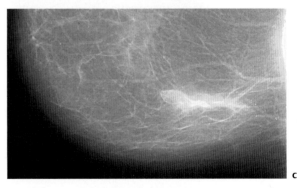

c

Fig. 8.**49 a – c**   **Resorption of a hematoma**
a Four weeks after excisional biopsy (for benign lesion): ill-defined oval mass with coarse spiculations
b Sonography shows a lesion with serrated contour and complex echo structure consistent with a hematoma
c Eight months later: almost complete resorption of the hematoma

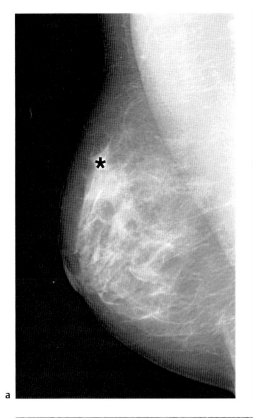

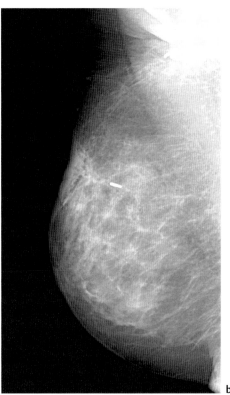

a   b

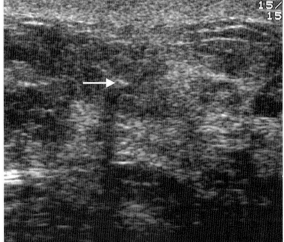

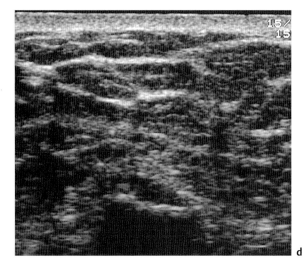

c   d

Fig. 8.50 a – d   Breast conservation therapy
a Lesion in the upper outer quadrant (*). Histology: IDC
b Lumpectomy with axillary node dissection. A surgical clip
  has been left behind at the site of the lumpectomy and in the
  axilla for postoperative radiation therapy

c Sonography shows skin thickening and blurring secondary to
  generalized edema. The clip can be recognized as small
  echogenic structure with a narrow but distinct acoustic
  shadow
d For comparison, the medial side of the same breast with normal skin thickness and sharply defined fatty and parenchymal structures

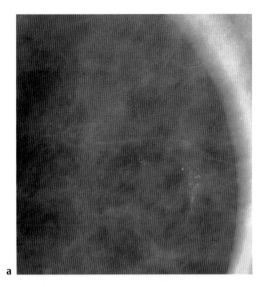

a

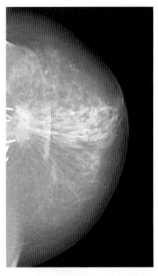

b

Fig. 8.**51 a, b** **Large scar with skin retraction after excisional biopsy for a cluster of microcalcifications.** Histology: DCIS
a Preoperative magnification view of the cluster of microcalcifications
b Postoperative mammogram with large scar

by an excessive production of collagen in the scar tissue. The complication is externally visible and should not pose any diagnostic difficulty.

Differential diagnosis of postirradiation skin edema

- Lymphatic obstruction caused by intralymphatic growth
- Bacterial infection (mastitis)
- Heart failure (cardiac decompensation)
- Dermatological disorder

■ Scar

A scar in the skin and fibroglandular tissue can present as local distortion of the architecture or stellate lesion (Fig. 8.**51**). If the scar induces skin retraction, a double contour appears on mammography, occasionally including nipple retraction. Without awareness of the clinical history, the image can easily be mistaken for a malignancy.

Differential diagnostic features

- Fat is often trapped in the scar, which produces a lucent area within the scar.
- As a scar lies in a single plane, its configuration changes in different projections, in contrast to a stellate malignancy, which generally extends in three dimensions.
- Cicatricial spiculation is usually slightly curved, shorter and coarser than malignant spiculation, which is straight and long.

■ Hematoma and Seroma

Hematomas and seromas arise frequently at the site of the excision if no drain is left behind, and often are larger than the excised lesion. They resorb very slowly and can persist for 6–12 months or, rarely, years. On the mammogram, they appear as circumscribed densities with well-defined borders or, in the presence of fresh scar tissue, with indistinct borders. Sonography can reveal fluid accumulation. Sonographically, a *hematoma* usually exhibits a well-demarcated complex lesion due to a mixture of blood clot and fibrosis, but it can be internally anechoic due to liquefaction. A *seroma* is a simple anechoic fluid collection within the scar and later develops hypoechoic compartments (Fig. 8.**52**). A scar can have densities that resemble a solid lesion with ill-defined borders, with or without sonographic shadowing. This usually represents a *foreign body reaction* (Fig. 8.**53**), but the diagnosis should always be confirmed by fine-needle or core-needle biopsy. Hematomas and seromas can degenerate into oil cysts or fat necrosis with calcification.

■ Fat Necrosis and Fibrosis

Any surgical procedure damages fat cells, leading to the release of fat that is removed by lipophages. Fat vacuoles develop and are encapsulated by fibroblasts. After about six months, calcium salts may be deposited in the scar tissue. This phenomenon develops not only after surgery but also after radiation therapy, bacterial or abacterial inflammation (plasma cell mastitis), or trauma (e.g., seatbelt injury).

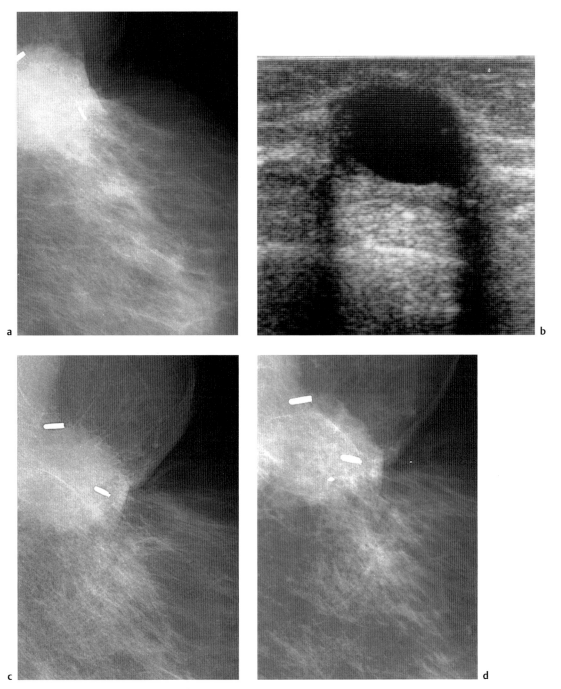

Fig. 8.**52 a – d**   **Delayed resorption of a postoperative seroma**

a Mammogram six months after breast conservation therapy shows an ill-defined lesion. The patient complains of brownish nipple discharge

b Sonography shows a fluid collection with a slightly thickened wall. Aspiration reveals the same brownish exudate constituting the nipple discharge. The cytological analysis found only macrophages

c Follow-up mammogram after two years shows a decrease in size of the lesion. The nipple discharge has ceased spontaneously

d Follow-up mammogram after three years shows further resorption. A small dystrophic calcification has appeared

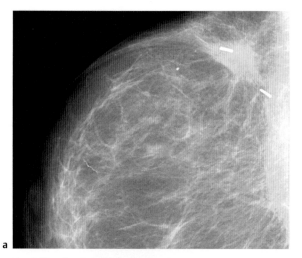

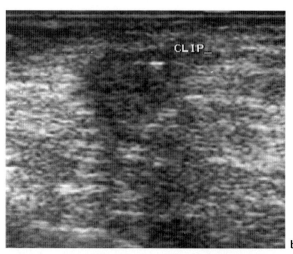

Fig. 8.53 a, b   Foreign body reaction
a Three years after breast conservation therapy, a newly developed density was visible at the site of the scar. Little trapped fat could be recognized in the scar. A local recurrence cannot be ruled out

b Sonography shows a solid mass around the surgical clip and does not add to the diagnosis. Histology: granuloma rich in macrophages

Various forms of calcification that can be distinguished radiographically

- *Liponecrotic microcysts and macrocysts*: Mostly solitary, rarely arranged in groups, and showing a central radiolucency or punctate or amorphous calcifications within a calcific ring. A macrocyst can be described as oil cyst with a calcified capsule.
- *Clustered amorphous calcifications around the scar*: Branching, rod-shaped, and punctate microcalcifications near the scar, which become coarse and lumpy on follow-up examinations. When they are located near calcified liponecrotic microcysts, differentiation from an intraductal carcinoma becomes easier.
- *Calcification of suture material*: This occurs in 1% of cases. It is characterized by the combination of linear calcification with a small central knot. (Fig. 8.**29**).

■ Radiotherapy

The described postsurgical changes and calcifications become more pronounced after irradiation, especially after iridium-192 implantation (Fig. 8.**54**). The changes progress in the first six months after radiotherapy. Chronic edema predominates for 6–12 months. In two-thirds of cases, these changes are resolved after two to four years, but at that time the breast has usually become smaller and firmer due to radiation fibrosis. The local skin thickening does not completely regress.

Scars and other postoperative and radiation-induced changes often lead to mammograms that are difficult to interpret. Furthermore, the painful breast does not always allow good compression and optimal positioning. For postoperative mammography, it may advantageous to replace the oblique view with a mediolateral view, as this often displays parenchymal remnants better. An exaggerated craniocaudal view ("Cleopatra view") can be a useful addition.

■ Locoregional Recurrence

A locoregional recurrence refers to a recurrent tumor at the surgical site or to metastases in the regional lymph nodes. It also includes tumor remnants. A recurrence develops in about 7–10% of cases, on average three years after the surgery (Fig. 8.**55**). Recurrences within the first seven years are usually located in the immediate vicinity of the scar. Thereafter, they also occur in the remaining parenchymal tissue. Despite the difficulties encountered with postoperative mammography, radiographic follow-up plays an important role:

- One third of recurrences are discovered by mammography only.
- Early diagnosis of locoregional recurrences is important for good cosmetic results of salvage operations.

The mammographic findings are usually similar to the primary tumor in locally recurrent DCIS, but may vary in IDC. Differentiation between recurrence and scar can be difficult. The most important differentiating criterion is the continuous decline of the density and architectural distortion found with scar tissue on follow-up examinations.

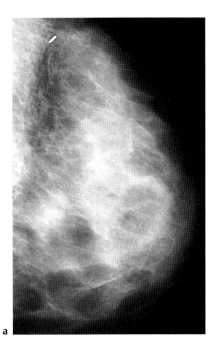

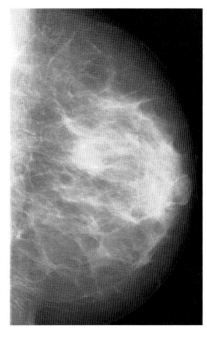

a

b

Fig. 8.**54 a, b   Increased breast density after radiation therapy**
a Follow-up mammogram one year after breast conservation therapy with ^{192}Ir implantation (50 Gy)
b Follow-up mammogram four years after irradiation: obvious decrease in the skin thickening and edema. Because of retraction at the site of the scar, the nipple no longer projects tangentially

---

Earliest signs of a recurrence

- Increase in size and density of the region of the scar
- Increase of the residual therapy-related skin thickening
- Development of malignant microcalcifications
- Appearance of a new solid lesion near the scar

MRI can be expected to play an increasing role in the future. When scar formation is completed after a period of 12–18 months, MRI permits a reliable distinction between connective tissue formation and a local recurrence (see chapter 7, p. 178).

If it is not certain whether the margins of the surgical specimen are free of tumor, especially in cases of invasive ductal carcinoma with extensive intraductal component, the first postoperative mammography should be performed four to six weeks after the operation and before commencement of radiation therapy. In all other cases, annual follow-up mammography is sufficient. The first follow-up mammogram is difficult to evaluate, but should serve as baseline study. Follow-up mammography of the contralateral breast is also important since the risk of a second primary breast carcinoma exists for the contralateral breast as much as for the operated breast.

■ Breast Reduction

Breast reduction is considered after contralateral mastectomy or breast conservation therapy or for aesthetic reasons. Breast parenchyma is removed from the inferior

aspect of the breast and the nipple-areola complex is moved upward. The resultant mammographic features are

- altered architecture of the breast;
- breast parenchyma located more inferiorly relative to the nipple-areola complex;
- interrupted continuity between nipple and fibroglandular tissue;
- secondary fat necrosis and dystrophic calcifications.

■ Breast Augmentation

Types of Implants

Various techniques can be used to reconstruct the breast after mastectomy.

The *TRAM flap* (*transverse rectus abdominis myocutaneous flap*) is gaining popularity as *silicone implants* have fallen into disfavor due to a series of complications. In the United States, silicone implants are no longer allowed for cosmetic indications, but implants consisting of a silicone capsule filled with a physiological saline solution may be applied for breast reconstruction. In the 1940s, silicone was introduced as inert substance and quickly found application in several medical fields. In the 1950s and 1960s, silicone material was injected directly into the breast for augmentation. Complications were soon recognized, consisting of the formation of painful masses and migration of silicone particles into the soft tissues of the thoracic wall. Silicone injections were banned and replaced by silicone implants. The classic silicone implant consists of a silicone envelope with a single lumen filled with a monomer silicone gel. It has an

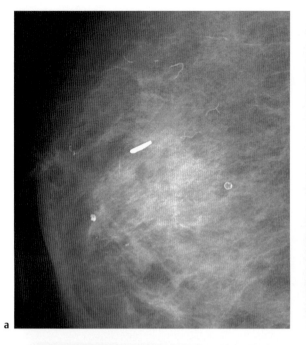

a

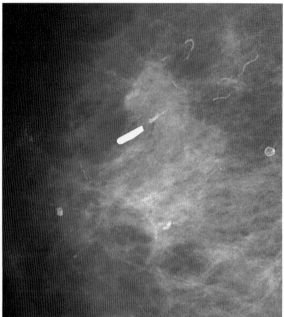

b

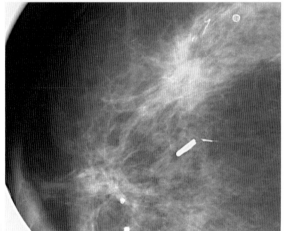

c

Fig. 8.**55a–c**   **Follow-up mammogram after breast conservation therapy**
a After four years, classical postradiation changes
b After five years, new ill-defined density superior to the surgical clip
c Magnification view shows a finding suspicious for local recurrence. Histology: IDC

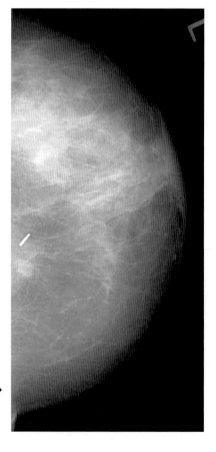

Fig. 8.**56**   **Locoregional recurrence.** Follow-up mammogram ▶ three years after breast conservation therapy (clip) shows a small spiculated nodule in the vicinity of the clip, suspicious for IDC. Histology: IDC

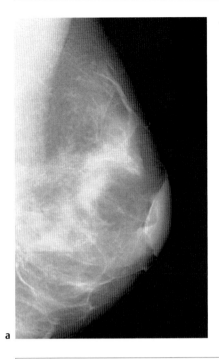

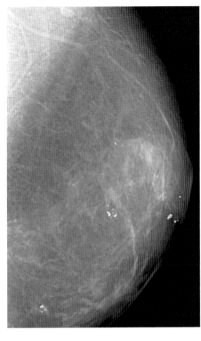

Fig. 8.57 a – c Mammographic appearance of breast reduction
a After breast reduction, architectural distortion in the lower aspect of the breast. Interrupted continuity between nipple and parenchyma
b After breast reduction, slight skin thickening and amorphous calcifications scattered along the course of the scar
c Diagram of the surgical technique of breast reduction: the incision around the nipple and areola is connected with the inframammary incision (keyhole incision). The excess breast tissue is removed and the nipple is superiorly repositioned

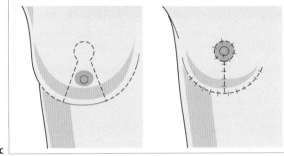

ellipsoid shape and conforms to the cosmetic requirements.

Almost invariably a fibrous capsule, which can shrink or calcify, develops around the silicone implant. The silicone gel sooner or later leaks through the semipermeable membrane constituting the envelope ("gel bleed"). These complications have led to the development of several types of new implants:

- *Implants with a polyurethane coating*: These were taken off the market very quickly because the coating led to granulomatous and inflammatory reactions and their break-down products proved to be carcinogenic in animal studies.
- *Implants with two compartments ("double lumen")*: The outer lumen consists of a silicone envelope filled with saline solution and the inner lumen filled with silicone gel. They are more susceptible to traumatic damage than the other types, but other complications are less frequent. They sometimes contain a valve for controlled expansion, e.g., for cosmetic reconstruction after mastectomy.

- *Completely radiolucent implants with soy oil (triglycerides)*.

Implants can be inserted through an inframammary or periareolar incision. They can be placed behind the glandular body or behind the pectoralis muscle. The latter procedure is more extensive but deters the development of a capsule. Removal of the implants uses the same approach but requires incision and opening of the fibrous capsule. The implant must be removed very carefully, using rubber-coated forceps to avoid rupture and spillage of silicone gel. Contraction and calcification of the capsule can lead to atrophy of the surrounding breast parenchyma, pectoralis muscle, ribs, and skin. It therefore often becomes necessary to perform a reconstruction with a TRAM flap or a mastopexy after removal of a breast implant.

Complications

Acute postsurgical complications are rare and include hematomas, seromas, or bacterial infections. As a side effect, these complications will lead to rapid encapsulation. It has become apparent that late complications associated with silicone prostheses are more widespread than originally thought.

Immunological disorders. Although silicone is practically chemically inert, it induces a foreign-body reaction. Silicone particles are resorbed by macrophages and surrounded by fibroblasts and lymphocytes. Silicone-specific antibodies have been demonstrated. Furthermore, silicone implants have been suspected to induce immunological disorders, but this is not supported by

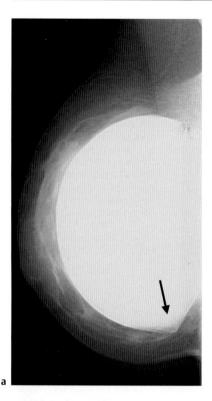

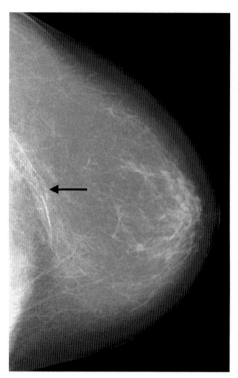

Fig. 8.**59**   Mammogram after removal of the implant. Remnants of the fibrous capsule can be recognized

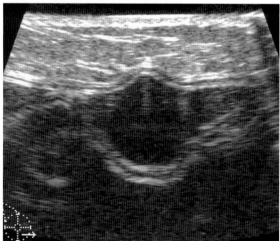

Fig. 8.**58 a, b   Silicone implant**
a Double-lumen implant. The outer compartment contains a saline solution. Grade 2 capsule formation: the prosthesis is palpable, but not visible. The patient felt a small mass in the lower inner quadrant, corresponding to a fold in the outer compartment of the implant (arrow)
b The fold was also sonographically visualized

with focal or diffuse calcification, the encapsulated implant becomes hardened and loses its oval shape. This complication occurs in 40% of implants. If it takes place within several weeks, it is known as firestorm fibrosis.

Four grades of capsule formation

- *Grade 1*: The breast feels as soft as a breast not operated upon.
- *Grade 2*: The breast is not as soft and the implant is palpable. A deformation of the breast is not noticeable.
- *Grade 3*: The breast is hardened and deformed, and the implant is palpable.
- *Grade 4*: The breast is hardened, painful, and deformed, and feels cold to the touch. External capsulotomy (vigorous manual compression) can correct these changes, but this can be complicated by hematoma, rupture, and silicone leakage.

recent epidemiological study. Studies to detect silicone migration, e.g., with MR spectroscopy, are still in the experimental stage.

Encapsulation. The thickness of the capsule around the implant can vary from 0.4 to 7.2 mm. It has an active contractile component, which causes shrinkage. Together

Silicon leakage. The silicone gel can leak through the semipermeable envelope, especially in regions of material fatigue, as occurring along folds. This leakage stimulates encapsulation. If the silicone particles remain inside the capsule, it is called an intracapsular leak. Conversely, if it extends outside, it is called an extracapsular leak.

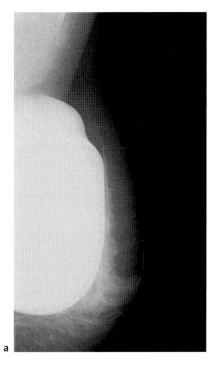

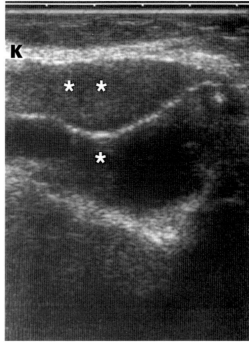

Fig. 8.**60 a, b   Intra-capsular silicone leakage**
a Single-lumen sili-cone implant with an irregular con-tour. This mammo-graphic finding is suspicious for a rupture, but fails to show free extra-capsular silicone gel
b The sonogram shows silicone gel within (*) and out-side (**) the sili-cone envelope, without signs of ex-tracapsular leakage

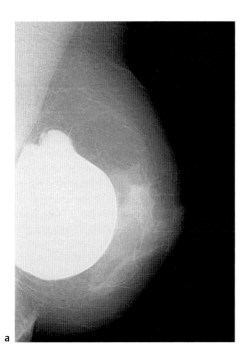

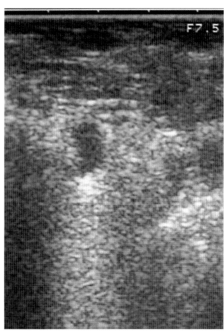

Fig. 8.**61 a, b   Extra-capsular silicone leakage**
a Ill-defined accumu-lation of gel outside the contour of the implant
b Sonography shows an ill-defined hypoechoic lesion, surrounded by echogenic noise ("snowstorm") caused by dis-persed small gel particles

Implant rupture. If the breast contour suddenly becomes irregular and mammography reveals free silicone gel outside the semipermeable envelope, the implant has ruptured. The rupture can be precipitated by trauma or manual capsulotomy, or can occur spontaneously and appear as incidental mammographic finding. The material can spread for quite a distance. Even discharge of silicone gel from the nipple has been described.

Additional breast pathology. Women with silicone implants for cosmetic reasons are usually young and not at a high risk of breast carcinoma. The implant itself does not increase the risk of malignancy. Patients with an increased risk for breast carcinoma should be advised against a silicone implant as it makes mammographic evaluation of the breast more difficult. This may lead to the detection of breast carcinoma at a more advanced stage in women with an implant than in women without an implant.

Mammography

Silicon implants do not present a contraindication for mammography but they compromise the imaging of the breast parenchyma since the implant is not radiolucent. Nevertheless, mammography represents the first step in evaluating a patient with breast complaints. Compression must be applied carefully if encapsulation is evident. The mammogram must be exposed manually since the automatic exposure control prolongs the exposure times because of the increased photon absorption in the radiodense silicone material.

The mammogram displays the radiodense silicone gel enclosed in the silicone envelope, which often shows superficial wrinkles, which are not pathologic. Implants filled with saline solution are less radiodense. The mammogram reveals the position of the implant behind the breast parenchyma or behind the pectoralis muscle. The fibrous capsule may appear as a curvilinear thickening around the implant, with or without calcifications. A contracted capsule is suspected when the hardened and rounded implant resists the usual compression. Low-grade, intracapsular silicone leakage or "gel bleed" is often not demonstrable. Extracapsular silicone leakage cannot be visualized until a sufficient amount of silicone gel has escaped.

A rupture inside a thick fibrous capsule can remain unnoticed as long as the contours are maintained. Most ruptures, however, become evident through a bizarre contour of the implant: the folded envelope floats in the center of the silicone gel, which is contained only by the fibrous capsule. Rupture and leakage are often symptomatic and induce painful granulomas and enlarged lymph nodes. These implants should be removed. After implant removal, the mammographic findings may return to normal, but the architecture often remains distorted by scarring and fat necrosis, with foreign-body reaction around silicone residues and suture material left behind.

Standard views always hide a portion of the breast parenchyma behind the implant (Fig. 6.**42**) and, consequently, are not suitable for screening. In patients with an implant, meticulous palpation is mandatory to determine the best mammographic approach:

- The lateral view often yields better result than the oblique view.
- A palpable lesion can be identified by a radiopaque marker for the supplementary magnification view.
- The Eklund view enables better compression of the breast by pulling the breast tissue forward and pushing the implant backward. This view is most suitable for subpectoral implants.

Additional Imaging Options

Sonography is especially useful for patients presenting with a palpable lesion (Fig. 8.**63**). It reliably differentiates between lesions arising from the implant and the breast parenchyma. Since imaging by mammography is limited, sonography is often the modality selected for distinguishing normal breast parenchyma, cysts, and solid lesions. Sometimes the implant bulges and produces an abnormal palpable finding. An *intact implant* has a smooth, echogenic anterior wall, which frequently produces reverberation echoes. The posterior wall is often incompletely visualized because silicone transmits sound at a lower velocity than does human tissue. Small surface wrinkles are often seen as thin, echogenic stripes that project 1–2 cm into the implant. The gel itself is anechoic, but echogenic aggregates appear with time, probably through physical or chemical transformations in the gel. The implant can be surrounded by a small amount of fluid. The contour can bulge through a locally weak area of the fibrous capsule, which does not necessarily indicate a defective implant. The capsule can be hardened like a contracture and still be barely demonstrable on sonography.

With an *intracapsular rupture,* the envelope collapses and appears sonographically as a collection of double lines within the silicone gel, arranged in either a straight or curvilinear fashion. The gel often contains echogenic aggregates. With an *extracapsular rupture*, the drops of silicon gel can be depicted as round hypoechoic lesions surrounded by hyperechoic connective tissue. Several small particles together produce a conspicuous difference in the acoustic impedance. The resultant defocusing of the sound waves creates the picture of a "snowstorm." This can hamper the evaluation of tissue located behind the lesion.

CT of the implant uses 5 mm slices and provides information about intracapsular ruptures, which appear as curvilinear, hypodense stripes inside the hyperdense silicone gel. Extracapsular leakage cannot be reliably visualized. Furthermore, CT is not genuinely suited for the evaluation of the breast parenchyma, especially when the delivered radiation dose is taken into consideration.

MRI, conversely, can reliably evaluate breast parenchyma and implants. There are many *silicone-selective MRI techniques*. A consensus about the best sequence has not yet been achieved. The sequences depend on the type of equipment used (see chapter 7, p. 172).

It is possible to distinguish the different types of implants. A double-lumen implant has a signal in the water compartment different from the signal in silicone compartment.

The fibrous capsule surrounds the implant as a rim of low signal intensity, measuring several millimeters in width. Capsular calcifications are not visualized. A rupture of the capsule is disclosed as interruption in the low-signal-intensity rim and a contracted capsule as unnatural or rounded configuration of the implant.

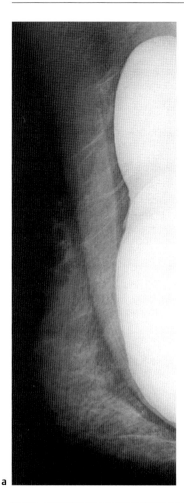

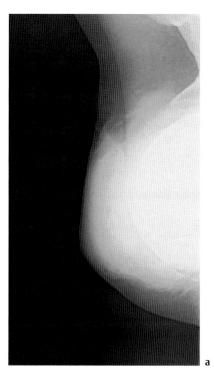

a

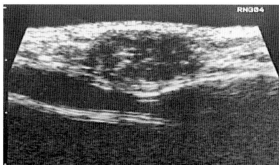

b

Fig. 8.**63 a, b   Additional breast pathology**
a Lesion in upper outer quadrant, barely discernible because of suboptimal technique. The lesion has an ill-defined contour
b Sonography shows a solid lesion with a heterogeneously hypoechoic structure and partially well-defined and partially ill-defined margins. Histology: IDC

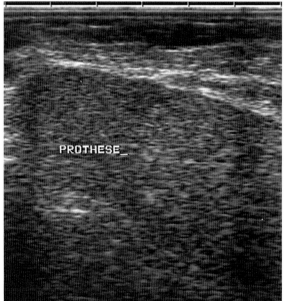

b

Fig. 8.**62 a, b   Subpectoral implant**
a Implant behind the pectoral muscle shows a rupture in the axillary region
b Sonography shows degenerated echogenic silicone gel

Wrinkles and radial folds are almost always visible as low-signal lines and should not be mistaken for an intracapsular rupture. Customarily, several planes are imaged, e.g., axial and coronal planes.

The characteristic image of an intracapsular rupture is a tangle of curvilinear low-signal structures within the silicone gel, lending it the name linguine sign. With an extracapsular rupture, macroscopic amounts of silicone gel are seen as foci of high-signal intensity outside the fibrous capsule. The distinction between gel leakage through an extracapsular rupture and extensive gel bleeding from an intact capsule is difficult. Gel bleeding often deposits free silicone gel exclusively between fibrous capsule and silicone envelope. An extracapsular rupture frequently coexists with an intracapsular rupture.

Sensitivity and specificity of detecting complications of implants are highest with MRI (see p. 176). However, MRI for the evaluation of breast complaints in a patient with an implant should always be preceded by mammography and sonography.

References

Strategy for Viewing the Mammogram:

Heywang-Köbrunner, S., I. Schreer: Bildgebende Mammadiagnostik. Thieme, Stuttgart 1996

Kopans, D. B.: Breast Imaging. Lippincott, Philadelphia 1989

Logan-Young, W., N. Yanes Hoffman: Breast Cancer, a Practiacal Guide to Diagnosis. Vol. 1: Procedures. Mt. Hope, Rochester 1994

Roebuck, E. J.: Clinical Radiology of the Breast. Heinemann, Oxford 1990

Tabár, L., P. B. Dean: Teaching Atlas of Mammography, 2nd ed. Thieme, Stuttgart 1985

Circumscribed Lesions:

Brenner, R. J., E. A. Sickles: Acceptability of periodic follow-up as an alternative to biopsy for mammographically detected lesions interpreted as probably benign. Radiology 171 (1989) 645–646

Cole-Beuglet, C., R. Z. Soriano, A. B. Kurtz: Fibroadenoma of the breast: sonomammography correlated with pathology in 122 patients. Amer. J. Roentgenol. 140 (1983) 369–375

Cupples, T. E., G. W. Eklund, G. Cardenosa: Mammographic halosign revisited. Radiology 199 (1996) 105–108

Dyess, D. L., C. O. Lorino, A. Grieco, J. J. Ferrara: Selective nonoperative management of solid breast masses. Amer. Surgn. 58 (1992) 437–440

Elson, B. C., M. A. Helvie, T. S. Frank, T. W. Wilson, D. D. Adler: Tubular carcinoma of the breast. Amer. J. Roentgenol. 161 (1993) 1173–1176

Evans, A. J., S. Pinder, I. O. Ellis, M. Sebbering et al.: Screening-detected and symptomatic ductal carcinoma in situ mammographic features with pathologic correlation. Radiology 191 (1994) 237–240

Evers, K., R. H. Troupin: Lipid cyst: classic and atypical appearances. Amer. J. Roentgenol. 157 (1991) 271–274

Feig, S. A.: The importance of supplementary mammographic views to diagnostic accuracy. Amer. J. Roentgenol. 151 (1988) 40–41

Feig, S. A.: Breast masses. Mammographic and sonographic evaluation. Radiol. Clin. N. Amer. 30 (1992) 67–92

Gershon-Cohen, J., L. Moore: Roentgenography of giant fibroadenoma of the breast (cystosarcoma phylloides). Radiology 74 (1960) 619–625

Gomez, A., J. M. Mata, L. Donoso, A. Rams: Galactocele: three distinctive radiographic appearances. Radiology 158 (1986) 43–44

Gordenne, W., F. Malchair: The peritumoral clear halo in mammography. Proc. VI Europ. Congr. Radiol. 1987 (S. 211) (abstract ERC)

Helvie, M. A., C. Paramagul. H. A. Oberman, D. D. Adler: Invasive lobular carcinoma. Imaging features and clinical detection. Invest. Radiol. 28 (1993) 202–207

Hoeffken, W., M. Lanyi: Röntgenuntersuchung der Brust. Thieme, Stuttgart 1973

Homer, M. J.: Imaging features and management of characteristically benign and probably benign breast lesions. Radiol. Clin. N. Amer. 25 (1987) 939–951

Ikeda, D. M., I. Andersson: Ductal carcinoma in situ: atypical mammographic appearances. Radiology 172 (1989) 661–666

Jackson, V. P., H. E. Reynolds: Stereotactic needle-core biopsy and finde-needle aspiration cytologic evaluation of nonpalpable breast lesions. Radiology 181 (1991) 633–634

Maes, R. M., D. J. Dronkers, J. H. C. L. Hendriks, M. A. O. Thijssen, H. W. Nab: Minimal signs in Mammography. Brit. J. Radiol. 70 (1997) 34–38

Meyer, J. E., E. Amin, K. K. Lindfors: Medullary carcinoma of the breast: mammographic and ultrasound appearance. Radiology 170 (1989) 79–82

Mitnick, J. S., D. F. Roses, M. N. Harris, H. D. Feiner: Circumscribed intraductal carcinoma of the breast. Radiology 170 (1989) 423–425

Muller, J.: The management of nonpalpable circumscribed breast masses. In Friedrich, M., E. A. Sickles: Radiological Diagnosis of Breast Diseases. Springer, Berlin 1997

Paulus, D. D.: Benign disease of the breast. Radiol. Clin. N. Amer. 21 (1983) 27–50

Paulus, D. D.: Lymphoma of the breast. Radiol. Clin. N. Amer. 28 (1990) 833–840

Rissanen, R. J., H. P. Makarainen, S. I. Mattila, E. L. Lindholm, M. I. Heikkinen, H. O. Kiviniemi: Breast cancer recurrence after mastectomy: diagnosis with mammography and US. Radiology 188 (1993) 463–467

Roebuck, E. J.: Clinical Radiology of the breast. Heinemann, Oxford 1990

Sickles, E. A.: Practical solutions to common mammographic problems: tailoring the examination. Amer. J. Roentgenol. 151 (1988) 31–39

Sickles, E. A.: Nonpalpable, circumscribed, noncalcified solid breast masses: likelihood of malignancy based on lesion size and age of patient. Radiology 192 (1994) 439–442

Stomper, P. C., S. Leibowich, J. E. Meyer: The prevalence and distribution of well-circumscribed nodules on screening mammography: analysis of 1500 mammograms. Breast Dis. 4 (1991) 197–203

Tabár, L., P. B. Dean: Teaching Atlas of Mammography, 2nd ed. Thieme, Stuttgart 1985

Calcifications:

Dongen, van J. A., I. S. Fentiman, J. R. Harris, R. Holland et al.: Insitu breast cancer: the EORTC consensus meeting. Lancet II (1989) 25–27

Holland, R., J. H. C. L. Hendriks, A. L. M. Verbeek et al.: Extent distribution and mammographic/histological correlations of breast ductal carcinoma in situ. Lancet 335 (1990) 483–485

Holland, R., J. H. C. L. Hendriks, A. L. M. Verbeek, M. Mravunac, J. H. Schuurmans Stekhoven: Extent, distribution, and mammographic/histological correlations of breast ductal carcinoma in situ. Lancet 335 (1990) 519–522

Holland, R., J. H. C. L. Hendriks: Microcalcifications associated with ductal carcinoma in situ: mammographic-pathologic correlation. Semin. diagn. Pathol. 11 (1994) 181–192

Holland, R., J. L. Peterse, R. R. Millis, V. Eusebi et al.: Ductal carcinoma in situ: A proposal for a new classification. Semin. diagn. Pathol. 11 (1994) 167–180

Kopans, D. B.: Breast Imaging. Lippincott, Philadelphia 1989

Kopans, D. B., P. I. Nguyen, F. G. Koerner et al.: Mixed form, diffusely scattered calcifications in breast cancer with apocrine features. Radiology 177 (1990) 807–811

Lanyi, M.: Formanalyse von 5641 Mikroverkalkungen bei 100 Milchgangskarzinomen: die Polymorphie. Fortschr. Röntgenstr. 139 (1983) 240

Lanyi, M.: Diagnosis and Differential Diagnosis of Breast Calcifications. Springer, Berlin 1986

Sickles, E. A.: Breast calcifications mammographic evaluation. Radiology 160 (1986) 289–293

Stomper, P. C., J. L. Connolly: Ductal carcinoma in situ of the breast: correlation between mammographic calcification and tumor subtype. Amer. J. Roentgenol. 159 (1992) 483–485

Tabár, L., P. B. Dean: Teaching Atlas of Mammography. Thieme, Stuttgart 1983

Architectural Distortion and Asymmetry:

Bird, R. E., T. W. Wallace, B. C. Yankaskas: Analysis of cancers missed at screening mammography. Radiology 184 (1992) 613–617

Ciatto, S., D. Morrone, S. Catarzi et al.: Radial scars of the breast: review of 38 consecutive mammographic diagnoses. Radiology 187 (1993) 757–760

Hilleren, D. J., I. T. Anderson, K. Lindholm, F. S. Linnell: Invasive lobular carcinoma: mammographic findings in a 10-year experience. Radiology 178 (1991) 149–154

Holland, R., J. H. C. L. Hendriks, M. Mravunac: Mammographically occult breast cancer. Cancer 52 (1983) 1810–1819

Le Gal, M., L. Ollivier, B. Asselain, M. Meunier et al.: Mammographic features of 455 invasive lobular carcinomas. Radiology 185 (1992) 705–708

Newstead, G. M., P. B. Baute, H. K. Toth: Invasive lobular and ductal carcinoma: mammographic findings and stage at diagnosis. Radiology 184 (1992) 623–627

Roebuck, E. J.: Clinical Radiology of the Breast. Heinemann, Oxford 1990

Schinz, H. R., W. E. Baensch, W. Frommhold, R. Glauner, E. Uehlinger, J. Wellauer: Lehrbuch der Röntgendiagnostik, 6. Aufl. II-2. Thieme, Stuttgart 1981

Sickles, E. A.: The subtle and atypical mammographic features of invasive lobular carcinoma. Radiology 178 (1991) 25–26

Tabár, L., P. B. Dean: Teaching Atlas of Mammography. Thieme, Stuttgart 1983

Trojani, M.: A Colour Atlas of Breast Histopathology. Chapman and Hall Medical, London 1991

Changes of the Skin:

Dershaw, D. D., M. P. Moore, L. Liberman, B. M. Deutch: Inflammatory breast carcinoma: mammographic findings. Radiology 190 (1994) 831–834

Tabár, L., P. B. Dean: Teaching Atlas of Mammography. Thieme, Stuttgart 1983

Tucker, A.: Textbook of Mammography. Churchill Livingstone, Edinburgh 1993

Lymph Nodes:

Dershaw, D. D., D. G. Selland, L. K. Tan, E. A. Morris, A. F. Abramson, L. Liberman: Spiculated axillary adenopathy. Radiology 201 (1996) 439–442

Egan, R. L.: Breast Imaging: Diagnosis and Morphology of Breast Diseases. Saunders, Philadelphia 1988

Kalisher, L., R. G. Peyster: Clinicopathological correlation of xerography in determining involvement of metastatic axilla-ry nodes in female breast cancer. Radiology 121 (1976) 333–335

Kopans, D. B.: Breast Imaging. Lippincott, Philadelphia 1989

Pamilo, M., M. Soiva, E. Lavast: Real-time ultrasound, axillary mammography and clinical examination in the detection of axillary lymph node metastases in breast cancer patients. J. Ultrasound Med. 8 (1989) 115–120

Mammographic Findings after Surgery and Radiation Therapy:

Brenner, R. J., J. M. Pfaff: Mammographic features after conservation therapy for malignant breast disease; serial findings standardized by regression analysis. Amer. J. Roentgenol. 167 (1996) 171–178

Caskey, C. I., W. A. Berg, U. M., et al.: Imaging spectrum of extracapsular silicone: correlation of US, MRI, mammographic, and histopathologic findings. Radiographics 19 (1999) S39–S51

Eklund, G. W., R. C. Busby, S. H. Miller: Improved imaging of the augmented breast. Amer. J. Roentgenol. 151 (1988) 469–473

Gabriel, S. E., W. M. O'Fallon, L. T. Kurland, C. M. Beard, J. E. Woods, L. J. Melton: Risk of connective-tissue disease and other disorders after breast implantation. New Engl. J. Med. 330 (1994) 1697–1702

Giess, C. S., D. M. Keating, M. P. Osborne, R. Rosenblatt: Local tumor recurrence following breast-conservation therapy: correlation of histopathologic findings with detection method and mammographic findings. Radiology 212 (1999) 829–835

Gorczyca, D. P., S. Sinha, C. Y. Ahn, N. D. DeBruhl et al.: Silicone breast implants in vivo: MR imaging. Radiology 185 (1992) 407–410

Hayes, M. K., R. H. Gold, L. W. Bassett: Mammographic findings after the removal of breast implants. Amer. J. Roentgenol. 160 (1993) 487–490

Lanyi, M.: Verkalkungen außerhalb des milchproduzierenden und -ableitenden Systems. In Lanyi, M.: Diagnostik und Differentialdiagnostik der Mammaverkalkungen. Springer, Berlin 1986 (S. 161)

Leibman, A. J., M. B. Kossoff, B. D. Kruse: Case report. Intraductal extension of silicone from a ruptured breast implant. Plast. reconstr. Surg. 89 (1991) 546–547

Mendelsohn, E. B.: Evaluation of the postoperative breast. Radiol. Clin. N. Amer. 30 (1992) 107–138

Rieber, A., E. Merkle, H. Zetler, et al.: Value of MR mammography in the detection of recurrent breast cancer. J. Comput. Assist. Tomogr. 21 (1997) 780–784

Steinbach, B. G., N. S. Hardt, P. L. Abbitt: Mammography: breast implants-types, Complications and adjacent breast pathology. Curr. Probl. diagn. Radiol. 12 (1993) 37–88

Stigers, K. B., J. G. King, D. D. Davey, C. B. Stelling: Abnormalities of the breast caused by biopsy: spectrum of mammographic findings. Amer. J. Roentgenol. 156 (1991) 287–291

Stomper, P. C., A. Recht, A. L. Berenberg, M. S. Jochelson, J. R. Harris: Mammographic detection of recurrent cancer in the irradiated breast. Amer. J. Roentgenol. 148 (1987) 39–43

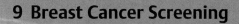

9 Breast Cancer Screening

D. J. Dronkers, J. H. C. L. Hendriks, B.–P. Robra and A. L. M. Verbeek

Toward the end of the 19th century, surgical techniques, such as radical mastectomy (Halsted), were developed that offer a chance for successful treatment of breast cancer. Until then, breast cancer was considered incurable and all treatments were actually palliative.

Further improvement in treatments reduced the breast cancer mortality to approximately 40–45%, a figure that has hardly changed in recent decades.

Since a 100% effective treatment for breast cancer does not exist and is not to be expected in the near future, prevention seems to be the only way to reduce breast cancer mortality further.

The possibilities of *primary prevention,* such as dietary changes, decreasing excess estrogen exposure, and first full-term pregnancy at a younger age, are limited and take a long time to show an effect. *Chemoprevention or -suppression* with tamoxifen or retinoids (vitamin A and its derivatives) for women with a high breast cancer risk are still in the experimental phase. *Pharmacological*

blockage of ovarian steroid production is under investigation. For women with a high breast cancer risk, *prophylactic bilateral mastectomy* is generally considered too radical.

Survival statistics of patients with different breast cancer stages have shown that the 10-year survival rates exceed 90% for tumors without axillary metastases and are even higher for tumors smaller than 1 cm.

Therefore, *secondary prevention* by means of early diagnosis seemed to be the only possible way for achieving further reduction of breast cancer mortality. Detecting the disease when it is still curable offers the opportunity to begin effective treatment before metastases develop, which ultimately should reduce mortality.

Of the methods available for early diagnosis, mammography ranks first beside clinical breast examination by specifically trained medical personnel and by the woman herself.

Results of Breast Cancer Screening Programs

Several randomized studies have shown that mammography screening, with or without clinical examination, can lead to systematic early diagnosis of the disease. Until now, definite proof of breast cancer mortality reduction has only been found in patients older than 50 years (Table 9.1).

In the first randomized screening program (HIP), the not-yet-optimal quality of mammography was possibly compensated to some extent by additional clinical ex-

amination. Most of the later studies were designed to evaluate the value of mammography without clinical examination. Many women discover their breast cancer by self-examination. Screening programs with clinical examination by experts and programs for encouraging self-examination have proved to be insufficient methods for early diagnosis since they did not affect breast cancer mortality (de Jong, 1979; Huguley et al., 1988). This is confirmed by data from mammography screening at

Table 9.1   Reduction of breast cancer mortality by mammography screening in randomized studies

Trial	Age group	Views	Screening-interval (months)	Number of screening rounds	Follow-up (years)	Mortality reduction expressed in RR	95% CI
HIP (1963–1969)	50–59	2 E, CBE	12	4	6	0.46	(0.25–0.84)
					10	0.69	(0.46–1.02)
					18	0.77	(0.55–1.08)
Malmö (1976–1986)	55–69	1 oder 2 E	18–24	5	8.8	0.79	(0.51–1.24)
					12	0.82	(0.57–1.19)
Two-county (1977–1985)	50–74	1 E	33	4	6	0.61	(0.44–0.84)
	50–59				8	0.60	(0.40–0.90)
	50–59				11	0.63	(0.45–0.88)
Edinburgh (1979–1988)	50–64	1 oder 2 E	24	4	7	0.80	(0.54–1.17)
					10	0.85	(0.62–1.15)
Stockholm (1981–1985)	50–64	1 E	28	2	7.4	0.57	(0.30–1.10)
					11	0.62	(0.38–1.00)
Göteborg (1982–1988)	50–59	2 E	18	4	7	0.91	(0.53–1.55)
Canada (1980–1987)	50–59	2 E, CBE	12	5	7	0.97	(0.62–1.52)

CI   Confidence interval
RR   relative risk (a RR of 0.60 means a mortality reduction of 40%)
E   mammography projections
CBE clinical breast examination

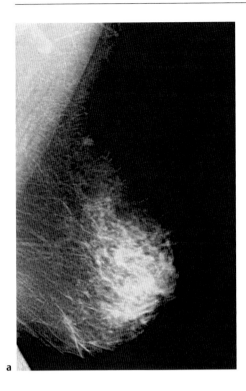 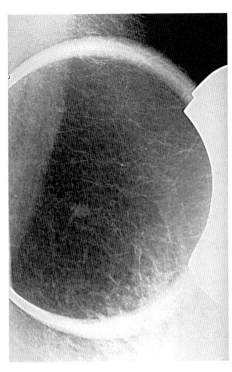

Fig. 9.**1** **Breast cancer screening of elderly women**. Ill-defined density of 6 mm in left breast of 75-year-old woman. Finding at initial screening. Histology: poorly differentiated IDC. Axillary nodes negative
a MLO view
b Magnification view

a

b

two-year intervals, which revealed that about 50% of all detected cancers are not palpable even on targeted clinical examination. This attests to the superiority of mammography over clinical examination.

In women under the age of 50 years, the sensitivity of mammography is lower than in postmenopausal women, due to the often still incomplete fatty involution of the glandular tissue at the earlier age. Furthermore, the breast cancer incidence in these younger women is lower than in women 50–70 years of age, and the average growth rate of breast cancer is higher in younger women. These factors contributed to the fact that it took many years before final conclusions could be drawn about the effectiveness of screening of women at this age. It seems that screening under the age of 50 years is beneficial but is less effective than screening in the age group between 50 and 70 years. It takes at least 10 years before any effect on mortality can be expected. Since the costs of screening are still high, the cost-effectiveness of screening in these younger women is poor. Moreover, for patients of this age the risk of cancer induction by the radiation dose might not be negligible.

For women 70–75 years old, breast cancer screening has been found to be effective (Fig. 9.**1**). Sensitivity and detection rate are high. Because of the increasing health consciousness of senior citizens, it can be expected that more women in this age group will participate in breast screening than before. It probably is cost-effective to extend breast screening programs to this age group.

European Guidelines

On the basis of controlled studies, experts of the European Union recommend the introduction of screening programs with a two-year interval for asymptomatic women over the age of 50 years. Since 1986, pilot projects have been initiated in several countries under the patronage of the European Union.

Nationwide screening programs have been established in the United Kingdom, The Netherlands, Finland, and Sweden. In these countries, mass screening is performed in specialized centers with strict quality control programs and double reading of all mammograms.

The European Commission has published official guidelines for quality assurance (see p. 83). These guidelines are established with the realization that a systematic program for early detection of breast cancer must have a high quality standard to be beneficial. The desired positive benefit/cost ratio can be achieved only by maintaining such a high quality throughout the entire screening process.

These guidelines and protocols address various aspects of the screening process, such as invitation to enroll, the medical diagnostic process (mammographic examination as such, role of radiographer and radiologist, cytology, histology), and the epidemiological analysis of the results. A separate protocol deals with the quality assurance of the technical aspects of mammography screening, with emphasis on quality control of the equipment.

Initiating a mass screening program requires access to an adequate medical infrastructure to guarantee optimal follow-up examinations and treatment. At the outset of a mass screening program, the aim should be clearly defined in terms of target group, detection rate, and positive predictive value. Proper facilities should be available for training the personnel. A quality-assurance protocol should be in place and comprehensive breast cancer registration should be operative. For monitoring the screening process epidemiological data such as incidence, stage, and mortality must be recorded.

The quantitative results of the ongoing evaluation must be used to reassess the primary screening process.

The program "Europe Against Cancer" has established a European Network of Reference Centers for Mammography Screening (EUREF) for training, coordination, and documentation. EUREF provides experts for the quality-assurance programs to be established with the various screening programs. In addition, EUREF should offer advice during the early phases of new screening programs.

European guidelines for treatment have not yet been established.

Theoretical Basis for Screening Programs

The main purpose of screening is detecting breast cancer in a curable stage, i.e., before the primary tumor has spread.

It is assumed that a tumor has no metastases in its initial stage. Metastasis begins at a certain moment in the development of a tumor, probably depending on the growth-related vascularization in and around the tumor. Although tumors with a diameter of 5 mm may already have metastasized and tumors with a diameter of several centimeters may not have, all studies suggest a strong correlation between size of the tumor and risk of metastases. It is believed that metastic spreading begins at the average diameter of about 1.5 cm.

Assuming an average tumor doubling time of 100 days, Gullino (1977) estimated that it takes at least nine years until or before a tumor has reached a diameter of 5 mm (Fig. 9.2).

In many cases, tumors of this size can be detected by mammography. It takes two additional years for the tumor to reach a diameter of 20 mm. Depending on the location of the tumor and the size of the breast, many tumors have become clinically palpable when they have reached this size.

Therefore, mammography offers the opportunity for detecting a tumor two years earlier than by clinical breast examination. This period, in which the tumor is preclinically detectable by mammography, is called the detectable *preclinical phase* or *sojourn time* (Fig. 9.3).

If the tumor is detected in this period by mammography, the gain in time for the diagnosis is called *lead-time*.

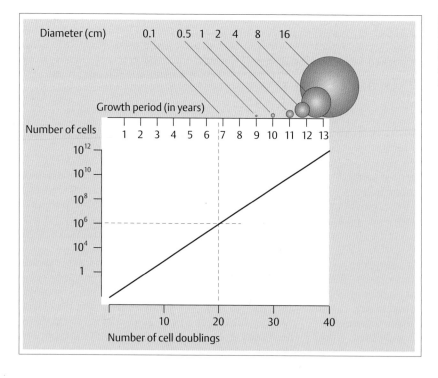

Fig. 9.2 **Natural growth of breast cancer.** Long preclinical period of breast cancer on the basis of an average tumor doubling time of 100 days (according to Gullino, 1977)

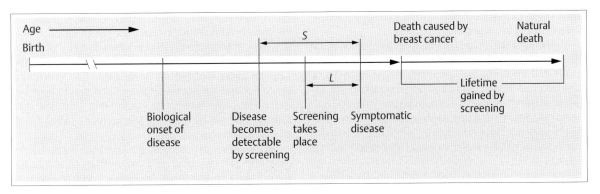

Fig. 9.**3** **Natural history of breast cancer** (adapted from Cole and Morrison, 1978)
S = sojourn time: the length of time that a lesion is potentially   L = lead time: the length of time by which detection by
   detectable in the pre-clinical phase   screening is brought forward

This gain in time is generally considered the essence of mammography screening.

Unfortunately, it has been proved that approximately 5% of all breast cancers larger than 1 cm are not visible on mammograms. These cancers are mammographically occult. This fact alone means that mammography misses one of 20 breast cancers.

Besides cancers that are mammographically occult for unknown reasons, there are factors known to contribute to false negative screening results. The major factor is mastopathy with its mammographically dense pattern of fibroglandular tissue. Cancers that manifest themselves exclusively as density may be hidden or barely show up in these dense breasts. Thus, mastopathy diminishes the sensitivity of mammography. Figure 9.**4** shows the age-specific incidence of mammographic density and breast cancer.

In mass mammography screening programs the consequence of a false negative screening outcome is the loss of the intended gain in time (early diagnosis) for participating women. If a cancerous lump is discovered by a participating woman in her breast, its average prognosis is comparable to that of a breast cancer in a non-participant, but the woman with a false-negative result is disadvantaged when the negative result discourages her from consulting a doctor after finding a lump at self-examination.

A similar phenomenon is such a confidence in the screening program that women wait for the next screening appointment after self-detection of a lump, instead of consulting a doctor. Theoretically, mammography screening could increase the mortality in these cases. This can be prevented by proper education, with emphasize on the importance of immediate consultation with a

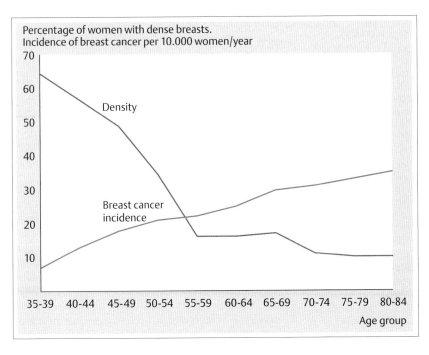

Fig. 9.**4** **Age-specific incidence of mammographic density and breast cancer** (adapted from van Gils et al., 1998; NCR, 1990)

physician when she herself discovers a lump, regardless of the result of the screening program.

Mammographic presentation of breast cancer is not always characteristic of a cancer, leading to false positive results and lowering the specificity to less than 100%. False positive results and their consequences (for instance, surgery because of a benign lesion) may be detrimental to participation in screening programs. The quality of a screening program is to be judged by sensitivity, specificity, positive predictive value, and detection rate (Fig. 9.**5**).

In a mammography screening program, the primary goal is to separate all participants into two groups:

- Women without any mammographic suspicion for breast cancer
- Women who have mammographic abnormalities suspicious for breast cancer

A mammography screening program offers no diagnosis but selects women requiring additional examination.

Mammographic screening is not a single event but an ongoing process. Participants should be examined periodically, with an interval of, for instance, two years for several decades.

Test result	Existing disease		Total
	Yes	No	
Positive	a	b	$a+b$
Negative	c	d	$c+d$
Total	$a+c$	$b+d$	$a+b+c+d$

Fig. 9.5   Characteristics of mammographic screening

Sensitivity: Sensitivity indicates the ability of mammography to identify women with breast cancer. Of all women with breast cancer ($a+c$), mammography detects only a number (a). The sensitivity is then $a/(a+c) \times 100\%$. c is the number of women with breast cancer who are not detected by screening, i.e., the screening is false negative. The percentage of false negatives is complementary to the sensitivity:
Sensitivity (in %) = 100% minus the proportion of false negative cases (in %)

Specificity: Specificity indicates the ability to identify women without breast cancer. Of all women without breast cancer ($b+d$), mammography only identifies group (d) as being without cancer, but group (b) has a positive screening result, i.e., a false positive result. The specificity is $d/(b+d) \times 100\%$. The percentage of false positives is complementary to the specificity:
Specificity (in %) = 100% minus the proportion of false positive cases (in %)

Positive predictive value: The positive predictive value of screening is the correct part of all positive findings, i.e., $a/(a+b) \times 100\%$.

Detection rate: The detection rate is the correct part of all true positive screening results per 1000 participants, i.e., $a/(a+b+c+d) \times 1000$ (in ‰)

In the initial screening of a particular age group, the number of detected breast cancers, the so-called prevalence, is approximately three times greater than the natural incidence in this group (Fig. 4.**2**). This reflects the gain in time realized by screening. The preclinical cancers found are not only cancers that would have become clinically detectable within one year but also cancers that would manifest themselves clinically only after one or two years.

In the subsequent screening rounds, the breast cancer detection rate is about 50% lower than in the initial screening. With an interval of two years, only tumors that became mammographically visible during the interval are found in the subsequent round, as long as the initial screening had a sufficiently high sensitivity. Theoretically, this number cannot be higher than twice the annual incidence in the age group undergoing screening. Indeed, it has been shown that subsequent screening rounds detect no more than twice the number of breast cancers expected from the natural incidence. Accordingly, the high detection rate in the initial screening falls back in subsequent screening to the level of the incidence before the screening program. Most of the screening-detected cancers have a more favorable stage than the cancers detected before the screening program.

As not all breast cancers have the same growth rate within the interval of two years, fast-growing tumors may develop from undetectable to clinically manifest tumors. These cancers constitute the main portion of the so-called *interval cancers,* which are cancers that become clinically manifest during the interval after negative previous screening. Interval cancers are fast-growing cancers (curve F in Fig. 9.**6**) that were not visible or missed on the preceding screening examination (curve M in Fig. 9.**6**).

Most tumors detected in subsequent screening were not mammographically visible two years earlier. Contrary to the initial screening, subsequent screening also detects less slowly growing tumors. A certain selection takes place on average, with subsequent screening rounds finding somewhat faster growing tumors than the first screening round. Consequently, tumors detected in subsequent screening have a slightly less favorable prognosis. The same also applies to interval carcinomas.

Discriminating between screen-positive and screen-negative mammograms can basically follow two different strategies:

- The premise of the first strategy is finding all detectable breast cancers. This means giving priority to the highest possible sensitivity. As a consequence, almost all women with an abnormal finding at mammography undergo further investigations, with no fewer than 50–100 of every 1000 participants called back for additional diagnostic procedures. The average number of detected breast cancers per 1000 screened women is high. Even with increasing use of percutaneous needle core biopsies, many women

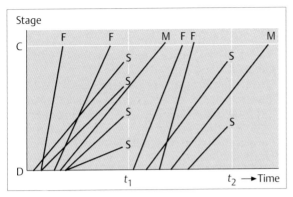

Fig. 9.6 Schematic representation of breast cancers occurring during the implementation of a screening program. Cancers become detectable by mammography at phase D and symptomatic at phase C. The first screening takes place at t_1 and the second screening at t_2. S signifies cancers detected at screening; F signifies fast growing cancers appearing in the interval between screens; M signifies cancers missed at screening and appearing in the interval between screening examinations (false-negative cases). Both M and F are called interval cancers (adapted from Brekelmans, 1995)

still undergo surgical biopsies. The positive predictive value is low as most surgical biopsies find a benign lesion.

- The premise of the second strategy is achieving a high specificity without compromising the sensitivity. This means subjecting only suspicious lesions to further investigations. The number of screen-positives per 1000 is lower and, consequently, also the number of unnecessary operations in these asymptomatic women. The positive predictive value of open biopsies is high and finding three cancers in four biopsies is not uncommon. The detection rate of this strategy is lower than the strategy of pursuing the highest sensitivity. Consequently, the number of interval cancers is also higher.

Conclusion

Screening aiming at maximum sensitivity
- All abnormalities are investigated further, therefore a high proportion of referrals.
- High percentage of false positives: many unnecessary operations and much anxiety.
- Lower percentage of false negatives, i.e., fewer interval cancers.

Screening aiming at high specificity and maintaining sufficient sensitivity
- Not all detected abnormalities are investigated further, therefore a low referral percentage.
- Lower percentage of false positives: fewer unnecessary operations and less anxiety.
- Slightly more interval cancers.

A high percentage of screen-positives and a low detection rate indicate a poor performance of the screening. A low percentage of screen-positives and a detection rate corresponding to the natural incidence indicate a good performance.

An additional important performance indicator of a screening program is the compliance rate of the target group. Without a system of inviting women by sending out personal invitations indicating time and place, it is difficult to achieve high attendance. Almost 80% of all women (in the target group 50–70 years of age) participate in the nationwide screening program in The Netherlands, which uses an invitation system based on the local population registration, with a reminder sent after several weeks to women who have not come for the screening examination. The entire screening program is financed by the national social security system.

The length of the interval between two screening rounds is crucial for effective screening. If the interval is short compared to the lead time, fast-growing tumors (which will rarely benefit from screening) are likely to be screen-detected. With an increasing interval, less fast-growing tumors are detected, and the proportion of slowly growing tumors among the tumors detected will increase. This is a reflection of a probabilistic distribution of tumor growth rates. If the interval is considerably longer than the lead time, most tumors that are detected will be slowly growing, and on average will have a better prognosis. It is doubtful whether such a screening program would reduce the mortality of breast cancer.

Most screening programs are offered to women over the age of 50 years. Experience has shown that the optimal length of the interval depends on the average age of the target group. This is a consequence of the average growth rate of breast cancer, which is higher in younger women than in older women (p. 35, Table **3.3**). Up to the age of 55 years, an interval of one year is recommended, beyond that age an interval of two years. For women over 70 years of age, an interval of three years might be sufficient.

Although not in all cases, early detection by mammography screening leads to a definite cure and, consequently, to a lower mortality. The exception applies to the following scenarios:

- For breast cancers that have already metastasized, screening is not beneficial.
- For very slowly growing cancers that do not develop into overt cancers during the woman's life span, screening may not be beneficial, especially when the woman dies from unrelated causes.
- Possibly for DCIS since it is not known whether all develop into invasive cancer.

Operational Models of Mammography Screening

<table>
<tr><td>

Starting points of mammography screening

- Participation should be restricted to asymptomatic women of a certain age group.
- The final result depends on
  - rate of participation;
  - quality of the screening program.

</td></tr>
</table>

Different models are available.

- *Invitation or not?*
  Without invitation, screening attendance remains a self-selection of women who are concerned about their health and are not a representative group of the population. Only if women of a targeted age group are personally invited and participate in a sufficient number, effective screening is achievable.
- *In specialized centers or not?*
  In The Netherlands, it was found that the quality of mammography was higher in specialized centers than in most hospitals and private offices.
- *Partially or completely subsidized or not subsidized?*
  To achieve a high rate of participation, subsidization by government or insurance companies seems to be essential.
- *Cancer registration or not?*
  To determine the number of interval cancers, a complete registration of all cancers is essential. Evaluating the interval cancers is an important quality criterion of the screening program.
- *Combination with clinical breast examination by specially trained personnel or not?*

Palpation can detect palpable, mammographically occult cancers.

- *Screening with or without further assessment?*
  Incorporation of further assessment in the screening program is especially advisable if no film processing is done at the place of the examination, which also means that no comparison with previous films is possible immediately following the examination when the woman is still present.

Assessment in the screening organization means that screening is offering a diagnosis, reducing the number of false positive as well as false negative findings and, therefore, leading to a higher sensitivity and specificity of the screening.

Screening without assessment means that screening is no more than selecting women for further examination. This is the least expensive way of screening since the cost of the referred diagnostic procedures is not included in the screening.

The examination itself can be performed in several ways:

- Mammography with two views (CC and MLO) per breast for initial and subsequent screening.
- As above, but only one view (MLO) in subsequent screening.
- As above, but review of the MLO in subsequent screening and comparison with previous films; the radiographer decides whether an additional CC is needed.
- Mammography exclusively with one view (MLO) per breast in all screening rounds.

Practical Advice on the Execution of a Screening Program

It is advisable to have previous films available for comparison when the mammographic films are obtained and again when they are read. The interpreting radiologist should be given the following information:

- Any breast complaints
- Previous operations or radiation
- Family history of breast cancer
- Estrogen replacement

It is also essential that the radiographer makes a notation of the existence and location of scars and skin lesions, such as papillomas, birthmarks, and warts.

It has been proved that double readings executed independently increase the sensitivity of mammography screening (Thurfjell, 1994). The two readers should reach a consensus as to the need for any referral for dis-

cordant findings. It is advisable that at least one of the readers be involved in the evaluation of screen-positives and interval cancers. This allows the continuous clinical feedback essential to achieve and maintain a high level of interpretative proficiency. A preceding initial reading by the radiographer may also contribute to higher sensitivity of the screening.

A woman with bloody nipple discharge, perimammillary eczema, or lump at the screening examination is strongly advised to visit her physician, even when the mammogram is negative. The same advice is given when the radiographer discovers one of these abnormalities during positioning or compression of the breasts.

Probably benign lesions found in otherwise screen-negative cases are not always reported to the woman or her physician, to reduce the frequently demanded excision for assurance. Not reporting palpable lesions may undermine the faith in the screening program, making this a questionable strategy.

Women with the following require a more dedicated examination than standard screening mammography can offer:

- Silicone breast implants
- Intramammary pacemakers
- Considerable postsurgical or posttraumatic breast deformations.
  These women need additional and/or special views and/or sonography.

If a screening program is selected with only one view in subsequent rounds, it is advisable to authorize the radiographers to decide in which cases a CC view is needed. The following are criteria for an additional CC view:

- Women who have not participated in the initial round

- New microcalcifications or an increased number of preexisting microcalcifications
- New density or progression of an existing density, including a new dense axillary lymph node
- Asymmetry, new or progressed
- Architectural distortion
- After surgery for breast cancer and breast reduction only once, and in cases of breast implants always (see also p. 121)
- When the woman was screen-positive in the previous round
- In cases of considerable mastopathy with possible local underexposure
- When previous films are unavailable for comparison
- Whenever the radiographer assumes that the interpretation of the mammograms might be difficult.

Interpretation, Double Reading

The reading of screening mammograms requires special training and expertise. At times, it can be very difficult or even impossible to distinguish between a benign and a malignant lesion. Each finding demands a yes or no decision, whereby a balance must be found between false positive and false negative results, positive and negative predictive values, and detection rate.

During the first years of a screening program, analysis of the results usually shows a learning process. The rate of positive findings of the initial screening decreases slightly and with it, though less pronounced, the biopsy rate. At the same time, the cancer detection rate might increase slightly. These trends reflect an improvement of the entire diagnostic process as evidence of the learning process. The improved quality ultimately leads to an increase in the positive predictive value.

A distinction must be made between initial and subsequent screenings when evaluating the screening program. The first category includes not only women who are examined for the first time but also women who skipped one or several screening rounds.

When all women of the target group in a certain region have been invited and examined, the age distribution of patients examined for the first time changes within a short period. Many newcomers are just over 50 years of age. These younger women have a lower breast cancer incidence, more dense breasts and tumors that on average have a higher growth rate. This results in a lower detection rate and a higher referral rate, leading to a decrease in the positive predictive value.

It was expected that the large number of mammograms of the mass screening program would reduce the current number of diagnostic mammograms in symptomatic women, in women after treatment for breast-cancer and as screening in women at high risk.

This was not observed in the Arnhem region (Netherlands) (Fig. 9.7). Although the screening program has induced a slight increase in the number of diagnostic mammograms (screen positives), the decrease in the number of diagnostic mammograms in women belonging to the target group, was fully compensated for by self-referral of women not belonging to the target group. This demand may be generated by the screening program.

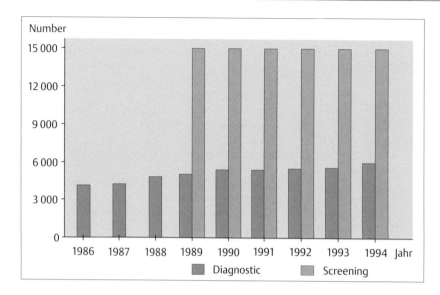

Fig. 9.**7**   **Yearly number of diagnostic mammograms in institutions before and during execution of mass screening program** (region of Arnhem 1986–1994)

Radiation Risk

Although the breast parenchyma belongs to the most sensitive tissues for radiation-induced cancer, it is doubtful whether the very low radiation dose of modern mammography is harmful. The present risk estimates are calculated on the basis of extrapolation of known radiation effects of doses over 1000 mGy. It is known that the risk of cancer induction in the breast correlates with the development and activity of the breast parenchyma. Therefore, the risk is highest during menarche and first full-term pregnancy. After that period, the sensitivity of the breast parenchyma steadily decreases resulting in a low risk for cancer induction over 50 years of age. Furthermore, the radiation dose delivered with mammography decreases with age due to involution of the breast parenchyma. Based on today's knowledge, the average radiation dose of approximately 1 mGy per mammographic exposure in women over 50 years is not expected to increase the breast cancer incidence. Should a risk exist, it is so small that it can be neglected considering the benefit of breast cancer screening.

Analysis of Cost-Benefit and Cost-Effectiveness

The cost-benefit of breast cancer screening is determined by comparing cost and benefit in a population undergoing screening with cost and benefit in a population not offered screening, with the most important benefit the reduction in breast cancer mortality (see Fig. 9.**8**).

In The Netherlands, the reduction of mortality is almost 50% for all participating women and 30% for women in the target group if the average participation rate is 70%. For the entire female population, the mortality is expected to be reduced by 16% in the year 2016. Together with a reduction of the mortality comes a reduction of the number of women with advanced breast cancer, improving quality of life and decreasing treatment costs. More women can be treated with breast conservation therapy instead of mastectomy.

The gain in quality of life and the cost savings achieved by treating fewer women with advanced disease justify the cost of screening, even when taking into account the considerable cost of quality control. In The Netherlands, the cost per life year gained is between US$ 3000 and 4000. This amount is lower than the costs of many other life-saving medical activities with established cost effectiveness, including screening for cervical cancer. Moreover, breast cancer screening has a positive effect on the quality of clinical mammography and probably also on the diagnosis and treatment of small nonpalpable breast lesions.

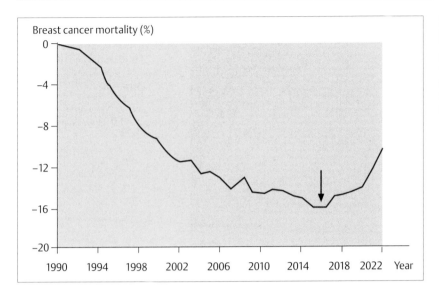

Fig. 9.8 **Expected reduction in mortality from breast cancer in The Netherlands due to mass screening (expected duration 1990–2016), shown as a percentage of breast cancer mortality without screening** (de Koning, 1993)

Interval Cancers

Interval cancer refers to a cancer that is diagnosed in the interval between a negative screening examination and the next scheduled examination of a screening program (Figs. 9.**9** and 9.**10**).

In The Netherlands, the number of interval cancers is approximately 1.0–1.5 per 1000 participants in two years. The average natural breast cancer incidence for women in the target group of 50–69 years is 2.25 per 1000, consequently 4.5 breast cancers per 1000 women will appear every two years. The subsequent two-year-interval screening rounds will detect 3–3.5 breast cancers per 1000 women. When adding the interval cancers, this number equals the number of the expected natural incidence. Of all breast cancers occurring in the target group, about 30% are interval cancers.

It is understandable that women with an interval cancer are quite disappointed in the screening program, especially when they learn that, in retrospect, the last screening mammography already showed a tiny abnormality. Such occurrences may lead to a lawsuit against the screening organization. Since interval cancers are inevitable in a mass screening program, it is important to state on the invitation to a screening program that a negative screening never offers an absolute guarantee of being free of (sub)clinical cancer.

It should also be emphasized that a routine screening examination, especially if confined to one view per breast, is a limited examination compared with clinical mammography.

Reviewing the mammograms preceding the detection of interval cancers represents an important learning experience, especially for radiologists undergoing training in screening mammography.

It is advisable to collect all interval cancers and to review them with outside experts. Basically, interval cancers can be divided into "true" interval cancers that even in retrospect were undetectable by mammography at the time of the preceding screening and cancers that retrospectively were visible on the screening mammogram, but were not called at the time of screening.

Classification of interval cancers

- Not visible at screening (even retrospectively)
- Minimal finding at screening, but below threshold for referral
- Tumor visible at screening:
  - Missed by both readers
  - Missed because of inadequate positioning
  - Missed due to poor technique (underexposure, inadequate film processing)
- Tumor "mammographically occult" at time of screening and when detected

---

In a review of previous mammograms of interval and screen-detected cancers, van Dijck et al. (1993) found that 15% of all interval cancers are retrospectively visible and must be classified as missed cancers. Subtle stellate distortions in the retromamillary region of dense breasts are notorious for being missed. In approximately 45% of the cases, no abnormality is visible even in retrospect (true interval cancer). In approximately 35% of cases, screening mammography retrospectively shows minimal changes where the tumor later develops. These may be a few nonspecific microcalcifications, a vague ill-defined density of less than 1 cm in diameter, a delicate architectural distortion, or a slight asymmetry. These minimal signs cannot be classified as suspicious since they are encountered in about 10% of all participants. Most

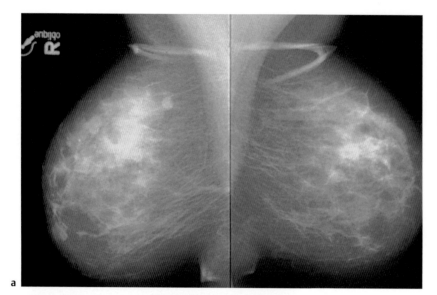

a

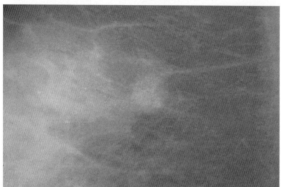

b

Fig. 9.**9 a, b   Interval cancer missed at screening**. Palpable tumor in the right breast 15 months after screening. Histology: IDC measuring 20 mm diameter; positive axillary lymph nodes
a MLO views. Screening
b Detail of (**a**). Upper part of the right breast

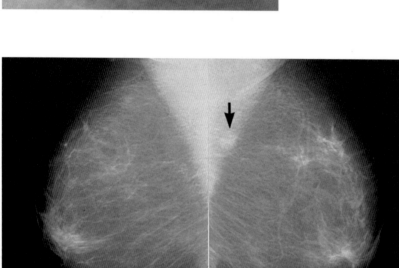

Fig. 9.**10   Interval cancer**. Cancer in the left breast, superimposed on pectoral muscle, missed at screening (arrow) in a woman of 52 years. Palpable lump nine months after screening. Histology: IDC; diameter 12 mm; negative axillary lymph nodes

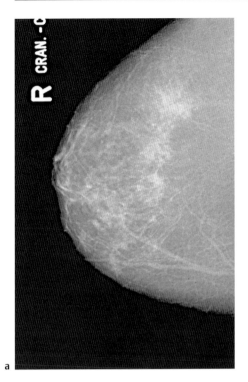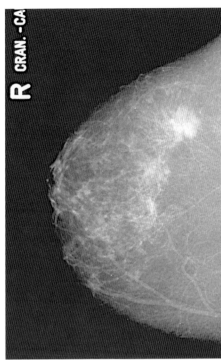

a

b

Fig. 9.**11 a, b** Minimal signs in the right breast at screening
a Screening in 1989
b Screening in 1991. One of the minimal signs has become more dense. Histology: IDC measuring 20 mm in diameter; negative axillary lymph nodes

minimal signs remain unchanged in the subsequent screening rounds, but they may disappear spontaneously or turn into a benign lesion. As found in the review of previous mammograms of interval cancers and screen-detected cancers, such minimal signs can also be the first sign of breast cancer.

The risk of minimal signs developing into an invasive cancer within two years is about 1%, which is small enough to classify minimal signs as nonspecific and not requiring referral.

This will avoid many unnecessary diagnostic procedures (among others, surgical biopsies) in 99 of 100 women, but denies 1 of 100 women the benefit of early diagnosis by screening.

The essential difference between the two screening strategies is the referral or nonreferral to diagnostic mammography if minimal signs are found at screening (Figs. 9.**11** – 9.**13**).

Mammographically occult tumors and technical failures account for 5% of interval cancers in quality-controlled screening. Most interval cancers occur in the final segment of the interval. With an increase of the interval from two to three years, interval cancers will increase and their occurrence rate in the last year of the extended interval concurs with the natural incidence. Interval cancers largely share the prognosis of clinically detected cancers and, consequently, have a less favorable prognosis than screen-detected cancers.

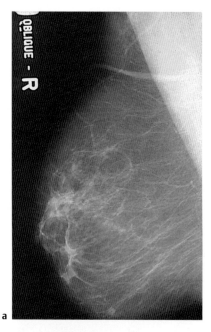

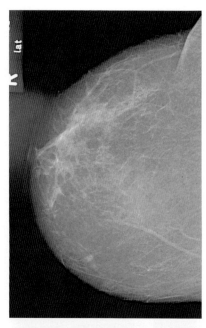

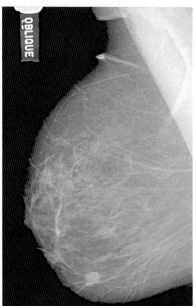

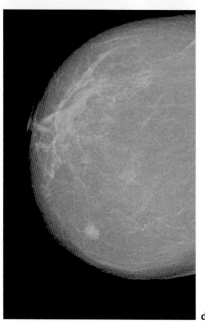

a

b

c

d

Fig. 9.**12 a – d**   **Minimal signs in the right breast**
a, b Screening
a MLO view, small round lesion in the lower part
b CC view. Small irregular lesion medial
c ,d Two years later, the lesion has grown. Histology: IDC measuring 9 mm in diameter; negative axillary lymph nodes

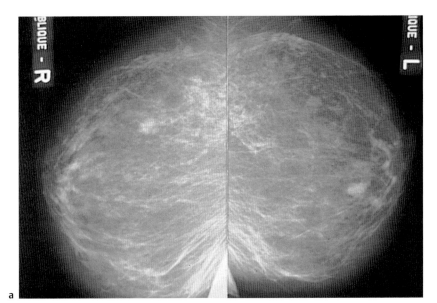

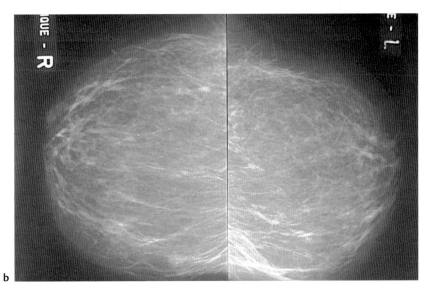

Fig. 9.13 a, b   Minimal signs in both breasts
a Screening 1991
b Screening 1995. Spontaneous regression of minimal signs

Conclusion

In mammography screening, organization, performance, clinical assessment, and evaluation must be of high quality to realize the desired goal of reducing mortality. Breast cancer is one of the main threats to health in civilized countries. Mammography screening makes a substantial contribution to the reduction of breast cancer mortality.

References

Andersson, I., K. Aspegan, L. Janzon, et al.: Mammographic screening and mortality from breast cancer: The Malmö mammographic screening trial. Brit. Med. J. 297 (1988) 943 – 948

Bassett, L. W., A. J. Hollatz-Brown, R. Bastani, J. C. Pearce, K. Hirji, L. Chen: Effects of a program to train radiologic technologists to identify abnormalities on mammograms. Radiology 194 (1995) 189 – 192

Brekelmans, C. T. M.: Natural History and Epidemiology of Interval Breast Cancer in the DOM Screening Programme. Thesis, Utrecht 1995

Cole, P., A. A. Morrison: Basic issues in cancer screening. In Miller, A. B.: Screening in cancer. UICC Technical Report Series 40 (1978) 7 – 39

Dijck, van J. A. A. M., A. L. M. Verbeek, J. H. C. L. Hendriks, R. Holland: The current detectability of breast cancer in a mammographic screening programme: a review of the previous mammograms of interval and screen-detected cancers. Cancer 72 (1993) 1933 – 1938

Europäische Leitlinien für die Qualitätssicherung im Mammographie-Screening. Juni 1996. Europäische Kommission, Brüssel 1996

Faulk, R. M., E. A. Sickles, R. A. Sollitto, S. H. Ohinsky, H. B. Galvin, S. D. Frankel: Clinical efficacy of mammographic screening in the elderly. Radiology 194 (1995) 193 – 197

van Gils, C. H., J. D. M. Otten, A. L. M. Verbeek, J. H. C. L. Hendriks: Breast parenchymal patterns and their changes with age. Brit. J. Radiol. 68 (1995) 1133 – 1135

Gullino, P. M.: Natural history of breast cancer. Progression from hyperplasia to neoplasia as predicted by angiogenesis. Cancer 39 (1977) 2697 – 2703

Harris, J. R., S. Hellman, I. C. Henderson, D. W. Kinne: Breast Diseases. Lippincott, Philadelphia 1987

Harris, J. R., M. E. Lippman, U. Veronesi, W. Willett: Breast cancer. New Engl. J. Med. 327 (1992) 319 – 329

Huguley, C. M., R. L. Brown, R. S. Greenberg, W. S. Clark: Breast self-examination and survival from breast cancer. Cancer 62 (1988) 1389 – 1396

Jong, de W.: Bevolkingsonderzoek op Borstkanker in Leiden 1975. Thesis, Leiden 1979

Kerlikowske, K., D. Grady, S. Rubin, K. C. Sandio, V. Ernster: Efficacy of screening mammography, a metaanalysis. J. Amer. med. Ass. 273 (1995) 149 – 154

Koning, de H.: The Effects and Costs of Breast Cancer Screening. Thesis, Rotterdam 1993

Kopans, D. B.: Mammography screening and the controversy concerning women aged 40 to 49. Radiol. Clin. N. Amer. 33 (1995) 1273 – 1291

Maes, R. M. D. J. Dronkers, J. H. C. L. Hendriks, M. A. O. Thijssen, H. W. Nab: Minimal signs in mammography. Brit. J. Radiol. 70 (1997) 34 – 38

Moskowitz, W.: Retrospective reviews of breast cancer screening: What do we really learn from them? Radiology 199 (1996) 615 – 620

Netherlands Cancer Registry (NCR) 1990

Shapiro, S., W. Venet, P. Strax, L.Venet: Periodic Screening for Breast Cancer: The Health Insurance Plan Project and Its Sequelae 1963 – 1986 The Johns Hopkins University Press, Baltimore 1988

Thurfjell, E. L., K. A. Lernevall, A. A. S. Taube: Benefit of independent double reading in a population-based mammography screening program. Radiology 191 (1994) 241 – 244

Verbeek, A. L. M., M. C. van den Ban, J. H. C. L. Hendriks: A proposal for short-term quality control in breast cancer screening. Brit. J. Cancer 63 (1991) 261 – 264

Wald, N. J., Ph. Murphy, Ph. Major, C. Parkes, J. Townsend, C. Frost: UK CCCR multicentre randomised controlled trial of one and two view mammography in breast cancer screening. Brit. med. J. 311 (1995) 1189 – 1193

10 Diagnosis of Breast Diseases in Males

Benign and Malignant Changes of the Male Breast

Th. Wobbes and L. V. A. M. Beex

Gynecomastia and breast cancer are the relevant pathological clinical conditions of the male breast. Gynecomastia is frequent and breast cancer is rare. Occasionally metastases may be detected in the male breast.

■ Gynecomastia

Gynecomastia is defined as enlargement of the male breast and may occur unilaterally or bilaterally. A distinction is made between gynecomastia spuria and gynecomastia vera. *Gynecomastia spuria* refers to an enlargement caused by fatty tissue and is frequently observed in obese men, while *gynecomastia vera* refers to an enlargement of the glandular breast tissue. Gynecomastia vera is commonly seen in boys during puberty (30–60% of all boys) and in older men (50–80 years) as senescent gynecomastia. In both age groups, gynecomastia is considered physiological. In boys, it generally resolves spontaneously after puberty.

However, gynecomastia may be a sign of a number of pathological conditions of endocrine and nonendocrine origin:

- Klinefelter syndrome
- Tumors of the adrenal gland
- Nonseminomatous germ cell tumors of the testis, producing HCG (human choriogonadotropin)
- Ectopic HCG-producing tumors (i.e., bronchial carcinoma)

Gynecomastia can be the first sign of these conditions and, if occurring outside the physiological age groups, should always be looked at with suspicion. Moreover, gynecomastia may occur in liver cirrhosis, caused by elevated estrogen plasma levels due to insufficient metabolic clearance of estrogens by the liver. Enlargement of the male breast can also be seen in obstructive pulmonary diseases, sarcoidosis, and ulcerative colitis. Not infrequently, drugs can induce gynecomastia: steroids, antiestrogens, alkylating anticancer drugs, digoxin, antihypertensive drugs, H_2 receptor blockers, and psychotherapeutic drugs. Finally, drug addiction with heroin and marijuana and alcohol abuse may give rise to gynecomastia. In a number of cases, no definite cause of gynecomastia can be elicited.

Even when gynecomastia is not associated with a serious condition, it can lead to psychological problems. Surgical removal is then an adequate solution. Sometimes the condition can also be treated for a certain period with an antiestrogen medication such as tamoxifen.

■ Breast Cancer

Breast cancer in males is a rare condition that comprises less than 1% of all male cancers. Of all breast cancers, 0.5–1% occur in males. The onset of the disease is 10 years later than in females at the mean age of 60 years.

Predisposing factors for male breast cancer

- Previous irradiation, for example in skin diseases
- In conjunction with elevated estrogen levels: Klinefelter-syndrome (XXY-chromosome), liver insufficiency
- Treatment with estrogens, for example in prostate cancer

Although gynecomastia is found in 40% of cases, a causal relationship seems to be unlikely, and gynecomastia is not considered to be a premalignant condition.

Familial occurrence is rare but, if found, has the same risk profile as observed in females. A close relationship between a mutation in the *BRCA 2* gene and male breast cancer has been established. In 10% of men with breast cancer, a second malignant tumor will be discovered in another organ of the body during their lifetime.

Clinical Characteristics of Male Breast Cancer

As in females, the clinical presentation of male breast cancer is a *painless swelling* behind or adjacent to the areola (70–80%). *Nipple retraction or infiltration* is found in 10% of cases. Even ulceration of the overlying skin can occur. *Bloody nipple discharge* has been described. Since the clinical picture of breast cancer is less pronounced in males than in females, primary treatment is often delayed for several months. In clinical practice, this means that most men present with a relatively advanced stage of disease (T3 b and T4), and a relatively high percentage have lymph node involvement (45–65%).

Most tumors are invasive ductal cancers, and ductal carcinoma in situ is found in less than 10% of patients. An invasive lobular carcinoma is a rare occurrence since no lobules are formed in the male breast. Bilaterality has also been described in males.

The clinical behavior of breast cancer in males is not different from that in females. Clinical studies have shown that the prognosis depends on the size of the primary tumor and lymph node status, as in females.

Treatment of the Primary Tumor and Axillary Lymph Nodes

The standard treatment is a modified radical mastectomy. In some institutions, however, a radical mastectomy (Halsted) is advised because of the relatively frequent involvement of the underlying pectoralis muscle. To avoid unnecessary mutilation, wide local excision of the tumor with surrounding muscle with a two-centimeter margin is sufficient, to be followed by postoperative radiation. In case of lymph node involvement, adjuvant chemotherapy is indicated.

There is no experience with sentinel lymph node biopsy in males. Theoretically, this procedure may also be of value in males. As in females, it might avoid complete axillary nodal dissection in case of histologically negative lymph nodes. In patients with a T4 tumor, only palliative treatment can be offered. The treatment of choice is wide local excision of the tumor followed by radiation of the thoracic wall and axilla, provided no distant metastases are found. An alternative treatment is, as in females, a combination of inductive chemotherapy, surgery, and radiotherapy to achieve maximal local control.

Palliative Treatment

With distant metastases, the disease follows the same course found in females. Males have a high chance of responding to hormonal treatment. In 80% of patients, the tumor has estrogen receptor activity. Hormonal treatment (orchidectomy, antiandrogens, LH-RH analogues, antiestrogens, aromatase inhibitors) leads to an objective response in 50% of patients. Hormone-independent tumors should be treated with chemotherapy. Lytic bone metastases should be considered for additional treatment with bisphosphonates.

Mammography of the Male Breast

D. J. Dronkers

Indications

Imaging of the male breast is usually restricted to an enlarged breast, a (painful) palpable lesion, or nipple discharge.

Positioning

See chapter 6.

The Normal Mammogram

The male breast mostly consists of fatty tissue. The normal mammogram shows only radiolucent tissue. In some cases converging structures are visible in the subareolar region. A rudimentary duct system exists but lobuli are not developed.

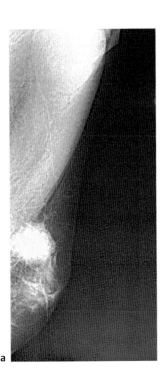
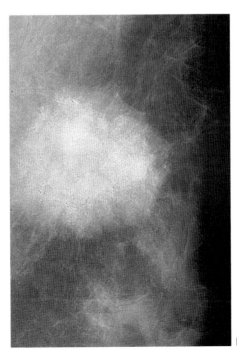

Fig. 10.**1 a, b   Male breast cancer**
a Ill-defined density in the left breast, in addition to central gynecomastia
b Magnification view of the ill-defined density. Histology: IDC

a

b

Breast Pathology

Gynecomastia

The first mammographic sign is a small discoid subareolar density representing glandular proliferation. In more advanced cases, the density is more extensive, predominantly in the upper outer quadrant. Sometimes the male mammogram of advanced gynecomastia does not differ from the normal female mammogram. Cysts, fibroadenoma, and lipoma are extremely rare in males. In pseudo-gynecomastia (gynecomastia spuria) the mammogram shows no increased density at all, indicating that the enlarged breast only consists of fatty tissue.

Breast Cancer

Breast cancer in males has the same mammographic appearance as in females. All lesions suspicious for breast cancer must be differentiated from unilateral gynecomastia. Breast cancer in males is usually excentric in location, in contrast to the more centrally located gynecomastia. Breast cancer can also occur in the subareolar region. The location of the lesion, therefore, can never establish benignancy or malignancy. Most breast cancers in males represent as more or less ill-defined nodular densities. Spicules and microcalcifications may be present. Although breast cancer can be mammographically distinguished from gynecomastia, it can never be excluded by mammography alone.

Metastases

Multiple well-defined densities in the male breast should first raise the suspicion of metastases of a primary cancer outside the breast, such as malignant melanoma, bronchial cancer, and prostate cancer. These lesions are preferentially located in the subcutaneous tissue.

References

Benign and Malignant Changes of the Male Breast:

Guinee, V. F., H. Olson, T. Moller, R. C. Shallenberger et al.: The prognosis of breast cancer in males. A report of 325 cases. Cancer 71 (1993) 154–161

Haraldsson, K., N. Loman, Q. X. Zang, O. Johansson, H. Olsson, A. Borg: BRCA2 germ-line mutations are frequent in male breast cancer patients without a family history of the disease. Cancer Res. 58 (1998) 1367–1371

Heller, K. S., P. P. Rosen, D. Schottenfeld, R. Ashikaria, D. W. Kinne: Male breast cancer: a clinicopathological study of 79 cases. Ann. Surg. 00 (1978) 60–65

Schön, M., M. Zaiac, P. M. Schlag: Mammakarzinom des Mannes, Risikofaktoren, Prognose, Therapie. Onkologie 18 (1995) 16–21

Yildirim, E., U. Berberoglu: Male breast cancer: a 22-year experience. Eur. J. Surg. Oncol. 24 (1998) 548–552

Mammography of the Male Breast:

Cooper, R. A., B. A. Guntie, L. Ramamurthy: Mammography in men. Radiology 191 (1994) 651–656

Dershaw, D. D., P. I. Borgen, B. M. Deutch, L. Liberman: Mammographic findings in men with breast cancer. Amer. J. Roentgenol. 160 (1993) 267–270

Kapdi, C. K., N. J. Parekh: The male breast. Radiol. Clin. N. Amer. 21 (1983) 137–148

11 Retrospective View of Diagnostic Radiology of the Breast

J. H. C. L. Hendriks and G. Rosenbusch

Diagnostic radiology of the breast began with the examination of breast specimens. In 1913, Dr. **Albert Salomon**, resident at the Royal Surgical University Clinic in Berlin, published "Beiträge zur Pathologie und Klinik der Mammakarzinome" (Contributions to the pathology and clinical aspects of breast carcinoma). In this study Salomon "tries to demonstrate the spread of the carcinoma by roentgenograms of amputated breasts." He describes the tumor shadow, carcinomatous strands, calcifications, radiating extensions, and cysts, as well as normal and metastatically involved lymph nodes. One of the conclusions of his study was that "Roentgenograms of excised specimens of the breast give demonstrable general pictures of the extent and shape of carcinomas, which, together with the histological examination of the suspicious margins of the specimen, demonstrate the necessity of performing the excision of the tumor at least three-finger breadths away from its palpable borders." The quality of his reproduced roentgenograms is still impressive.

In 1927, **O. Kleinschmidt** from the clinic of E. Payr in Leipzig reported that some X-ray pictures of the breasts of some patients had been made. An X-ray picture of a breast carcinoma is reproduced in his publication.

"A roentgenologic study of the breast" by **Stafford L. Warren** (Rochester, 1930) was another pioneering work. Warren describes the roentgenological appearance of the normal breast and analyzes different pathologies. He recommends the examination of both breasts and performs stereoscopic examinations. Warren concludes from his studies that the roentgenological pictures of benign and malignant tumors resemble the gross findings and are sufficiently characteristic of the particular tumor. This examination therefore is of definite clinical importance. Technical data for his radiographs were 50–60 kV, 70 mA, 2.5 s exposure time, Kodak superspeed film, dual intensifying screens, and Potter–Bucky grid.

In the following years, studies were published, for instance by W. Vogel, also from the clinic of E. Payr on "X-ray demonstration of breast tumours" (1932), by **I. H. Lockwood** (1932, 1933) and by **J. Gershon-Cohen and A. Strickler** (1938) on the X-ray examination of the normal breast. These authors recommend improvement of the X-ray-technique to detect early carcinomas. The basis of every reading has to be knowledge of the normal breast under different physiological circumstances.

In 1930, **Emil Ries** introduced another method: he succeeded in detecting a tumor by injection of lipiodol into the lactiferous ducts. This method was improved by **N. Frederick Hicken** and called mammography (1937). This was the first time the term "mammography" was mentioned. Today, mammography refers to the radiographic examination of the breast without contrast media.

As early as 1951, **R. Leborgne** (Montevideo) called for the radiographic examination of the breast as part of the clinical examination for the evaluation of breast pathology. Leborgne stated that many cases of malig-

nant breast tumors have multiple punctate calcifications in the tumor itself or in the immediate surrounding of the tumor shadow. These calcifications differ from those of vessels or ducts and also from those of benign tumors. He used 20–30 kV, 5 mAs per 1 cm thickness of the compressed breast, a target-film distance of 60 cm, and plain (no screen) films. The basis was always a CC view of the diseased breast with the woman standing, followed by a spot-view using a long metallic cone with a narrow diameter. The cone was attached to the X-ray tube and served for compression. Leborgne was the first to use local compression in mammography, a technique that led to mammography with general compression. If a tumor was suspected in the upper breast, the examination was completed with a lateral view.

Beginning in 1951, **Charles Gros** and his co-workers (Strasbourg) published papers on mammography. They thoroughly analyzed the normal and pathological pictures of the breast and correlated them with clinical and histological findings. They succeeded in demonstrating clinically undetectable breast cancers, leading to the definite breakthrough of mammography. Gros contributed immensely to the improvement of the radiographic technique. He designed the first dedicated mammography unit, which was introduced as "Senographe" by CGR in France (1967). The X-ray tube had an anode made of molybdenum instead of tungsten, taking advantage of the characteristic low-energy radiation of molybdenum of about 28 kVp. The increased contrast between parenchyma, fat and calcifications improved the visibility of fine structures. In addition, the focal spot was reduced to 0.7 mm. The built-in compression device lowered radiation scatter, reduced motion artifacts and provided a more uniform exposure, producing images with more detail. Many radiologists from different countries learned mammography from Ch. Gros in Strasbourg, France. In 1963, he published his experience in the comprehensive text *Les maladies du sein*.

In 1960, **R. L. Egan** (Houston) asked for further improvement of the radiographic technique: low kilovoltage, high milliamperage, and fine-grain films and intensifying screens. Establishment of the name "mammography" for the radiographic examination of the breast goes back to him. His book on mammography was a standard text for many years.

Die Röntgenuntersuchung der Brust (Mammography: Technique, Diagnosis, Differential Diagnosis, Results) was published by **W. Hoeffken and M. Lanyi** in 1973 and *Teaching Atlas of Mammography* by **L. Tabár and P. B. Dean** in 1983. Both books are still consulted today.

In 1986, **M. Lanyi** provided the fundamentals for understanding microcalcifications for recognizing carcinoma in situ with his monograph *Diagnostik und Differentialdiagnostik der Mikroverkalkungen* (Diagnosis and Differential Diagnosis of Microcalcifications).

J. Gershon-Cohen introduced the double-film technique in 1960. A 0.5 mm thick aluminum foil was placed between two films, which were exposed simultaneously. The upper film was better for interpreting the posterior thick parts of the breast and the lower film better for interpreting the anterior thin parts.

A new high-detail film-screen combination was introduced in 1972: high-resolution screens, which were brought into tight contact with a single-emulsion film by producing a vacuum in an airtight plastic cassette. **M. Friedrich and P. Weskamp** studied grids with film-screen combinations, leading to grid-mammography in the mid-1980s. Together with compression, automatic exposure control, and dedicated film processing, a relatively stable film quality was achieved. The film-screen combination used today requires 50–100 times less exposure than in earlier years of mammography.

In the 1960s, xeroradiography came into use, promoted by **John N. Wolfe** (Detroit). Electrostatic recording produces an image with accentuated contours, rendering calcifications easily detectable. This method was practiced for many years, especially in the United States. It was eventually abandoned after further improvement of the conventional radiographic technique and because of its relatively high radiation dose.

The isodense technique, or fluidography, of **W. Dobretsberger** (1962) examines the patient prone with the breast in an alcohol-water solution, which compensates the different radiation attenuation by the breast. This method did not advance because of its cumbersome setup and poor image quality.

The considerable individual variations in the composition of breast tissue necessitate rather different exposures for breasts of the same size. The photo-timed automatic exposure control can reproduce an optimal exposure of the film in most examinations. With a test exposure just before the final exposure, some systems select the optimal kVp or anode material and filter for the appropriate radiation quality.

The introduction of the motorized foot control of the compression device improved mammographic positioning because the technician has both hands free for positioning the breast during the initial phase of the breast compression.

Replacement of the classic high-voltage generators by smaller converter or high-frequency generators reduced weight and volume of the system. This also made it feasible to build compact systems suitable for mobile screening stations.

Different methods were developed for localizing nonpalpable and only mammographically visible lesions for histological analysis. **G. D. Dodd** and co-workers carried out the first needle localization in 1965. In l976, **H. A. Frank** and co-workers introduced a localization set, consisting of a needle containing a hookwire. After insertion into the breast, the needle is withdrawn and the wire remains in place by the hook. Localization sets with improved anchoring devices followed later. In 1977, **J. Bolmgren, B. Jacobsen, and B. Nordenström** from the Karolinska Institute in Stockholm, Sweden, developed the first device for stereotaxy, which later became the Mammotest. The patient lies prone on a table with an opening for the breast to be examined. The X-ray tube

and stereotactic device are beneath the table. Add-on devices for mammographic units were developed later. Stereotaxy enables quicker and more precise localization, for preoperative marking as well as for percutaneous needle biopsy. The latter has become important for histological analysis since the introduction of the biopsy pistol by **P. G. Lindgren** from Uppsala, Sweden.

The assumption that surgery can curatively remove a breast carcinoma in its early stage and that mammography can detect nonpalpable carcinomas led to the concept of mammography as a screening method for breast carcinoma, especially since a reduction of the mortality of breast carcinoma has not been observed with the introduction of improved therapeutic methods. In 1961, **J. Gershon-Cohen, M. B. Hermel, and S. M. Berger** reported periodically performed mammography in asymptomatic women. The HIP-study (Health Insurance Plan) in New York was carried out from 1963 to 1969 and found a reduction in breast cancer mortality in women over the age of 50 years.

J. Wolfe in 1965 in the United States and **L. Tabár** and co-workers in 1985 in Sweden reported on mammographic screening. Tabár used a single oblique view for screening. Meanwhile in several European countries such as Sweden, The Netherlands, and Great Britain, national mammography screening programs were successfully introduced. Special centers for training of physicians, technicians and pathologists were established. Mandated technical and medical quality assurance programs guarantee a high standard. The reduction of the mortality from breast carcinoma found in different studies justifies mammographic screening.

In 1977, **E. A. Sickles, K. Doi, and H. K. Genant** reported their experience with magnification mammography. Today‹s X-ray-tubes for mammography are usually equipped with a dual focal spot, one larger focal spot with a nominal size of 0.3 mm for survey and one smaller with a nominal size of 0.15 mm for magnification.

The development of small-part transducers made sonography an important supplementary method to mammography in the 1980s, especially for the differentiation between cystic and solid lesions. Sonography is also suitable for guiding biopsies.

MRI of the breast, especially when performed with gadolinium-DTPA, is another important addition to the diagnosis of breast diseases, as shown by the work published by **S. Heywang-Köbrunner**.

With the diagnosis of early breast carcinoma possible today, breast-conservation treatment has received important emphasis.

References

Bolgrem, J., B. Jacobsen, B. Nordenström: Stereotaxic instrument for needle biopsy of the mamma. Amer. J. Roentgenol. 129 (1977) 121–125

Dobretsberger, W.: Mammadiagnostik mittels Isodenstechnik. Radiol. Austriaca 13 (1962) 239

Dodd, G. D., K. Fry, W. Delany: Pre-op localization of occult carcinoma of the breast. In Nealon, T. F.: Management of the Patient With Breast Cancer. Saunders, Philadelphia 1965 (p. 88–113)

Egan, R. L.: Experience with mammography in tumor institution: evaluation of 1000 studies. Radiology 75 (1960) 894–900

Egan, R. L.: Mammography. Thomas, Springfield 1964

Egan, R. L.: Fundamentals of technique and positioning in mammography. Oncology 23 (1969) 99–112

Frank, H. A., F. M. Hall, M. L. Steer: Preoperative localizations of nonpalpable breast lesions demonstrated by mammography. New Engl. J. Med. 295 (1976) 259–260

Friedrich, M., P. Weskamp: Komplexe Bewertung film-mammographischer Abbildungssysteme. Teil I: Methodische Grundlagen. Fortschr. Röntgenstr. 140 (1984) 585–596

Friedrich, M., P. Weskamp: Komplexe Bewertung film-mammographischer Abbildungssysteme. Teil II: Vergleich von 18 Systemen mittels Signal-Rausch-Matrix. Fortschr. Röntgenstr. 140 (1984) 707–716

Gershon-Cohen J., A. Strickler: Roentgenologic examination of normal breasts; its evaluation in demonstrating early neoplastic changes. Amer. J. Roentgenol. 40 (1938) 189–210

Gershon-Cohen, J., M. B. Hermel, S. M. Berger: Detection of breast cancer by periodic X-ray examinations: a five-year survey. J. Amer. med. Ass. 176 (1961) 1114–1116

Gershon-Cohen, J., H. Ingleby: Roentgenography of cancer of the breast. Amer. J. Roentgenol. 68 (1952) 1–7

Gershon-Cohen, J., H. Ingleby: Carcinoma of the breast. Roentgenographic technique and diagnostic criteria. Radiology 60 (1953a) 68–76

Gershon-Cohen, J., H. Ingleby, M. B. Hermel: Roentgenographic diagnosis of calcification in carcinoma of the breast. J. Amer. med. Ass. 29 (1953b) 676–677

Gershon-Cohen, J., H. Ingleby, M. B. Hermel: Accuracy of preoperative x-ray diagnosis of breast tumor. Surgery 35 (1954) 766–771

Gershon-Cohen, J., H. Ingleby, M. B. Hermel: Occult carcinoma of the breast. Arch. Surg. 70 (1955) 385

Gros, Ch. M.: Les Maladies du Sein. Masson, Paris 1963

Gros, Ch. M., M. Sigrist: La radiographie de la mamelle. Annuel congres des médecins électro-radiologique de culture latine, Brüssel 1951a

Gros, Ch. M., M. Sigrist: La radiographie et la transillumination de la mamelle. Strasbourg méd. (1951b) 1–15

Heywang-Köbrunner, S.: Contrast-Enhanced MRI of the Breast. Karger, Basel 1990

Hicken, N. F.: Mammography: roentgenologic diagnosis of breast tumors by means of contrast media. Surg. Gynecol. Obstet. 64 (1937) 593–603

Hoeffken, W., M. Lanyi: Röntgenuntersuchung der Brust. Thieme, Stuttgart 1973

Kleinschmidt, O.: Brustdrüse. In Zweifel, P., E. Payr: Die Klinik der bösartigen Geschwülste. Hirzel, Leipzig 1927

Lanyi, M.: Diagnostik und Differentialdiagnostik der Mammaverkalkungen. Springer, Heidelberg 1986

Leborgne, R.: Diagnosis of tumors of the breast by simple roentgenography, calcifications in carcinomas. Amer. J. Roentgenol. 65 (1951) 1–11

Lindgren, P. G.: Percutaneous needle biopsy; a new technique. Acta radiol. diagn. 23 (1982) 653–656

Lockwood, I. H.: The value of breast radiography. Radiology 3 (1932) 202–207

Lockwood, I. H.: Roentgen-ray evaluation of breast symptoms. Amer. J. Roentgenol 29 (1933) 145–155

Lockwood, I. H., W. Stewart: Roentgen study of physiologic and pathologic changes in mammary gland. J. Amer. med. Ass. 99 (1932) 1461–1466

Ries, E.: Diagnostic lipiodol injection into milkducts followed by abscess formation. Amer. J. Obstet. Gynecol. 20 (1930) 414–416

Salomon, A.: Beiträge zur Pathologie und Klinik der Mammakarzinome. Arch. klin. Chir. 103 (1913) 573–668

Shapiro, S., W. Venet, P. Strax, L. Venet: Evaluation of periodic breast screening with mammography: methology and early observations. J. Amer. med. Ass. 195 (1966) 731–738

Sickles, E. A:, K. Doi, H. K. Genant: Magnification film mammography: image quality and clinical studies. Radiology 125 (1977) 69–76

Tabár, L., P. B. Dean: Teaching Atlas of Mammography. Thieme, Stuttgart 1983

Tabár, L., C. J. G. Fagerberg, A. Gad et al.: Reduction in mortality from breast cancer after mass screening with mammography. Randomized trial from the Breast Cancer Screening Working Groups of the Swedish National Board of Health and Welfare. Lancet I (1985) 829–832

Verbeek, A. L. M., J. H. C. L. Hendriks, R. Holland: Reduction of breast cancer mortality through mass screening with modern mammography. Lancet I (1984) 1222–1226

Vogel, W.: Die Röntgendarstellung von Mammatumoren. Arch. klin. Chir. 171 (1932) 618–626

Warren, S. L.: A roentgenologic study of the breast. Amer. J. Roentgenol. 24 (1930) 113–124

Wolfe, J. N.: Mammography as a screening examination in breast cancer. Amer. J. Roentgenol. 84 (1965) 703–708

Wolfe, J. N.: Xerography of the breast. Radiology 91 (1968) 231–240

Index